English-Spanish
Spanish-English
MEDICAL
Dictionary

Diccionario
MÉDICO
inglés-español
español-inglés

Notice

Medicine is an ever-changing science. As new research and clinical experience broaden our knowledge, changes in treatment and drug therapy are required. The authors and the publisher of this work have checked with sources believed to be reliable in their efforts to provide information that is complete and generally in accord with the standards accepted at the time of publication. However, in view of the possibility of human error or changes in medical sciences, neither the editors nor the publisher nor any other party who has been involved in the preparation or publication of this work warrants that the information contained herein is in every respect accurate or complete, and they disclaim all responsibility for any errors or omissions or for the results obtained from use of the information contained in this work. Readers are encouraged to confirm the information contained herein with other sources. For example and in particular, readers are advised to check the product information sheet included in the package of each drug they plan to administer to be certain that the information contained in this work is accurate and that changes have not been made in the recommended dose or in the contra-indications for administration. This recommendation is of particular importance in connection with new or infre-quently used drugs.

MEDICAL Dictionary

Diccionario MÉDICO
inglés-español
español-inglés

Tercera Edición

Glenn T. Rogers, MD

McGraw-Hill
Medical Publishing Division

New York   Chicago   San Francisco   Lisbon   London   Madrid
Mexico City   Milan   New Delhi   San Juan   Seoul   Singapore
Sydney   Toronto

The McGraw·Hill Companies

English-Spanish Spanish-English Medical Dictionary, Third Edition

1 2 3 4 5 6 7 8 9 0   DOC/DOC   0 9 8 7 6

ISBN-13: 978-0-07-143186-6
ISBN-10: 0-07-143186-1

This book was set in Times Roman.
The editors were Jason Malley and Robert Pancotti.
The production supervisor was Phil Galea.
The cover designer was Margaret Webster-Shapiro.
RR Donnelley was printer and binder.

This book is printed on acid-free paper.

Cataloging-in-Publication data for this title is on file with the Library of Congress.

To my wife, Cynda, and our children,

Valle and Casey

CONTENTS / MATERIAS

PREFACE TO THE THIRD EDITION

This edition represents the first major revision of this dictionary since it was originally published in 1991. The entire text of the dictionary was reviewed term by term with the goal of improving translations wherever possible, and approximately 5,000 new terms were added. Readers wanted more technical terms and these were added. Colloquialisms and regionalism were a strength of this book from the start, and with this edition health professionals should have no trouble finding words with which to communicate with their Spanish-speaking patients—whether their patients come from a *ranchito* and possess very little education or whether they happen to be quite sophisticated and knowledgeable.

Also added were many terms consisting of more than one word, some technical, some not. These compound terms and phrases are more difficult to collect systematically than single words and are often missing in dictionaries. Examples of terms included here which are difficult to find elsewhere include: 'bird flu,' 'doctor-patient confidentiality,' 'developmental milestone,' 'learning disability,' 'to sober up,' 'growth spurt,' 'highly active antiretroviral therapy (HAART),' 'hormone-replacement therapy,' and 'to throw one's back out.' More than ever health providers seem to find themselves addressing psychosocial issues such as depression, drug use, sexuality (safe or otherwise), domestic abuse, homelessness, and lack of health insurance, and I have included terms that should facilitate the comfortable and natural discussion of these issues. Many new drug names were added, bringing the total number of drugs listed to over 500. Translations of drug names include common terms as well as the term recommended by the World Health Organization in its Proposed International Nonproprietary Names List #88.

Another exciting feature of this new edition is the accuracy of the translations. An obstacle to progress in medical Spanish translation has been the fact that medical Spanish is less standardized than medical

English and there has never been an adequate and widely-accepted Spanish-only medical dictionary to set the standard. U.S.-based translators often offer terms that make sense literally but which are not the terms actually used by Spanish-speaking health professionals or patients. For instance 'radiation therapy' is often translated as 'terapia por radiación,' but the term actually used is 'radioterapia.' In order to ensure the best possible translations, the approach taken in this edition was to compare term frequencies in large Spanish databases using sophisticated computer searches. All technical terms were compared against a database consisting of the titles of all medical articles originating in Spanish, and both technical and non-technical terms were compared against large lay databases in key Spanish-speaking countries. This method generated hundreds and sometimes even thousands of citations, ensuring high statistical validity, and furthermore the lay database searches could be made context-specific allowing for checks on accuracy and breadth of meaning. As an example of how this method works, 'terapia por radiación' appeared 6 times in the titles of medical articles and 18 times in the large lay databases, while 'radioterapia' appeared 733 times in the titles of medical articles and upwards of 10,000 times in the same large databases.

As with previous editions the text remains grammatically rigorous, and there are denotations for gender, parts of speech, irregular inflections, region, subject, and level of usage. Where use of a translation is not straightforward, example phrases are provided. To the extent possible, translations are crafted to satisfy the Substitution Rule—that is, they can be inserted directly into a sentence in place of the term being translated. The Appendix has revised sample dialogues applicable to a medical history and physical, nursing, pediatrics and dentistry; and two new sections on radiology and discussing code status have been added. Previous readers may notice that the book's trim size is slightly smaller; this was accomplished by using thinner paper and trimming margins. The book should fit all the more easily into a coat pocket and is designed to be carried into an exam room and used on the spot.

Many people deserve thanks for making this project possible. First, I would like to thank my family and any friends I have left for putting up with my general absence during the last two and a half years. I would like to thank my patients for putting up with my reduced hours and my colleagues for pinch-hitting for me. I would like to thank my editor,

Jason Malley, and the staff at McGraw-Hill for their support and for tolerating several failed deadlines with regard to this edition. For help with the actual text I owe special thanks to Jose De La Torre, Wayra Salazar and Alisson Sombredero for their insightful criticism and un-flagging enthusiasm. Other physicians who helped with the manuscript and deserve thanks include Melvyn Braiman, Melissa Islas, Roberto Lopez, Jaime Morataya, Johanna Paola Reina, Nulbix Quintana, and Juan Carlos Sarol.

Glenn Rogers
Potter Valley, CA

PRÓLOGO A LA TERCERA EDICIÓN

Esta edición constituye la primera gran revisión de este diccionario desde su publicación inicial en 1991. El contenido completo del diccionario fue revisado término por término, con el fin de mejorar en todo lo posible las traducciones y se agregaron aproximadamente 5.000 nuevos términos. La mayoría de los términos añadidos son términos técnicos. Gran parte de la literatura médica mundial se escribe en inglés y, por lo tanto, los profesionales hispanos de la salud que deseen acceder a esta fuente inagotable de información encontrarán en esta publicación un recurso muy valioso. Con el propósito de conservar el tamaño pequeño y útil del libro, se excluyeron términos técnicos muy especializados— términos como periampular, aortoesofágico, y enantiómero. Las traducciones inglesas de estos términos derivados en gran parte del griego y del latín por lo general son fáciles de reconocer, y con un conocimiento moderado del inglés y un poco de práctica, se pueden traducir del español al inglés, gracias a la manera consistente en que se traducen las raíces que los componen.

Otro atributo importante de este libro es el gran número de términos coloquiales que contiene—términos que frecuentemente no se incluyen en los diccionarios médicos o técnicos. Los profesionales de la salud que tengan contacto con pacientes angloparlantes o que pretendan ejercer en los Estados Unidos, tendrán la satisfacción de saber lo que quieren decir sus pacientes cuando dicen, "I've got a charley horse in my leg," "I threw my back out ," o "Doc, I've been slamming speed."

Un problema común de la nomenclatura médica que enfrenta esta edición es el gran número de términos que se aplican a una sola acepción. Los términos que se encuentran en este diccionario son los más utilizados, como se ha comprobado por medio de búsquedas sofisticadas en Internet, en grandes bases de datos médicas y legas, en español y en inglés. Estas búsquedas se pueden restringir conforme a varios contextos, y el uso repetido de tales búsquedas para la mayoría de los términos en este libro ha resultado en un grado sumamente alto de precisión en la traducción.

La inclusión de términos formados por más de una palabra constituye otra ventaja de este diccionario. Estos términos compuestos y locuciones son más difíciles de recopilar que aquellos de una sola palabra y por eso se omiten en muchos diccionarios. Algunos ejemplos de términos incluidos en este diccionario que son difíciles de encontrar en otras fuentes, son: 'bajarle la regla,' 'contacto visual,' 'contener la respiración,' 'gripe aviar,' 'hito del desarrollo,' 'secreto médico,' 'terapia hormonal sustitutiva,' 'trastorno del aprendizaje,' y 'tratamiento antirretroviral de gran actividad (TARGA).'

El trabajo social y el reconocimiento de problemas sociales se han vuelto cada vez más importantes en el campo de la medicina y por lo tanto se han incluido aquí términos que facilitarán una discusión natural y cómoda de temas como el uso de drogas, factores de riesgo para el VIH y la violencia doméstica. Este diccionario contiene los nombres de aproximadamente 500 medicamentos, cuya traducción incluye términos comunes tanto como el nombre recomendado por la Organización Mundial de la Salud en su lista de denominaciones comunes internacionales para sustancias farmacéuticas.

Al igual que en las ediciones anteriores, el texto preserva su rigor gramatical y contiene indicaciones de género, inflexiones irregulares y categoría gramatical, así como indicadores de uso regional, campo y nivel de uso. En casos en los que el uso de la traducción no es de fácil comprensión, se incluyen frases como ejemplos. Los lectores de las ediciones anteriores tal vez notarán que el tamaño del libro es un poco más pequeño. Esto se logró usando papel más delgado y márgenes mas estrechos. El libro cabe fácilmente en un bolsillo y puede usarse cómodamente en el consultorio y transportarse en los viajes.

Muchas personas merecen mi agradecimiento por hacer posible este proyecto. Ante todo, quisiera agradecer a mi familia y a cualquier amigo que aún me quede, por soportar mi ausencia durante los últimos dos años y medio. Quisiera agradecer a mis pacientes por tolerar mi horario reducido y a mis colegas por tomar mi lugar cuando lo necesitaba. Quisiera darle las gracias al personal de Mc Graw-Hill por su apoyo y por disculpar que no cumpliera con muchas fechas límite acordadas. Me gustaría agradecerle especialmente a Jose De La Torre, Wayra Salazar y a Alisson Sombredero por su ayuda técnica con las traducciones y por su inagotable entusiasmo. Otros médicos que merecen agradecimiento son Melvyn Braiman, Melissa Islas, Roberto López, Jaime Morataya, Johanna Paola Reina, Nulbix Quintana y Juan Carlos Sarol.

Glenn Rogers
Potter Valley

PREFACE TO THE FIRST EDITION

Good medicine requires a good history. Few experiences are more frustrating for the health practitioner than to greet a patient and realize that the practitioner and the patient have no common language. For the patient, the experience must be equally frustrating and also frightening. Stories abound regarding the mishaps that occur due to ineffective communication. One such story, which appeared in the Oakland Tribune, involves an Oakland woman who returned to her native Mexico to die, believing she had leukemia. In fact, her doctors had told her she was anemic.

The rapid growth of the Spanish-speaking population presents a special challenge to health workers in the United States. Courses in medical Spanish are now available at many medical centers, and more than a dozen books have been published which offer medical Spanish instruction in the form of sample phrases, exercises, and the like. Notably absent has been a comprehensive medical Spanish dictionary to reinforce these other efforts. This dictionary is the first of its kind.

With over fourteen thousand entries, this dictionary contains virtually every health-related term likely to occur in a conversation between a health worker and a Spanish-speaking patient. There are technical terms which could be important to certain patients (e.g., 'white blood cell count,' 'glucose monitor'), common terms (e.g., 'stomachache,' 'to go to the bathroom'), recently coined terms, colloquialisms, and slang. The colloquialisms form an important feature of this dictionary, as they are used frequently by Hispanics to describe their ailments and can be quite frustrating when offered in response to the practitioner's carefully-crafted textbook Spanish. Many of these colloquialisms are recorded here for the first time.

Another unique feature of this dictionary is its focus on Spanish as it is spoken in the United States. The great majority of Spanish-speaking people in this country come from Mexico, Central America, Cuba, Puerto Rico, and the Dominican Republic, and translations have been chosen which will be best understood by the people of these areas. Terms peculiar to a particular country carry regional labels.

Over thirty doctors from eleven Spanish American countries assisted with the extensive verification and editing of this dictionary. Four Latin dentists reviewed the dental terms. Translations are based on current usage at major Spanish American medical centers and in the Spanish American medical literature. Multiple revisions were made to ensure completeness and accuracy.

Many people helped with various aspects of the production of this book. I would like to thank my wife Cynda Valle Rogers for her patience, Richard Blum for his help with the data management, and my parents for wiring me money to pay my Mexico City hotel bill when my credit card was suddenly and inexplicably declined. I would also like to thank Peter Beren, José de la Torre, Victor Guerrero, Antonio Gutiérrez, Gabriel Lerman, Camilo Leslie, Victor Marrero, Allan Ortejarai, Dan Poynter, Rolando Valdez, Gustavo Valero, and Vicente Valero.

PRÓLOGO A LA PRIMERA EDICIÓN

La mayoría de la literatura médica de importancia aparece en inglés y el estudiante de medicina, médico u otro practicante de la salud que quiere acceder a ella debe saber inglés médico básico. Un obstáculo a esta meta ha sido la falta de un práctico diccionario médico bilingüe. Hasta ahora no ha existido ninguno suficientemente extenso, preciso, económico y de tamaño conveniente. Este diccionario viene a llenar ese espacio vacío.

Abarcando más de 14.000 términos, este diccionario contiene la mayoría de los términos que se encuentran en artículos médicos. Además, contiene muchos modismos, los cuales podrían ser muy útiles para los que quieren practicar su profesión en Los Estados Unidos o que tienen contacto con pacientes de habla inglesa. Las formas irregulares de los plurales, comparativos, superlativos, pretéritos y participios pasados aparecen al igual que indicaciones de las funciones gramaticales y del nivel lingüístico. Para aquellos médicos que intentan presentarse al "FLEX" o a los "National Boards" este diccionario será indispensable.

Más de treinta médicos y otros especialistas han asistido en la redacción de este diccionario para asegurar la exactitud de las traducciones. Su tamaño conveniente lo hace ideal para ser llevado al hospital o a la biblioteca. Los principiantes del inglés médico podrán usar el diccionario para aumentar su vocabulario, mientras que los estudiantes más avanzados lo podrán usar como referencia. El propósito de este diccionario es llegar a servir como una autoridad para todo lo vinculado a la traducción médica.

Muchos me han ayudado en la realización de esta obra. Quisiera dar gracias en particular a mi esposa Cynda Valle Rogers por su paciencia, a Richard Blum por su consejo sobre computadoras, y a mis padres por haberme enviado con prontitud dinero para pagar la cuenta de mi hotel en México, D.F., cuando mi tarjeta de crédito fue repentina e inexplicablemente rechazada. Quiero dar gracias también a Peter Beren, José de la Torres, Victor Guerrero, Antonio Gutiérrez, Gabriel Lerman,

Camilo Leslie, Victor Marrero, Allan Ortejarai, Dan Poynter, Rolando Valdez, Gustavo Valero, y Vicente Valero.

HOW TO USE THIS DICTIONARY

Terms are listed in alphabetical order. For the purposes of alphabetization, ampersands, apostrophes, hyphens, periods, and spaces are ignored. Upper case and lower case letters are treated alike. Alphabetization in the Spanish-English section is essentially the same but with the addition of the letter 'ñ' which immediately follows 'n'. As a general rule material to be translated appears in bold, translations appear in regular typeface, and all other material appears in italics.

For terms with multiple meanings only those meanings which apply in some way to medicine are translated. For instance, under 'throw' the reader will find 'to throw up' and 'to throw one's back out', but not the usual meaning of the word 'throw'.

Chemical names consisting of more than one word are listed in their entirety and alphabetized according to the first word. Also alphabetized this way are certain terms such as 'black widow' which have meanings different from the sum of their parts. Other terms consisting of more than one word are listed as subheadings under the dominant word (usually a noun, often terminal), assuming that the dominant word is an entry in its own right. This system lends itself to lists; for example, all the syndromes are listed under 'syndrome' and all the arteries are listed under 'artery'.

Where the entry term is repeated in a subheading, the entry term is replaced by a long dash:

> prophylaxis *n* profilaxis *f*; **postexposure** — profilaxis
> postexposición

Dashes are not used to replace the entry term when the entry term is pluralized, inflected, combined with another term by a hyphen, or used in an example phrase. Run-ons are listed in strict alphabetical order save that plurals are treated as though they were singular.

Entries are followed by an indication of the part of speech. In the Spanish-English section, noun entries are followed by '*m*' if they are masculine, by '*f*' if they are feminine, and by '*mf*' if they vary according to context, as with 'cardiólogo -ga' and 'adolescente.' The indications '*mpl*' and '*fpl*' apply to masculine plural nouns and feminine plural nouns respectively. The indication '*m&f*' applies to a few Spanish nouns, such as 'enzima,' which may be considered masculine or feminine.

In the English-Spanish section gender is indicated for masculine Spanish nouns which do not end in 'o' and feminine nouns which do not end in 'a'. In the case of translations containing more than one noun, gender is indicated only for those nouns which appear as the first word in the translation. Gender is not indicated where it can be inferred from modifying adjectives.

Abbreviations for region, subject, and level of usage appear in italics between parentheses: '(*form*)' applies to terms used frequently in writing but which may not be understood by many Spanish-speaking patients; '(*fam*)' applies to terms used frequently in speech, but which might seem overly familiar or inappropriate in certain settings; and '(*vulg*)' applies to terms which should generally be avoided by health practitioners who do not have a solid feeling for Hispanic culture.

Parenthetical labels always appear after the term they modify but not necessarily immediately after. Consider the following example:

expectant *adj* (*obst, fam*) embarazada, esperando (*fam*)

In this case the label '(*obst, fam*)' applies to the entry term 'expectant' and indicates that only the obstetrical meaning of this word is being considered and that its use in this context is colloquial. The label '(*fam*)' applies to the translation 'esperando' and indicates that it also is a colloquial term.

Often multiple translations are offered for a particular entry term and these are usually ordered from most formal to least formal. Other factors which could affect this order include frequency of usage, accuracy of translation, and universality (application to all countries where Spanish is spoken). Translations which are synonyms are separated by commas, while translations of different meanings of the same entry term are separated by semicolons.

Where entries have more than one possible meaning, restrictive labels are used to indicate which meaning is being translated (as in the example 'expectant' noted above). In a similar fashion restrictive labels may follow a translation to indicate which of several possible meanings applies. An example would be:

báscula *f* scale *(for weighing)*.

In this example the label indicates that 'báscula' applies to a scale for weighing and not, say, to a sliding fee scale or a scale from 1 to 10.

Optional portions of an entry for a translation are enclosed in parentheses but are not italicized, distinguishing them from restrictive labels and glosses. Consider:

finger *n* dedo (de la mano)...

Here the parentheses indicate that in context 'dedo' may be used to mean finger, but that out of context it may be necessary to use the entire translation 'dedo de la mano' (in order to distinguish it from 'dedo del pie' or 'toe').

For drug names the World Health Organization's Proposed International Nonproprietary Names List #88 was consulted. In most cases the WHO-recommended name is listed first. In the few cases where another term is more commonly used, the more common term is listed first and the WHO-recommended name is listed afterward with the label '(OMS)' (Organización Mundial de la Salud). Where the label '(OMS)' does not appear therefore, it can be assumed that the first-listed name is the WHO-recommended name.

CÓMO USAR ESTE DICCIONARIO

Los términos aparecen en orden alfabético, sin que se consideren el signo '&', los apóstrofes, guiones, puntos y espacios. No se diferencia entre mayúsculas y minúsculas. El orden alfabético en la parte español-inglés es esencialmente el mismo que en la parte inglés-español pero con el agregado de la letra 'ñ' que viene inmediatamente después de la 'n'. Como regla general el material que va a ser traducido aparece en letra negrita, las traducciones aparecen en tipo regular y todo otro material está escrito en letra itálica.

En el caso de términos con más de un significado, sólo aparecen traducidos los significados que se aplican de alguna manera al campo médico. Por ejemplo, bajo 'throw' el lector encontrará 'to throw up' y 'to throw one's back out,' pero no el significado usual de la palabra 'throw.'

Los nombres químicos compuestos de más de una palabra aparecen en orden alfabético de acuerdo a la primera palabra. Del mismo modo aparecen listadas locuciones como 'viuda negra,' que tienen significados diferentes al de la suma de los significados de sus miembros. Otras locuciones aparecen en el artículo de la palabra dominante (usualmente un sustantivo), asumiendo que la palabra dominante funcione como entrada independiente en el diccionario. Este sistema se presta para realizar listas; por ejemplo, todos los síndromes aparecen bajo la palabra 'síndrome' y todas las arterias bajo la palabra 'arteria.'

En los casos en que la entrada se repite en una locución, la entrada se remplaza por una raya larga:

prophylaxis *n* profilaxis *f*; **postexposure** — profilaxis postexposición

No se usan rayas para remplazar a la entrada cuando ésta es plural, está conjugada, se encuentra combinada con otra palabra por medio de un guión, o es usada dentro de un ejemplo de uso. Las locuciones de un artículo aparecen en riguroso orden alfabético excepto que las palabras en plural se consideran como si estuvieran en singular.

Los vocablos cabeza de artículo están acompañados de indicadores de categoría gramatical. En la parte español-inglés, a los sustantivos les sigue una '*m*' si son masculinos, una '*f*' si son femeninos, y una '*mf*' si varían de acuerdo al contexto, como en el caso de 'cardiólogo -ga' y 'adolescente.' Los indicadores '*mpl*' y '*fpl*' se refieren a sustantivos masculinos plurales y sustantivos femeninos plurales respectivamente. El indicador '*m&f*' se aplica a algunos sustantivos en español, como 'enzima,' que pueden considerarse como masculino o femenino. En la parte inglés-español sólo se indica el género de los sustantivos masculinos en español que no terminan en 'o' y de los sustantivos femeninos que no terminan en 'a.' En el caso de traducciones que contienen más de un sustantivo, sólo se indica el género de los sustantivos si estos se encuentran al principio de la locución. No se indica el género cuando éste pueda inferirse por los adjetivos que modifican al sustantivo. En cuanto a los verbos, las formas transitivas se indican con '*vt*' y las formas intransitivas con '*vi*.' En la parte español-inglés se usa '*vr*' para indicar todas las formas que terminan en 'se.'

Los indicadores de región, campo, y grado de formalidad aparecen en letra itálica entre paréntesis: '(*form*)' se aplica a términos que se utilizan con frecuencia por escrito pero que pueden no ser comprendidos por muchos pacientes; '(*fam*)' se refiere a términos que se emplean frecuentemente en el lenguaje hablado, pero que pueden expresar una excesiva familiaridad o pueden parecer poco apropiados en ciertas situaciones; y '(*vulg*)' se aplica a términos que deben evitar los profesionales de la salud que no tienen un conocimiento amplio de la cultura hispana. Estos indicadores siempre aparecen después del término que modifican pero no necesariamente inmediatamente después. Por ejemplo:

expectant *adj* (*obst, fam*) embarazada, esperando (*fam*)

En este caso el indicador '(*obst, fam*)' se refiere al artículo 'expectant' e indica que sólo se está considerando su significado relacionado con la obstetricia y que su uso en este contexto es coloquial. El indicador '(*fam*)' se refiere a la traducción 'esperando' e indica que también es un término coloquial.

Con frecuencia, se incluyen varias traducciones para una misma entrada, usualmente ordenadas de más formal a menos formal. Otros factores que pueden afectar este orden incluyen frecuencia de uso, exactitud de la traducción, y universalidad (uso en todos los países donde se habla el español). Las traducciones que son sinónimos están separadas por comas, mientras que las traducciones de diferentes significados de la misma entrada aparecen separadas por puntos y comas. En los casos en que las entradas tienen más de un significado posible, se utilizan aclaraciones entre paréntesis para indicar a cuál de sus significados corresponde la traducción (como en el caso antes señalado de 'expectant'). De manera similar, aclaraciones entre paréntesis a veces siguen una traducción para indicar cuál de varios significados posibles es el que se aplica. Un ejemplo sería:

angiogram *n* angiografía (*estudio imagenológico*)

En este ejemplo la aclaración entre paréntesis indica que 'angiogram' se refiere al estudio imagenológico y no a la técnica imagenológica. Partes opcionales de una entrada o de una traducción aparecen entre paréntesis pero no están escritas en letra itálica, lo que las distingue de las aclaraciones entre paréntesis. Considere el ejemplo siguiente:

finger *n* dedo (de la mano)

Aquí los paréntesis indican que dentro de un contexto 'dedo' puede usarse para decir 'finger,' pero que fuera de contexto puede ser necesario usar la traducción completa 'dedo de la mano' (para distinguirla de 'dedo del pie').

Las traducciones de los nombres de medicamentos están ordenadas de más usada a menos usada y siempre incluyen el nombre recomendado por la Organización Mundial de la Salud en su lista #88 de denominaciones internacionales para sustancias farmacéuticas. Cuando no hay indicador, quiere decir que la primera traducción es también el nombre recomendado por el OMS. A veces el nombre recomendado por el OMS sigue otro nombre más común en cual caso al nombre recomendado por el OMS le sigue el indicador '(*OMS*).'

MEDICAL SPANISH TIPS

- The most important advice I can give to anyone learning a foreign language is to try to master the pronunciation at an early stage. This has a double benefit. Not only will you be understood more easily, but you will be better able to identify and retain words and phrases of the foreign language as you hear them. This will greatly accelerate the learning process. As you hear the foreign language being spoken by a native speaker, repeat key phrases over and over in your mind—or even aloud if possible—comparing your pronunciation to the immediate memory of the correctly spoken sounds. Experiment with your tongue, lips, and palate to create sounds which may be unfamiliar to you. Take a deep breath and pronounce the soft 'i' of the English word 'sin,' then slowly modulate it to the 'ee' of 'seen.' Go back and forth between these two sounds. Somewhere in between is the '*i*' as it sounds in Spanish, for example in '*cinco*.' Pronounce the English 'd' sound over and over again and gradually modulate it to the 'th' of 'the.' Somewhere in between is the Spanish '*d*.' Pronounce the English 'h' sound over and over again and gradually modulate it to the English 'k.' Somewhere in between is a close facsimile of the Spanish '*j*.' Exercises like these will improve your pronunciation rapidly.

- On the subject of pronunciation, note that Spanish vowels are short and pure. Never linger on a vowel as in English. Say the sentence, "No way!" with feeling and notice how the vowel sounds are drawn out. This rarely happens in Spanish; Spanish is much more staccato in its delivery. Note also that there is no schwa sound in Spanish. The schwa sound is the 'uh' sound so often given to unaccented syllables in English. For example the first, third, and fifth syllables of 'acetazolamide' are schwa sounds. In Spanish, vowels retain their characteristic sounds whether or not they are accented. 'Acetazolamida' is pronounced ah-ceh-tah-zoh-lah-MEE-dah, not uh-ceh-tuh-zoh-luh-MEE-duh. It is often helpful first to practice a word without consonants. 'Acetazolamida' without consonants would be ah-eh-ah-oh-ah-EE-ah. When you have mastered the vowel changes for a given word, it is usually a simple matter to fill in the consonants. Learn to say *cah-BEH-sah*, not *cuh-BEH-suh*; *meh-dee-SEE-nah*, not *meh-duh-SEE-nuh*.

- When referring to a part of the body in Spanish, it is common to use the definite article instead of the possessive adjective, provided it is clear whose body is involved. The Spanish definite articles, recall, are *el* and *la*. *¿Le duele la cabeza?* is the best translation of "Does your head hurt?" *¿Le duele su cabeza?* is redundant in Spanish.

- The indirect object* is used much more often in Spanish than in English. Health workers are frequently doing things to patients and this often involves the use of *le* or, in familiar speech, *te*.

  > *Quiero tomarle el pulso*...I want to take your pulse.
  > *Voy a escucharle el corazón*...I'm going to listen to your heart.
  > *Tenemos que operarte la pierna*...We need to operate on your leg.

  This phrasing often sounds less brusque than *Quiero tomar su pulso, Voy a escuchar su corazón,* etc.

- English-speaking people are often confused by the choices available for the direct object in Spanish. *Te* is always correct when speaking informally, for instance to a child.

  > *Voy a examinarte, hijo.*.I'm going to examine you, young man.

When speaking formally, most Spanish speakers use *lo* for males and *la* for females.

> *Voy a examinarlo, señor*..I'm going to examine you, sir.

* Recall that a *direct* object may be any type of object and receives the direct action of the verb, while the *indirect* object is always a person (or other living being) *to* whom or *for* whom the action is being performed.

> *Voy a examinarla, señora*..I'm going to examine you,
> ma'am.

There are a few exceptions to this rule; for instance, the verb *pegar*, when it means 'to hit' takes *le* for a direct object.

> *¿Le pegó?*..Did it hit you?

Some Spanish speakrs will use *le* for *all* (formal) second person direct objects, male or female.

> *Voy a examinarle, señor*..I'm going to examine you, sir.
> *Voy a examinarle, señora*..I'm going to examine you,
> ma'am.

This style is common in Mexico.

- Some verbs require that the subject and object be inverted when translating between English and Spanish. The Spanish student is likely to encounter this for the first time when learning to translate the verb 'to like.' "I like coffee" would be *Me gusta el café*. The subject and object are inverted. This particular construction is a stumbling block to fluency and even advanced students often have to think for a couple seconds in order to conjugate the verb correctly and choose the correct object pronouns.

> *Me falta el aire*..I am short of breath.
> *Les falta el aire*..They are short of breath.

Le salieron los dientes..His teeth came in.
Me dieron náuseas..I got nauseated.
¿Le salieron moretones?..Did you get bruised?
Te falta hierro..You're low on iron.

Notice that the English subject corresponds to the Spanish *indirect* object in all these cases.

- Many Spanish verbs are used in the reflexive form when applied to medicine. The use of the reflexive pronoun *se* turns the action of the verb back on the verb's subject.

  Orinó..He urinated.
  Se orinó..He urinated on himself.

  Corté el pan..I cut the bread.
  Me corté el dedo..I cut my finger.

  Puede vestirla..You can dress her.
  Puede vestirse..You can get dressed (literally 'dress yourself').

  La enfermera le va a inyectar..The nurse will give you an injection.
  La enfermera le va a enseñar como inyectarse..The nurse will teach you how to inject yourself.

A reflexive construction is often used when an English-speaking person would use the past participle preceded by 'to get' or 'to become.'

  Se cansa..He gets tired..He becomes tired.
  Se mejoró..She got better.
  Se dislocó..It became dislocated.
  Se infectó..It became infected..It got infected.

- Most Spanish nouns which end in *-o* are masculine and most which end in *-a* are feminine; however, there are some important exceptions in medical Spanish. For instance, most Spanish words which end in *-ma* are derived from Greek and retain their original masculine gender.

> *un problema médico*..a medical problem
> *el electrocardiograma*..the electrocardiogram

Other medical terms which end in *-a* and are masculine include *aura, día, cólera* (the disease), *herbicida, insecticida, pesticida, raticida, espermaticida* and *vermicida*.

The word *mano*, which comes from the Latin *manus*, retains its original feminine gender—despite the fact it ends in *-o*.

> *Tengo las manos frías*..My hands are cold.

A source of confusion to Spanish students is the construction '*el agua.*' Although *agua* is feminine (and requires feminine modifiers), *el* is used instead of *la* to avoid the awkward double *ah* sound of '*la agua.*' This rule applies to any word which begins with an accented *ah* sound.

> *el agua fría*..the cold water
> *terapista del habla*..speech therapist

This rule also applies to the indefinite article.

> *un afta*..a canker sore
> *un arma blanca*..a sharp weapon

This rule does not apply to plural forms, since the double *ah* sound is then broken up by an *s* sound.

> *las aguas frías*..the cold waters
> *unas aftas*..some canker sores

Other medical Spanish terms which begin with an accented *ah* sound include *ámpula, área, asma,* and *hambre.*

- When comparing quantities, use *de.*

  > *más de dos pastillas*..more than two pills
  > *menos de una taza*..less than a cup

  In all other situations use *que.*

  > *más alto que tu hermano*..taller than your brother
  > *más que pesabas hace dos meses*..more than you weighed
  >   two months ago
  > *menos que siempre*..less than usual
  > *menos que nunca*..less than ever

- Health practitioners should be aware that the Spanish word *alcohol* is often considered a synonym for 'hard liquor.' Many Hispanic beer and wine drinkers will answer no in all sincerity to the question *¿Toma alcohol?* A slightly broader question would be *¿Toma bebidas alcohólicas?* And then to avoid all misunderstandings, you could follow a negative answer with *¿Cerveza?..¿Vino?*

SPANISH PRONUNCIATION

a   Like the English **a** in **father** (e.g., *padre*, *cama*).

b   Similar to the English **b**. At the beginning of a breath group or following an *m* or *n*, the Spanish *b* sounds like the **b** in **bite** (e.g., *boca*, *embarasada*). In all other situations the Spanish *b* lies somewhere between the English **b** and the English **v** (e.g., *tubo*, *jarabe*). Allow a little air to escape between slightly parted lips as you make this latter sound.

c   Like the English **c**. Before *a*, *o*, or *u* it is hard (e.g., *cara*); before *e* or *i* it is soft (e.g., *ácido*). (In Castilian Spanish, *c* preceding **e** or **i** is pronounced like the **th** in **bath**, but this form of Spanish is rarely spoken by Latin Americans.) The Spanish *ch* sounds like the English **ch** in **child**.

d   Similar to the English **d**. At the beginning of a breath group or following *l* or *n*, the Spanish *d* sounds like the English **d** in **dizzy** (e.g., *dosis*, *venda*). In all other situations the Spanish *d* lies somewhere between the English **d** and the **th** in **there** (e.g., *mudo*, *nacido*). Allow a little air to escape between the tip of your tongue and upper teeth as you make the latter sound.

e   Similar to the **ey** in **they** (e.g., *peso*, *absceso*), unless followed by a consonant in the same syllable, in which case it is closer to the **e** in **sepsis** (e.g., *esperma*, *recto*).

f   Like the English **f**.

g   When followed by *a*, *o*, *u*, or a consonant, the Spanish *g* is similar to the English **g** in **gout** (e.g., *gota*, *grasa*). Allow a little air to escape between your tongue and palate as you make this sound. When followed by *e* or *i*, the Spanish *g* is similar to the **h** in **hot** shaded slightly toward the English **k** (e.g., *gen*, *gingiva*).

h   Silent (e.g., ***hombre***, ***almohada***).

i   Like the **i** in **saline** or **latrine** (e.g., ***orina***, ***signo***, ***sífilis***). Preceding another vowel, the Spanish *i* sounds like the English **y**. ***Siesta*** is pronounced *SYES-tah*, ***sodio*** is pronounced *SO-dyoh*, ***viudo*** is pronounced *VYOO-doh*, etc. Following another vowel, *i* forms individual diphthongs: *ai* sounds like the **y** in **cry** (e.g., ***aire***, ***aislar***); *ei* sounds like the **ay** in **tray** (e.g., ***aceite***, ***afeitar***); *oi* sounds like the **oy** in **boy** (e.g., ***toxoide***, ***coloide***); and *ui* sounds like the **ui** in **suite** (e.g., ***cuidado***, ***ruido***).

j   The Spanish *j* is pronounced the same as the Spanish *g* followed by *e* or *i* (e.g., ***jugo***, ***bajar***). See above.

k   Like the English **k**. (*k* is not included in the Spanish alphabet and appears only in foreign words.)

l   Similar to the English **l** (e.g., ***lado***, ***pelo***). The Spanish *l* is articulated rapidly, never drawn out as in English. The Spanish *ll* is pronounced somewhere between the **ll** of **million** and the **y** of **yes**.

m   Like the English **m**.

n   Like the English **n**.

ñ   Like the **ni** in **bunion** (e.g., ***baño***, ***sueño***).

o   Similar to the English **o** in **coma**.

p   Like the English **p** in **spit**. Hold your hand in front of your mouth as you say **spit** and then **pit**. Note that less air is expelled in pronouncing **spit**. The Spanish *p* is not aspirated, which means little air should be expelled. It is a shorter, more explosive sound than the English **p**.

q   Like the English **k**. The Spanish *q* is always followed by *u*, but lacks the **w** sound of the English **qu**. ***Quinina*** is pronounced *kee-NEE-nah*, not *kwee-NEE-nah*. The **kw** sound of **quit** is represented in Spanish by *cu*, as in ***cuarto***, ***cuidado***, etc.

r   Similar to the **tt** of **butter**. At the beginning of a word the Spanish *r* is trilled. The Spanish *rr* is always trilled.

s   Like the English **s**. Before voiced consonants, the Spanish *s* sounds like the English **z** (e.g., *rasgar*, *espasmo*).

t   Like the English **t** in **stent**. Hold your hand in front of your mouth as you say **stent** and then **tent**. Note that less air is expelled in pronouncing **stent**. The Spanish *t* is not aspirated, which means little air should be expelled. It is a shorter, more explosive sound than the English **t**, made by quickly tapping the tip of the tongue against the back of the upper front teeth.

u   Like the English **u** in **flu** or **rule**. Be sure not to pronounce it like **you** (unless it follows an *i*—see below). The Spanish *u* has a **w** sound when it precedes another vowel (e.g., *agua*, *cuello*), except in the case of *gue*, *gui*, *que*, and *qui*, when it is silent (e.g., *inguinal*, *quebrar*). The **w** sound is retained in *güe* and *güi* (e.g., *agüita*, *ungüento*). The diphthong *au* sounds like the **ow** of **brow** (e.g., *aura*, *trauma*). The diphthong *iu* sounds like the **u** in **acute** or **use** (e.g., *viudo*, *diurético*).

v   Identical to the Spanish *b*. See above.

x   Like the English **x** in **flex**. Before consonants, the Spanish *x* is often pronounced like the English **s** (e.g., *extra*, *expediente*).

y   Similar to the English **y** (e.g., *yeso*, *yodo*). An exception is the word *y* (= **and**), which is pronounced like the **ee** in **see**.

z   Like the English **s** (e.g., *nariz*, *brazo*).

ABBREVIATIONS / ABREVIATURAS

abbr	abbreviation	abreviatura
adj	adjective	adjetivo
adv	adverb	adverbio
Amer	Latin America	Latinoamérica
anat	anatomy	anatomía
Ang	Anglicism	anglicismo
ant	antiquated	anticuado
arith	arithmetic	aritmética
bot	botany	botánica
CA	Central America	Centroamérica
card	cardiology	cardiología
Carib	Caribbean	caribe
chem	chemistry	química
comp	comparative	comparativo
conj	conjunction	conjunción
Cub	Cuba	Cuba
dent	dentistry	odontología
derm	dermatology	dermatología
El Salv	El Salvador	El Salvador
esp	especially	especialmente
Esp	Spain	España
euph	euphemism	eufemismo
f	feminine	femenino
fam	familiar	familiar
form	formal	formal
fpl	feminine plural	femenino plural
frec.	frequently	frecuentemente
ger	gerund	gerundio
Guat	Guatemala	Guatemala
Hond	Honduras	Honduras
gyn	gynecology	ginecología
interj	interjection	interjección
inv	invariant	invariable
m	masculine	masculino
mf	masculine or feminine	masculino o femenino

m&f	masculine and feminine	masculino y femenino
mfpl	masculine or feminine, plural	masculino o femenino, plural
math	mathematics	matemática
Mex	Mexico	México
micro	microbiology	microbiología
mpl	masculine plural	masculino plural
n	noun	nombre *o* sustantivo
neuro	neurology	neurología
Nic	Nicaragua	Nicaragua
npl	noun plural	nombre plural
obst	obstetrics	obstetricia
OMS	World Health Organization	Organización Mundial de la Salud
ophth	ophthalmology	oftalmología
ortho	orthopedics	ortopedia
path	pathology	patología
ped	pediatrics	pediatría
pharm	pharmacology	farmacología
physio	physiology	fisiología
pl	plural	plural
pp	past participle	participio pasado
PR	Puerto Rico	Puerto Rico
pref	prefix	prefijo
prep	preposition	preposición
pret	preterite	pretérito
psych	psychology	psicología
SA	South America	Sudamérica
SD	Santo Domingo	Santo Domingo
stat	statistics	estadística
super	superlative	superlativo
surg	surgery	cirugía
US	United States	Estados Unidos
V.	See	Véase
vi	verb, intransitive	verbo intransitivo
vr	verb, reflexive	verbo reflexivo
vt	verb, transitive	verbo transitivo
vulg	vulgar	vulgar
zool	zoology	zoología

ENGLISH-SPANISH

INGLÉS-ESPAÑOL

A

AA *V.* **Alcoholics Anonymous.**
abacavir *n* abacavir *m*
abdomen *n* abdomen *m*, barriga, vientre *m* (*esp. Esp*), estómago (*fam*)
abdominal *adj* abdominal
abdominoplasty *n* (*pl* -ties) abdominoplastia
ability *n* (*pl* -ties) capacidad *f*, habilidad *f*, — **to drive** capacidad para manejar
ablation *n* ablación *f*
abnormal *adj* anormal
abnormality *n* (*pl* -ties) anormalidad *f*, (*esp. congenital*) anomalía
abort *vt, vi* abortar
abortifacient *n* abortivo
abortion *n* aborto (provocado), interrupción voluntaria del embarazo (*form*); **habitual** — aborto habitual; **partial birth** — aborto de nacimiento parcial; **spontaneous** — aborto espontáneo; **therapeutic** — aborto terapéutico; **threatened** — amenaza de aborto; **to have an** — tener un aborto
above *adj* encima de; (*number*) superior a (*form*), por encima de, arriba de (*Amer*); **Keep your feet elevated above the level of your heart**.. Mantenga los pies elevados encima del nivel del corazón..**Your sugar is above 500**..Su azúcar está por encima de (superior a, arriba de) 500.
abrasion *n* abrasión *f* (*form*), raspadura (*fam*)

abrasive *adj & n* abrasivo
abscess *n* absceso
absence *n* ausencia, falta
absent *adj* ausente
absenteeism *n* ausentismo, absentismo (*Esp*)
absent-minded *adj* distraído, olvidadizo
absorb *vt* absorber
absorbable *adj* (*suture*) reabsorbible
absorbent *adj* absorbente
absorption *n* absorción *f*
abstain *vi* abstenerse; **to — from sex** abstenerse del sexo
abstinence *n* abstinencia
abuse *n* (*substance, sexual*) abuso, (*physical, mental*) maltrato; **child** — maltrato infantil; **drug** — abuso de drogas; **drug of** — droga de abuso; **elderly** — maltrato a las personas mayores; **physical** — maltrato físico; **psychological** — maltrato psicológico; **sexual** — abuso sexual; **substance** — abuso de sustancias, abuso de drogas o alcohol; *vt* abusar, maltratar
abuser *n* abusador -ra *mf*; **drug** — drogadicto -ta *mf*, persona que abusa de drogas
abusive *adj* abusivo
acalculous *adj* alitiásico
acanthosis nigricans *n* acantosis *f* nigricans
acarbose *n* acarbosa
access *n* acceso; — **to treatment** acceso a tratamiento; **venous** — acceso venoso; **wheelchair** — acceso

para silla(s) de ruedas

accessible *adj* accesible; **wheel-chair-accessible** con acceso para sillas de ruedas

accident *n* accidente *m*; **by** — sin querer; **cerebrovascular** — accidente cerebrovascular; **traffic** — accidente de tránsito, accidente de tráfico (*esp. Esp*), choque *m* (*fam*); **work** — accidente de trabajo

accidental *adj* accidental; — **death** muerte *f* accidental

acclimated *adj* aclimatado; **to become** — aclimatarse

accumulate *vt, vi* acumular(se)

accumulation *n* acumulación *f*

accuracy *n* exactitud *f*, precisión *f*

accurate *adj* exacto, preciso

acenocoumarol *n* acenocumarol *m*

acetabulum *n* acetábulo, cotilo

acetaminophen *n* paracetamol *m*

acetate *n* acetato

acetazolamide *n* acetazolamida

acetic acid *n* ácido acético

acetone *n* acetona

acetylsalicylic acid *n* ácido acetil-salicílico

achalasia *n* acalasia

ache *n* dolor *m*, dolor persistente; *vi* doler

achondroplasia *n* acondroplasia

acid *adj & n* ácido; **fatty** — ácido graso (*V. también* **fatty acid**.); **gastric** *o* **stomach** — ácido gástrico, ácido del estómago

acidity *n* acidez *f*

acidophilus *n* Lactobacillus acidofilus, acidofilus *m*

acne *n* acné *m&f* — **rosacea** acné rosácea; **cystic** — acné quístico; [*Note: feminine usage is correct from a historical and etymological viewpoint but masculine usage has become almost universal save with* acné rosácea.]

acoustic *adj* acústico

acquire *vt* adquirir

acquired *adj* adquirido

acromegaly *n* acromegalia

acrophobia *n* acrofobia

acrylamide *n* acrilamida

acrylic *adj & n* acrílico

act *n* acto; *vt, vi* **to** — **out** expresar

(*emociones o impulsos reprimidos*) sin comprender los motivos

ACTH *abbr* **adrenocorticotropic hormone**. *V.* **hormone**.

actinic *adj* actínico

actinomycosis *n* actinomicosis *f*

action *n* acción *f*

activate *vt* activar

activator *n* activador *m*; **tissue plasminogen — (tPA)** activador tisular del plasminógeno

active *adj* activo; **sexually** —sexualmente activo; **Are you sexually active?**..¿Es Ud. sexualmente activo?..¿Ha tenido relaciones sexuales recientemente?

activity *n* (*pl* **-ties**) actividad *f*; **activities of daily living** actividades de la vida diaria; **strenuous** — actividad fuerte

actually *adv* en realidad, realmente

acuity *n* agudeza; **visual** — agudeza visual

acupressure *n* acupresión *f*, tipo de masaje empleando presión de los dedos sobre ciertas áreas con el fin de curar

acupuncture *n* acupuntura

acute *adj* agudo

acyclovir *n* aciclovir *m*

Adam's apple *n* nuez *f* de Adán, manzana de Adán (*esp. Mex*)

adapt *vt, vi* adaptar(se)

adaptation *n* adaptación *f*

add *vt* añadir, agregar; (*arith*) sumar; **Add this medicine to your others** ..Añada esta medicina a las otras ...**Add a teaspoon of salt**.. Agregue una cucharadita de sal...**Can you add 7 and 16?**.. ¿Puede sumar 7 y 16?

addict *n* adicto -ta *mf*; **drug** — drogadicto -ta *mf*; **heroin** — adicto a la heroína

addicted *adj* adicto; **to get** *o* **become** — volverse adicto

addiction *n* adicción *f*; **drug** — drogadicción *f*; **heroin** — adicción a la heroína

addictive *adj* adictivo, que crea dependencia, que crea hábito

additive *adj & n* aditivo

address *n* dirección *f*, domicilio

adefovir *n* adefovir *m*

adenitis *n* adenitis *f*

adenocarcinoma *n* adenocarcinoma *m*

adenoidectomy *n* (*pl* -**mies**) adenoidectomía

adenoids *npl* adenoides *fpl*

adenoma *n* adenoma *m*; **villous** — adenoma velloso

adenomatous *adj* adenomatoso

adenovirus *n* adenovirus *m*

adequate *adj* adecuado, suficiente

ADHD *abbr* **attention deficit-hyperactivity disorder.** *V.* **disorder.**

adherence *adj* adherencia; — **to treatment** adherencia al tratamiento

adherent *adj* adherido

adhesion *n* adherencia, brida

adhesive *adj & n* adhesivo

adjust *vt* (*chiropractice, etc.*) ajustar; *vi* adaptar; **well-adjusted** bien adaptado

adjustable *adj* ajustable, regulable

adjustment *n* (*chiropractice, etc.*) ajuste *m*

adjuvant *adj* adyuvante

administer *vt* (*a drug, etc.*) administrar

administration *n* administración *f*; **Food and Drug Administration (FDA)** Administración de Alimentos y Drogas

admission *n* ingreso, admisión *f*

admit *vt* (*pret & pp* **admitted**; *ger* **admitting**) (*to the hospital*) ingresar, admitir (al hospital), hospitalizar, internar

Admitting *n* (*area of hospital*) Ingresos

adolescence *n* adolescencia

adolescent *adj & n* adolescente *mf*

adopt *vt* adoptar

adoption *n* adopción *f*

adoptive *adj* adoptivo; — **parents** padres adoptivos

adrenal *adj* suprarrenal; *n* (*fam*) glándula suprarrenal, suprarrenal *f* (*fam*)

adrenalectomy *n* (*pl* -**ties**) adrenalectomía, suprarrenalectomía

adrenaline *n* adrenalina

adsorbent *adj* adsorbente

adult *adj & n* adulto -ta *mf*

adulterated *adj* adulterado

adulthood *n* edad adulta, vida adulta

advance *n* avance *m*

advanced *adj* avanzado

advance directive *n* directiva anticipada, documento que indica de antemano la atención médica deseada en caso de coma u otra incapacidad para expresarse; (*living will*) testamento vital, testamento en vida

advantage *n* ventaja

adverse *adj* adverso

advice *n* consejo

advise *vt* aconsejar(se)

advisory *n* aviso; **health** — aviso sanitario (*form*), aviso sobre peligro para la salud pública

advocate *n* defensor -ra *mf*; **patient** — defensor del paciente

AED *abbr* **automated external defibrillator.** *V.* **defibrillator.**

aerobic *adj* (*metabolism*) aeróbico; (*micro*) aerobio

aerobics *npl* aeróbic *m*, aeróbicos, ejercicios aeróbicos; **low impact** — aeróbic (aeróbicos, ejercicios aeróbicos) de bajo impacto

aerosol *n* aerosol *m*

aerosolized *adj* en aerosol

affect *n* (*psych*) afecto; *vt* afectar

affected *adj* afectado; — **by** afectado por

affection *n* afecto, cariño

affectionate *adj* afectuoso, cariñoso

affliction *n* aflicción *f*, mal *m*, padecimiento (*esp. Mex*)

aflatoxin *n* aflatoxina

afraid *adj* **to be** — tener miedo; **Are you afraid of injections?**...¿Les tienes miedo a las inyecciones?

after *prep* después de, siguiente; — **a week** después de una semana; — **meals** después de las comidas; **the day** — el día siguiente; *adv* después

afterbirth *n* secundinas, placenta y membranas expulsadas después del parto

afternoon *n* tarde *f*

aftertaste *n* sabor *m* que deja la comida, bebida, o medicamento

against medical advice, contra el

consejo del médico

agammaglobulinemia *n* agammaglobulinemia

age *n* edad *f*; **bone** — edad ósea; **child-bearing** — edad fértil; **gestational** — edad gestacional; **middle** — mediana edad; **old** — vejez *f*, tercera edad (*euph*)

agency *n* (*pl* **-cies**) agencia

agent *n* agente *m*; **Agent Orange** agente naranja

aggravate *vt* agravar, empeorar

aggression *n* agresión *f*

aggressive *adj* agresivo

agile *adj* ágil

aging *n* envejecimiento

agitated *adj* agitado; **to become** — agitarse

ago *adj* hace; **two weeks ago**..hace dos semanas

agonal *adj* agónico

agony *n* dolor intenso, angustia extrema

agoraphobia *n* agorafobia

agree *vi* to — with (*medication, etc.*) caer(le) bien (a uno); **This pill didn't agree with me**..Esta pastilla no me cayó bien.

agression *n* agresión *f*, hostilidad *f*

agricultural *adj* agrícola

aid *n* ayuda, socorro, auxilio; *vt* ayudar, asistir

aide *n* auxiliar *mf*, ayudante *mf*; **nurse** — auxiliar de enfermería

AIDS *abbr* **acquired immunodeficiency syndrome**. *V.* **syndrome**.

ailment *n* enfermedad *f*, achaque *m*, padecimiento (*esp. Mex*)

air *n* aire *m*

airbag *n* airbag *m*, bolsa de aire (*esp. Mex*)

airborne *adj* de transmisión aérea (*form*), transmitido por el aire

air conditioning *n* aire acondicionado

airsickness *n* mareo (en avión)

airway *n* vía aérea (*frec. pl*)

akathisia *n* acatisia

alanine *n* alanina

albendazole *n* albendazol *m*

albinism *n* albinismo

albino *adj* albino; *n* (*pl* **-nos**) albino -na *mf*

albumin *n* albúmina

albuminuria *n* albuminuria

albuterol *n* salbutamol *m*

alcohol *n* alcohol *m*, bebidas alcohólicas (*incluyendo vino y cerveza*); **Do you drink alcohol?**.. ¿Toma Ud. bebidas alcohólicas? ¿vino? ¿cerveza? **denatured** — alcohol desnaturalizado; **rubbing** — alcohol para fricciones, alcohol isopropílico

alcoholic *adj & n* alcohólico -ca *mf*; **recovering** — alcohólico en recuperación

Alcoholics Anonymous (AA) *n* Alcohólicos Anónimos

alcoholism *n* alcoholismo

aldosterone *n* aldosterona

aldosteronism *n* aldosteronismo

alendronate *n* alendronato

alert *adj* alerta; *n* alerta; **health** — alerta sanitaria (*form*), alerta sobre peligro para la salud pública

alfalfa *n* (*bot*) alfalfa

algae *npl* algas

alginate *n* alginato

alienated *adj* alienado, aislado emocionalmente

alienation *n* alienación *f*, aislamiento emocional

align *vt* alinear

alignment *n* alineación *f*

alimentary *adj* alimentario

alive *adj* vivo, con vida

alkaline *adj* alcalino; — **phosphatase** fosfatasa alcalina

alkalosis *n* alcalosis *f*

alkaptonuria *n* alcaptonuria

alky *n* (*pl* **-kies**) (*vulg*) alcohólico -ca *mf*, borracho -cha *mf* (*fam*)

allergen *n* alergeno *or* alérgeno

allergic *adj* alérgico; **Are you allergic to any medicine?**..¿Es Ud. alérgico a algún medicamento?

allergist *n* alergólogo -ga *mf*, alergista *mf*, médico -ca *mf* especialista en alergias

allergy *n* (*pl* **-gies**) alergia; **seasonal** — alergia estacional

alleviate *vt* aliviar

allopath *n* alópata *mf*

allopathic *adj* alopático

allopathy *n* alopatía

allopurinol *n* alopurinol *m*
almotriptan *n* almotriptán *m*
aloe *n* (*bot*) aloe *m*, sábila, acíbar *m* (*esp. Esp*)
alopecia *n* alopecia
alovudine *n* alovudina
alpha *n* alfa; — **fetoprotein** alfafetoproteína; — **hydroxy acids** ácidos alfa hidróxidos
alprazolam *n* alprazolam *m*
alteplase *n* alteplasa
alternate *adj* alterno; — **days** días alternos; un día sí, un día no; *vt, vi* alternar
alternative *n* alternativa
altitude *n* altura, altitud *f*; **high** — gran altura *or* altitud
alum *n* alumbre *m*
aluminum *n* aluminio; — **hydroxide** hidróxido de aluminio
alveolar proteinosis *n* proteinosis *f* alveolar
alveolus *n* (*pl* -li) alvéolo *or* alveolo
always *adv* siempre; **almost** — casi siempre
amalgam *n* (*dent*) amalgama
amantadine *n* amantadina
ambidextrous *adj* ambidiestro *or* ambidextro
amblyopia *n* ambliopía, disminución *f* de la agudeza visual en un ojo sin lesión orgánica
ambulance *n* ambulancia
ambulate *vi* (*form*) deambular (*form*), caminar
ambulation *n* (*form*) deambulación *f* (*form*)
ambulatory *adj* ambulatorio
ameba *n* (*pl* -bae *o* -bas) ameba, amiba (*Mex*)
amebiasis *n* amebiasis *f*, amibiasis (*Mex*)
amebic *adj* amebiano, amibiano (*Mex*)
amenable *adj* sensible; — **to treatment** sensible al tratamiento
amenorrhea *n* amenorrea
amiloride *n* amilorida
amino acid *n* aminoácido
aminophylline *n* aminofilina
amiodarone *n* amiodarona
amitriptyline *n* amitriptilina
amlodipine *n* amlodipino, amlodipi-

na (*esp. SA*)
ammonia *n* amoníaco *or* amoniaco
ammonium *n* amonio; — **carbonate** carbonato de amonio
amnesia *n* amnesia
amniocentesis *n* (*pl* -ses) amniocentesis *f*
amnionitis *n* amnionitis *f*
amniotic *adj* amniótico; — **fluid** líquido amniótico
amoeba *V.* ameba.
amount *n* cantidad *f*
amoxacillin *n* amoxacilina
amphetamine *n* anfetamina
amphotericin B *n* anfotericina B
ampicillin *n* ampicilina
amprenavir *n* amprenavir *m*
ampule *n* ampolla, ámpula (*Mex, Cub*)
ampulla of Vater *n* ampolla de Vater
amputate *vt* amputar
amputation *n* amputación *f*; **above-the-knee** — amputación por encima de la rodilla; **below-the-knee** — amputación por debajo de la rodilla
amputee *n* amputado -da *mf*
amylase *n* amilasa
amyloidosis *n* amiloidosis *f*
amyotrophic *adj* amiotrófico
ANA *abbr* **antinuclear antibodies**. *V.* **antibody**.
anabolic *adj* anabólico
anaerobic *adj* (*metabolism*) anaeróbico; (*micro*) anaerobio
anal *adj* anal
analgesia *n* analgesia, supresión *f* de sensación dolorosa en el paciente consciente; **patient-controlled** — analgesia controlada por el paciente
analgesic *adj & n* analgésico
analysis *n* (*pl* -ses) análisis *m*; (*psych, fam*) psicoanálisis *m*, análisis *m* (*fam*); **semen** — análisis de semen
analyst *n* (*psych, fam*) psicoanalista *mf*, analista *mf* (*fam*)
analyze *vt* analizar; (*psych, fam*) psicoanalizar
analyzer *n* analizador *m*
anaphylactic *adj* anafiláctico
anaphylactoid *adj* anafilactoide
anaphylaxis *n* anafilaxia

anastomosis *n* anastomosis *f*
anatomical, anatomic *adj* anatómico
anatomy *n* anatomía
ancestor *n* antepasado
androgen *n* andrógeno
andropause *n* andropausia
anemia *n* anemia; **aplastic** — anemia aplásica; **hemolytic** — anemia hemolítica; **iron deficiency** — anemia ferropénica (*form*), anemia por deficiencia de hierro; **pernicious** — anemia perniciosa; **sickle cell** — anemia falciforme *or* de células falciformes, drepanocitosis *f*; **sideroblastic** — anemia sideroblástica
anemic *adj* anémico
anencephaly *n* anencefalia
anergy *n* anergia
anesthesia *n* anestesia; **epidural** — anestesia epidural; **general** — anestesia general; **local** — anestesia local; **regional** — anestesia regional; **spinal** — anestesia espinal
anesthesiologist *n* anestesiólogo -ga *mf*, médico -ca *mf* especialista en anestesia
anesthesiology *n* anestesiología
anesthetic *adj & n* anestésico; **general** — anestésico general; **local** — anestésico local
anesthetist *V.* nurse anesthetist.
anesthetize *vt* anestesiar, quitar la sensación de dolor
aneurysm *n* aneurisma *m*; **abdominal aortic** — aneurisma de aorta abdominal; **dissecting** — aneurisma disecante; **mycotic** — aneurisma micótico
angel dust *n* (*fam*) fenciclidina (PCP), polvo de ángel (*fam*)
angelica *n* (*bot*) angélica
anger *n* ira, enojo; — **management** manejo de ira
angiitis *n* vasculitis *f*, angeítis *f*
angina *n* angina (de pecho); **unstable** — angina inestable; **vasospastic** *o* **Prinzmetal's** — angina vasoespástica *or* de Prinzmetal
anginal *adj* anginoso
angiodysplasia *n* angiodisplasia
angioedema *n* angioedema *m*
angiogram *n* angiografía (*estudio imagenológico*)
angiography *n* angiografía, arteriografía (*técnica imagenológica*)
angioma *n* angioma *m*
angiomatosis *n* angiomatosis *f*; **bacillary** — angiomatosis bacilar
angioplasty *n* (*pl* -ties) angioplastia; **percutaneous transluminal coronary** — (**PTCA**) angioplastia transluminal percutánea coronaria
angiosarcoma *n* angiosarcoma *m*
angiotensin *n* angiotensina
angle *n* ángulo
angry *adj* enojado; **to get** — enojarse, enfadarse (*esp. Esp*)
anguish *n* angustia
aniline *n* anilina
animal *adj & n* animal *m*
ankle *n* tobillo
anklebone *n* hueso del tobillo
ankylosing spondylitis *n* espondilitis *f* anquilosante
ankylosis *n* anquilosis *f*
annoying *adj* molesto, fastidioso
annual *adj* anual
annular *adj* anular
anointing of the sick, extremaunción *f*, santos óleos
anomaly *n* (*pl* -lies) anomalía; **congenital** — anomalía congénita
anorexia *n* anorexia; — **nervosa** anorexia nerviosa
anorexiant *adj & n* anorexígeno
anovulation *n* anovulación *f*
anovulatory *adj* anovulatorio
ant *n* hormiga
antacid *adj & n* antiácido
antagonist *n* antagonista *m*; **calcium** — antagonista del calcio
anterior *adj* anterior
anthelmintic *adj & n* antihelmíntico
anthracosis *n* antracosis *f*
anthrax *n* carbunco, ántrax *m* (*Amer, Ang*)
antianginal *adj & n* antianginoso
antianxiety *adj* ansiolítico, que calma la ansiedad
antiarrhythmic *adj & n* antiarrítmico
antiasthmatic *adj & n* antiasmático
antibacterial *adj & n* antibacteriano
antibiotic *adj & n* antibiótico; **broad-spectrum** — antibiótico de amplio espectro

antibody *n* (*pl* **-dies**) anticuerpo; **antibodies against your own sperm**.. anticuerpos contra sus propios espermatozoides; **anti-mitochondrial antibodies** anticuerpos antimitocondriales; **anti-nuclear antibodies (ANA)** anticuerpos antinucleares; **antiphospholipid antibodies** anticuerpos antifosfolípidos

anti-cancer *adj* antineoplásico (*form*), anticanceroso

anticholinergic *adj* & *n* anticolinérgico

anticoagulant *adj* & *n* anticoagulante *m*; **lupus —** anticoagulante lúpico

anticoagulate *vt* tratar con anticoagulante, anticoagular

anticonvulsant *adj* & *n* antiepiléptico, anticonvulsivante *m*

antidepressant *adj* & *n* antidepresivo; **tricyclic —** antidepresivo tricíclico

antidiabetic *adj* antidiabético

antidiarrheal *adj* & *n* antidiarreico

antidote *n* antídoto

antidrug *adj* antidroga

antiemetic *adj* & *n* antiemético

antiepileptic *adj* & *n* antiepiléptico

anti-flu *adj* antigripal

antifreeze *n* anticongelante *m*

antifungal *adj* & *n* antifúngico, antimicótico

antigen *n* antígeno; **carcinoembryonic —** antígeno carcinoembrionario; **prostate-specific — (PSA)** antígeno prostático específico

antihistamine *adj* & *n* antihistamínico

antihypertensive *adj* & *n* antihipertensivo

antiinflammatory *adj* antiinflamatorio

antimalarial *adj* & *n* antipalúdico

antimicrobial *adj* & *n* antimicrobiano

antimonial *n* antimonial *m*

antioxidant *adj* & *n* antioxidante *m*

antiperspirant *adj* & *n* antitranspirante *m*

antipsychotic *adj* & *n* antipsicótico

antipyretic *adj* & *n* antipirético, antitérmico (*esp. Esp*)

anti-reflux *adj* antirreflujo

antiretroviral *adj* & *n* antirretroviral *m*, antirretrovírico

antiseptic *adj* & *n* antiséptico

antiserum *n* (*pl* **-ra**) antisuero

antismoking *adj* antitabaco, antitabáquico

antisocial *adj* antisocial

antispasmodic *adj* & *n* antiespasmódico

antithrombotic *adj* antitrombótico

antitoxin *n* antitoxina

antiviral *adj* & *n* antiviral *m*, antivírico

anus *n* (*pl* **anuses**) ano

anxiety *n* ansiedad *f*, angustia; **performance —** ansiedad de desempeño

anxiolitic *adj* & *n* ansiolítico

anxious *adj* ansioso, nervioso

aorta *n* aorta

aortic *adj* aórtico

apathetic *adj* apático

apathy *n* apatía

Apgar *n* (*fam*) *V.* **Apgar score.**

aphasia *n* afasia, dificultad *f* para hablar debida a una lesión del cerebro

aphrodisiac *n* afrodisíaco *or* afrodisiaco

aphthous *adj* aftoso

aplastic *adj* aplásica

apnea *n* apnea; **sleep —** apnea del sueño

apparatus *n* (*pl* **-tuses**) aparato

appear *vi* aparecer(se)

appearance *n* apariencia, aspecto

appendectomy *n* (*pl* **-mies**) apendicectomía

appendicitis *n* apendicitis *f*

appendix *n* (*pl* **-dices** *o* **-dixes**) apéndice *m*

appetite *n* apetito

apple *n* manzana

application *n* aplicación *f*; (*for insurance, etc.*) solicitud *f*

applicator *n* aplicador *m*; **cotton —** aplicador de algodón

apply *vt* (*pret* & *pp* **applied**) aplicar

appointment *n* cita

approach *n* abordaje *m*; **surgical —** abordaje quirúrgico

appropriate *adj* adecuado, apropiado; **the most appropriate treatment**..el tratamiento más adecuado

approximately *adv* aproximadamente

apraxia *n* apraxia

apron *n* delantal *m*; **lead** — delantal de plomo

aptitude *n* aptitud *f*

aqueous *adj* acuoso; — **humor** humor acuoso

arch *n* arco; — **of the foot** arco del pie; **fallen** — pie plano

ARDS *abbr* **adult respiratory distress syndrome.** *V.* **syndrome.**

area *n* (*geographic*) área, zona, región *f*; (*of body*) región *f* (*form*), zona, parte *f* (*fam*)

arginine *n* arginina

argon *n* argón *m*

aripiprazole *n* aripiprazol *m*

arm *n* brazo; **upper** — brazo superior, parte alta del brazo

armadillo *n* armadillo

armamentarium *n* arsenal terapéutico

armpit *n* (*fam*) axila, sobaco (*fam*)

armrest *n* reposabrazos *m*

arnica *n* (*bot*) árnica

aromatherapy *n* aromaterapia

around *adv* alrededor; aproximadamente; *prep* alrededor de; — **your arm** alrededor del brazo

arousal *n* (*from sleep*) (el) despertar; (*sexual*) excitación *f* (*sexual*)

arouse *vt* (*from sleep*) despertar; (*sexually, etc.*) excitar

arrest *n* paro; **cardiac** — paro cardíaco; **respiratory** — paro respiratorio

arrhythmia *n* arritmia

arsenic *n* arsénico

artemisinine *n* artemisinina

arterial *adj* arterial

arteriosclerosis *n* arteriosclerosis *f*

arteriovenous *adj* arteriovenoso

arteritis *n* arteritis *f*; **Takayasu's** — arteritis de Takayasu; **temporal** *o* **giant cell** — arteritis de células gigantes

artery *n* (*pl* -**ries**) arteria; **brachial** — arteria humeral *or* braquial; **carotid** — arteria carótida; **circumflex (coronary)** — arteria coronaria circunfleja; **coronary** — arteria coronaria; **femoral** —

arteria femoral; **iliac** — arteria ilíaca, arteria iliaca (*esp. Mex*); **left anterior descending (coronary)** — arteria (coronaria) descendente anterior; **left (main) coronary** — arteria coronaria izquierda; **mesenteric** — arteria mesentérica; **popliteal** — arteria poplítea; **radial** — arteria radial; **right coronary** — arteria coronaria derecha; **subclavian** — arteria subclavia

arthritic *adj* artrítico

arthritis *n* artritis *f*; **juvenile** — artritis juvenil; **rheumatoid** — artritis reumatoide

arthrogram *n* artrografía (*estudio imagenológico*)

arthrography *n* artrografía (*técnica imagenológica*)

arthroplasty *n* (*pl* -**ties**) artroplastia

arthroscopic *adj* artroscópico

arthroscopy *n* (*pl* -**pies**) artroscopia, artroscopía (*Amer, esp. spoken*)

artificial *adj* artificial

asbestos *n* asbesto, amianto

asbestosis *n* asbestosis *f*

ascariasis *n* ascariasis *f*, ascaridiasis *f*

ascending *adj* ascendente

ascites *n* ascitis *f*

ascorbic acid *n* ácido ascórbico

ASCUS *abbr* **atypical squamous cells of undetermined significance.** *V.* **cell.**

ASD *abbr* **atrial septal defect.** *V.* **defect.**

aseptic *adj* aséptico

asleep *adj* dormido; **to fall** — dormirse, quedarse dormido; **My foot fell asleep.**..Se me durmió el pie.

asparagine *n* asparagina *or* asparragina

asparagus *n* espárrago

aspergillosis *n* aspergilosis *f*

asphyxia *n* asfixia

asphyxiate *vt, vi* asfixiar(se)

aspirate *vt* (*to breathe in*) aspirar; (*to remove fluid with a syringe*) aspirar, sacar líquido con una jeringa

aspiration *n* aspiración *f*; **needle** — aspiración con aguja

aspirin *n* aspirina

assault *n* asalto, agresión *f*; **sexual —** agresión sexual

assay *n* análisis *m*, prueba

assertiveness *n* asertividad *f*

assessment *n* valoración *f*, evaluación *f*

assist *vt* asistir

assistance *n* ayuda, asistencia

assistant *n* asistente *mf*, auxiliar *mf*, ayudante *mf*; **medical —** asistente médico, persona entrenada para ayudar al médico en el consultorio o en la clínica; **nursing —** auxiliar de enfermería; **physician's —** (*US*) persona entrenada para diagnosticar y tratar enfermedades sencillas bajo la supervisión de un médico

assisted living *n* residencia para ancianos que ofrece servicios médicos tanto como asistencia para comer, vestirse, bañarse, etc.

assistive *adj* que asiste; **— device** bastón *m*, andador *m*, u otro dispositivo para asistir con las actividades de la vida diaria

associated *adj* asociado

astemizole *n* astemizol *m*

asthenia *n* astenia

asthma *n* asma

asthmatic *adj & n* asmático -ca *mf*

astigmatism *n* astigmatismo

astringent *adj & n* astringente *m*

asylum *n* asilo; **insane —** (*ant*) hospital psiquiátrico, manicomio (*ant*)

asymptomatic *adj* asintomático

asystole *n* asistolia

ataxia *n* ataxia

ataxic *adj* atáxico

atazanavir *n* atazanavir *m*

ate *pret de* **eat**

atenolol *n* atenolol *m*

atheroma *n* ateroma *m*

atherosclerosis *n* aterosclerosis *f*

athlete *n* deportista *mf*, atleta *mf*

athlete's foot *n* tinea pedis (*form*), pie *m* de atleta, infección *f* por hongos de los pies

athletic *adj* atlético; **— supporter** suspensorio

atopic *adj* atópico

atorvastatin *n* atorvastatina

atovaquone *n* atovacuona

atria *pl de* **atrium**

atrial *adj* auricular

atrioventricular *adj* auriculoventricular

atrium *n* (*pl* **atria**) (*of the heart*) aurícula

atrophy *n* atrofia; *vi* (*pret & pp* **-phied**) atrofiarse

atropine *n* atropina

attach *vt* ligar, conectar

attack *n* crisis *f*, ataque *m*; **anxiety —** crisis de angustia *or* ansiedad, ataque de nervios (*fam*); **asthma —** crisis asmática *or* de asma (*form*), ataque de asma (*fam*); **heart —** infarto de miocardio (*form*), ataque cardíaco, ataque al corazón (*fam*); **panic —** ataque *or* crisis de pánico, crisis de angustia *or* ansiedad; **transient ischemic — (TIA)** accidente *or* ataque isquémico transitorio (AIT), isquemia cerebral transitoria (*esp. Mex*)

attend *vt* (*a clinic, class, etc.*) asistir a; (*a patient*) atender, tratar, cuidar

attention *n* atención *f*

attenuated *adj* atenuado

attitude *n* actitud *f*

atypical *adj* atípico

audiogram *n* audiograma *m*

audiologist *n* audiólogo -ga *mf*, especialista *mf* en la audición

audiology *n* audiología, estudio de los trastornos de la audición

audiometer *n* audiómetro

audiometric *adj* audiométrico

audiometry *n* audiometría

auditory *adj* auditivo

augmentation *n* aumento; **breast —** aumento de mamas, cirugía para aumentar el tamaño de los senos

aunt *n* tía

aura *n* aura

autism *n* autismo

autist *n* (*form*) autista *mf*

autistic *adj* autista; **— person** autista *mf*

autoclave *n* autoclave *f*

autoimmune *adj* autoinmune

autoimmunity *n* autoinmunidad *f*

autologous *adj* autólogo

automobile *n* automóvil *m*, coche *m*, carro (*Amer*)

autonomy *n* autonomía; **patient —**

autonomía del paciente
autopsy *n* (*pl* **-sies**) autopsia, necropsia
autoregulation *n* autorregulación *f*
autosomal *adj* autosómico
autumn *n* otoño
auxiliary *adj* auxiliar
available *adj* disponible
average *adj* promedio (*esp. Amer, inv*), medio (*esp. Esp*); **the — height** la estatura promedio, la estatura media; *n* promedio, media (*form*); **above —** encima del promedio; **below —** debajo del promedio; **on —** como promedio
aversion *n* aversión f

avocado *n* aguacate *m*
avoid *vt* evitar; **You should avoid salt.**.Debe evitar la sal.
avoidance *n* evitación *f*, (el) evitar
awake *adj* despierto
aware *adj* consciente
awareness *n* consciencia
axes *pl de* **axis**
axilla *n* (*pl* **-lae**) axila
axillary *adj* axilar
axis *n* (*pl* **axes**) eje *m*
azathioprine *n* azatioprina
azelaic acid *n* ácido azelaico
azithromycin *n* azitromicina
AZT *n* AZT *m*

B

babble (*ped*) *n* balbuceo; *vi* balbucear
babesiosis *n* babesiosis *f*
baby *n* (*pl* **-bies**) bebé *mf*, criatura (*fam*)
baby-sitter *n* persona que cuida niños, niñero -ra *mf*
bacille Calmette-Guérin (BCG) *n* bacilo de Calmette-Guérin (BCG)
bacillus *n* (*pl* **-li**) bacilo
bacitracin *n* bacitracina
back *adj* de atrás; *adv* atrás; *n* espalda; (*of the hand*) dorso (*form*), la parte de atrás (*de la mano*); **the back of**..la parte de atrás de; **low — pain** dolor *m* lumbar (*form*), dolor de la espalda baja, dolor de la parte baja de la espalda; **upper —** parte alta de la espalda, espalda superior
backache *n* dolor *m* de espalda
backbone *n* columna vertebral, columna (*fam*)

backup *n* respaldo; **surgical —** respaldo quirúrgico
backward *adv* hacia atrás
baclofen *n* baclofeno, baclofen *m*
bacteremia *n* bacteriemia
bacteria *pl de* **bacterium**
bacterial *adj* bacteriano
bactericidal *adj* bactericida
bacterium *n* (*pl* **-ria**) (*frec. pl*) bacteria
bad *adj* (*comp* **worse**; *super* **worst**) malo; **Salt is bad for you.**.La sal es mala para Ud....**bad for your health** malo *or* nocivo para su salud...**a bad cold**..un resfriado fuerte ...**I have a bad back.**.Padezco problemas de la espalda.
bag *n* bolsa; **— of waters** bolsa de aguas, bolsa de las aguas (*esp. Esp*); **doctor's —** maletín del

médico; **hot-water** — bolsa de agua caliente; **to have bags under one's eyes** (*due to lack of sleep, etc.*) tener los ojos hinchados
bake *vt* hornear, cocer al horno
baker *n* panadero -ra *mf*
balance *n* equilibrio
balanced *adj* equilibrado, balanceado
balanitis *n* balanitis *f*
bald *adj* calvo
baldness *n* calvicie *f*; **frontal** — calvicie frontal; **vertex** — calvicie del vértice (*form*), calvicie de la parte superior de la cabeza
ball *n* pelota, (*soccer*) balón *m*; (*of cotton*) torunda
balloon *n* (*of a catheter*) balón *m*
balls *npl* (*fam*) testículos, huevos (*esp. Mex, fam*), cojones *mpl* (*vulg*)
balm *n* bálsamo, crema; **lip** — crema para los labios, bálsamo labial (*esp. Esp*)
banana *n* plátano
band *n* cinta, banda, (*around waist*) faja; (*orthodontics*) banda (*que se coloca alrededor de un diente*); *npl* (*fam*) aparato (de ortodoncia), corrector *m* dental (*esp. Esp*), brackets *mpl* (*fam*), frenos *or* frenillos (*Amer, fam*)
bandage *n* (*material*) venda, (*once placed*) vendaje *m*; **adhesive** — vendaje adhesivo, venda adhesiva, cura, (*small*) curita (*Amer*), tirita (*Esp*); **compression** — vendaje compresivo; **elastic** — venda elástica, vendaje elástico; **figure-of-eight** — vendaje en ocho; **pressure** — vendaje compresivo
Band-Aid *n* (*marca*) small adhesive bandage. *V.* **bandage**.
bank *n* banco; **blood** — banco de sangre; **food** — banco de alimentos; **organ** — banco de órganos
barb *n* lengüeta
barbecue *n* barbacoa; *vt* asar a la parrilla, asar a la barbacoa (*esp. Mex*)
barbed wire *n* alambre *m* de púas
barber *n* peluquero -ra *mf*, barbero
barbiturate *adj & n* barbitúrico
bare *adj* desnudo, descubierto
barefoot *adj* descalzo
barf (*fam*) *V.* **vomit**.

bariatric *adj* bariátrico
barium *n* bario
bark *n* (*bot*) corteza
barotrauma *n* barotrauma *m*
barrel *n* (*of a syringe*) cilindro; — **chest** tórax en tonel
barrier *n* barrera; **placental** — barrera placentaria
basal *adj* basal, (*at rest*) en reposo
basal ganglia *npl* ganglios basales
base *n* (*chem, pharm, etc.*) base *f*; (*of an ulcer*) base, fondo (*de una úlcera*); **data** — base de datos; **oil-based, water-based, etc.** a base de aceite, a base de agua, etc.
baseball *n* beisbol *m*
baseline *adj* basal; — **value** valor *m* basal; *n* (*behavior, physical exam*) estado habitual *or* normal (*para el paciente*); **Is he back to baseline?** ..¿Ha vuelto a lo normal?
bashful *adj* tímido
basic *adj* básico
basin *n* palangana, vasija; **emesis** — riñonera, recipiente para contener vómito(s)
basketball *n* (*sport*) baloncesto, basquetbol *m* (*Amer*)
bassinet *n* moisés *m*, cuna portátil
bat *n* (*zool*) murciélago
bath *n* baño; **sitz** — baño de asiento; **sponge** — baño de esponja; **steam** — baño de vapor; **to take a** — bañarse
bathe *vt, vi* bañar(se)
bathroom *n* cuarto de baño, baño; **to go to the** — ir al baño
bathtub *n* bañera, tina (de baño), bañadera (*Cub*)
battered *adj* maltratado, golpeado
battle n lucha; — **against cancer** lucha contra el cancer
BCG *V.* **bacille Calmette-Guérin**.
beam *n* (*of light, X-rays, etc.*) haz *m*
beans *npl* frijoles *mpl* (*Amer*), judías (*Esp*)
bear *vt* (*pret* **bore**) (*pp* **borne**) tolerar, aguantar, soportar; (*to give birth to*) dar a luz; **child-bearing age** edad fértil; **to — down** pujar; **Bear down as if you were having a bowel movement**..Puje como si estuviera defecando (haciendo

popó, etc.); **to — weight** soportar peso; **You shouldn't bear weight with your left leg for two weeks**..No debe soportar peso con su pierna izquierda durante dos semanas.

bearable *adj* tolerable, aguantable

beard *n* barba

beat *n* (*of the heart*) latido; *vi* (*pret* **beat**; *pp* **beaten** *o* **beat**) latir

beclomethasone *n* beclometasona

bed *n* cama, lecho; **— rest** reposo en cama; **hospital —** cama hospitalaria; **nail —** lecho ungueal; **to stay in —** guardar cama; **vascular —** lecho vascular

bedbug *n* chinche *f*

bedclothes, bedding *npl* ropa de cama

bedpan *n* bacinilla, pato (*Amer*), cómodo (*Mex*), chata

bedrail *n* baranda

bedridden *adj* encamado, incapaz de abandonar la cama

bedroom *n* dormitorio, cuarto, recámara (*esp. Mex*)

bedsheet *n* sábana

bedside *adj* de cabecera; **— manner** comportamiento con un enfermo; *n* **at the —** a la cabecera

bedsore (*fam*) **pressure sore**. *V.* **sore**.

bedtime *n* hora de acostarse

bedwetting *n* enuresis *f* (*form*), (el) mojar la cama

bee *n* abeja; **Africanized** *o* **killer —** abeja africanizada *or* asesina

beef *n* carne *f* de res (*esp. Amer*), carne de vaca (*esp. Esp*)

beeper *n* biper *m* (*Amer*), buscapersonas *m* (*Esp, SA*)

beer *n* cerveza

before *adv* antes; **Have you ever had these pains before?**..¿Ha tenido estos dolores antes? *conj* antes de que; **before you take this medicine**..antes de que tome esta medicina; *prep* antes de; **— meals** antes de las comidas

begin *vt, vi* comenzar, empezar

behavior *n* conducta, comportamiento

behind *adj* atrasado; **Is he behind in school?**..¿Está atrasado en sus estudios? *n* (*fam*) nalgas, trasero (*fam*); *prep* detrás de; **The bullet is behind your heart**..La bala está detrás de su corazón.

belch *vi* eructar

belief *n* creencia

belladonna *n* (*bot*) belladona

belly *n* (*pl* **-lies**) abdomen *m*, barriga (*fam*), vientre *m* (*esp. Esp*)

bellyache *n* dolor *m* de barriga

bellybutton *n* (*fam*) ombligo

below *adv* abajo; *prep* por debajo de, inferior a (*form*); **— 200** inferior a 200, por debajo de 200; **— the waist** por debajo de la cintura

belt *n* cinturón *m*, cinto

benazepril *n* benazepril *m*

bend *n* curva, ángulo; *vt* (*pret & pp* **bent**) doblar; **Bend your knee**.. Doble la rodilla; **to — one's head down** bajar *or* agachar la cabeza; *vi* doblarse; **to — over** *o* **down** agacharse, doblarse; **Bend over**.. Agáchese (Dóblese.)

bends *npl* **the —** enfermedad *f* por descompresión

beneficial *adj* beneficioso

benefit *n* beneficio, bien *m*; **for your —** para su beneficio, por su bien

benign *adj* benigno

bent *pret & pp de* **bend**

benzene *n* benceno

benzoate *n* benzoato

benzodiazepine *n* benzodiazepina *or* benzodiacepina

benzoin *n* benzoína

benzoyl peroxide *n* peróxido de benzoílo

beriberi *n* beriberi *m*

beta *n* beta; **beta-blocker** betabloqueante *m*, betabloqueador *m* (*esp. Mex*); **beta-hemolytic** beta-hemolítico

betamethasone *n* betametasona

better (*comp de* **good** *y* **well**) *adj & adv* mejor; **to get —** (*patient*) recuperarse, (*pain*) aliviarse, (*wound*) sanar, (*disease*) mejorarse, quitarse; **to make —** mejorar, aliviar

between *prep* entre; **between your teeth**..entre los dientes

bevel *n* (*of a needle, etc.*) bisel *m*

bezoar *n* bezoar *m*

bib *n* babero

bicarbonate *n* bicarbonato

biceps *n* bíceps *m*

bicuspid *adj & n* bicúspide *m*

bicycle *n* bicicleta; **stationary** — bicicleta estática; **to ride a** — ir *or* montar en bicicleta

bifocal *adj* bifocal; *npl* (*fam*) lentes *mpl* (*fam*) bifocales, bifocales *mpl* (*fam*)

big *adj* (*comp* **bigger**; *super* **biggest**) grande; (*sibling*) mayor; **How big was it?**..¿Qué tan grande era? — **sister** (*fam*) hermana mayor; **to get bigger** crecer, ponerse más grande

bile *n* bilis *f*

biliary *adj* biliar

bilingual *adj* bilingüe

bilirubin *n* bilirrubina

bill *n* (*doctor's*) honorarios, cuenta (*del médico*)

bind *vi* (*pret & pp* **bound**) (*clothing, etc.*) apretar

binge *n* (*alcohol*) borrachera (*esp. por varios días seguidos*); (*food*) atracón *m*, período de comer en exceso; **binge-eating** trastorno por atracón, (el) comer en exceso periódicamente; *vi* beber en exceso periódicamente; comer en exceso periódicamente

bioactive *adj* bioactivo

biochemical *adj* bioquímico

biochemistry *n* bioquímica

biodegradable *adj* biodegradable

bioengineering *n* bioingeniería

biofeedback *n* biorretroalimentación *f*

biohazard *n* riesgo biológico

biohazardous *adj* que presenta riesgo biológico

bioimpedance *n* bioimpedancia

biological *adj* biológico; — **mother** madre biológica

biological clock *n* reloj biológico

biology *n* biología

biomechanics *n* biomecánica

biomedical *adj* biomédico

bioprosthesis *n* (*pl* -ses) bioprótesis *f*

biopsy *n* (*pl* -sies) biopsia; **bone marrow** — biopsia de médula ósea; **breast** — biopsia de mama;

excisional — biopsia escisional *or* excisional; **fine needle aspiration** — punción *f* aspiración con aguja fina, biopsia por aspiración con aguja fina (*esp. Mex*); **incisional** — biopsia incisional; **hepatic** *o* **liver** — biopsia hepática (*form*), biopsia de hígado; **punch** — biopsia de piel, biopsia cutánea (*esp. Esp*); **prostatic** — biopsia prostática (*form*), biopsia de próstata; **renal** — biopsia renal (*form*), biopsia de riñón; **skin** — biopsia de piel, biopsia cutánea (*esp. Esp*); **stereotactic** — biopsia estereotáxica

biorhythm *n* ritmo biológico

biostatistics *n* bioestadística

biotechnology *n* biotecnología

bioterrorism *n* bioterrorismo

BiPAP *abbr* **bi-level positive airway pressure**. *V*. **pressure**.

bipolar *adj* bipolar

bird *n* ave *f*, pájaro

birth *n* nacimiento; (*childbirth*) parto; — **control** anticoncepción *f*, control *m* de la natalidad, método anticonceptivo; **Do you use birth control?**..¿Usa algún método anticonceptivo? — **weight** peso al nacer; **breech** — parto de nalgas; **(blind, deaf, etc.) from** — (ciego, sordo, etc.) de nacimiento; **natural** — parto natural; **to give** — dar a luz, aliviarse (*Mex, fam*), parir (*esp. Carib, fam*); **She gave birth to a baby girl**..Dio a luz a una niña.

birthday *n* cumpleaños *m*; **Happy birthday!**..¡Feliz cumpleaños!

birthing *n* parto asistido por un médico o partera con intervención mínima y en un ambiente natural y hogareño

birthmark *n* marca de nacimiento

bisexual *adj* bisexual

bismuth *n* bismuto

bisoprolol *n* bisoprolol *m*

bisphosphonate *n* bisfosfonato

bite *n* (*of food*) bocado; (*wound*) mordedura; (*of an insect*) picadura; (*dent*) mordida; *vt, vi* (*pret* **bit**; *pp* **bitten** *o* **bit**) morder; (*insect*) picar; **Bite down**..Apriete los dientes.

bitter *adj* amargo

black *adj* negro; **to — out** desmayarse, perder el conocimiento *or* la conciencia

black-and-blue *adj* (*fam*) que tiene muchos moretones, severamente magullado, que tiene muchos cardenales (*Esp*)

black cohosh *n* (*bot*) Cimicifuga racemosa o Actaea racemosa, planta medicinal nativa de los Estados Unidos

black eye *n* ojo morado

blackhead *n* espinilla, barro

blackish *adj* negruzco

black lung *n* (*fam*) antracosis *f*, enfermedad de los pulmones producida por el polvo de carbón

blackout *n* (*loss of consciousness*) desmayo, pérdida del conocimiento; (*lapse of memory*) laguna mental; (*due to alcohol*) laguna mental de horas o días (*debida al tomar alcohol en exceso*)

black widow *n* viuda negra

bladder *n* vejiga; **hyperactive —** vejiga hiperactiva; **neurogenic —** vejiga neurogénica, vejiga neurógena (*esp. Esp*); **overactive —** (*fam*) vejiga hiperactiva

blade *n* hoja (*de navaja, cuchillo, etc.*)

bland *adj* (*food*) blanda, sin sazón

blanket *n* manta, frazada (*Amer*), cobija (*esp. Mex*), friza (*PR, SD*); **electric —** manta térmica *or* eléctrica

blastomycosis *n* blastomicosis *f*

bleach *n* blanqueador *m*, cloro

bleed *n* hemorragia, sangrado (*fam*); **(upper, lower) GI —** hemorragia digestiva (alta, baja); *vi* (*pret & pp* **bled**) sangrar

bleeding *adj* sangrante; **— ulcer** úlcera sangrante; *n* hemorragia, sangrado; **dysfunctional uterine —** hemorragia uterina disfuncional; **menstrual —** sangrado menstrual

bleomycin *n* bleomicina

blepharitis *n* blefaritis *f*

blepharoplasty *n* (*pl* **-ties**) blefaroplastia

blew *pret de* **blow**

blind *adj* ciego

blindness *n* ceguera; **color —** daltonismo (*form*), dificultad *f* para diferenciar ciertos colores; **night —** ceguera nocturna

blink *n* parpadeo; *vi* parpadear

blister *n* ampolla; **fever —** fuego, calentura (*frec. pl*), ampolla en los labios debida al herpes

bloated *adj* (*swollen*) hinchado; (*uncomfortably full*) distendido, hinchado (*fam*); **to feel —** tener distensión abdominal (*form*), sentirse distendido, hincharse(le) (a uno) el estómago, tener gases

bloating *n* hinchazón *f*; (*abdominal*) distensión *f* abdominal, hinchazón del estómago (*fam*)

block *n* bloqueo; **bundle branch —** bloqueo de rama; **heart —** bloqueo cardíaco; **nerve —** bloqueo nervioso; *vt* (*pharm, physio*) bloquear, (*anat, surg*) obstruir

blockage *n* obstrucción *f*, bloqueo

blocked *adj* obstruído (*form*), bloqueado, tapado (*fam*)

blocker *n* bloqueante *m*, bloqueador *m* (*esp. Mex*), antagonista *m*; **angiotensin receptor —** antagonista de los receptores de la angiotensina II; **beta-blocker** beta-bloqueante *m*, betabloqueador *m* (*esp. Mex*); **calcium channel —** antagonista del calcio; **H₂ blocker** antihistamínico H₂; **neuro-muscular —** bloqueante neuromuscular, bloqueador neuromuscular (*esp. Mex*)

blond *adj* rubio; *n* rubio -bia *mf*, güero -ra *mf* (*Mex*)

blonde *n* rubia, güera (*Mex*)

blood *n* sangre *f*; **arterial — gas** gasometría arterial, gases *mpl* arteriales; **— poisoning** septicemia (*form*), infección *f* de la sangre; **— pressure** *V*. **pressure**; **— pressure monitor** *V*. monitor

bloodborne *adj* de transmisión sanguínea (*form*), transmitido por la sangre

bloodshot *adj* rojo (*el ojo*)

bloodstream *n* torrente sanguíneo

blood thinner *n* (*fam*) anticoagulante *m*

bloody *adj* sanguinolento, con sangre; — **discharge** secreción sanguinolenta, secreción con sangre; — **nose** (*fam*) hemorragia nasal (*form*), sangrado nasal, sangrado por la nariz (*fam*); — **show** (*obst*) sangrado vaginal (*antes de la expulsión del feto*)

blot *n* blot *m*, tipo de prueba médica muy precisa; **Western —, Southern —,** etc. Western blot, Southern blot, etc.; *vt* (*pret & pp* **blotted**; *ger* **blotting**) secar por presión con material absorbente

blotch *n* mancha, roncha (*de la piel*)

blouse *n* blusa

blow *n* golpe *m*; **psychological —** golpe psicológico; *vt, vi* (*pret* **blew**; *pp* **blown**) soplar; **Blow as hard as you can**..Sople lo más fuerte que pueda; **to — one's nose** sonarse la nariz, soplarse la nariz (*Carib*)

blue *adj* azul; (*fam, sad*) triste; *npl* **the —** (*fam*) melancolía, tristeza

bluish *adj* azulado

blunt *adj* (*object*) romo, sin filo; (*trauma*) cerrado

blur *vi* (*pret & pp* **blurred**; *ger* **blurring**) (*one's vision*) empañarse, borrarse (*la visión*)

blurred, blurry *adj* borroso; — **vision** visión borrosa

blush *vi* ruborizarse, sonrojarse, ponerse colorado

BM *V.* **bowel movement**.

BMI *abbr* **body mass index**. *V.* **index**.

board and care *n* (*US*) residencia para ancianos o minusválidos en que se ofrece comidas y cuidados básicos como bañar, vestir, etc.

board-certified *adj* (*US*) que ha aprobado un examen estatal en su campo

body *adj* corporal; *n* (*pl* **bodies**) cuerpo, organismo; — **heat** calor *m* corporal; — **language** lenguaje *m* corporal; — **odor** olor *m* corporal; **foreign —** cuerpo extraño; **upper —** parte *f* superior del cuerpo

bodybuilder *n* culturista *mf*, fisicoculturista *mf*

bodybuilding *n* culturismo, fisicoculturismo

bodywork *n* trabajo corporal

bodyworker *n* masajista *mf*, practicante *mf* de trabajo corporal

boil *n* forúnculo (*form*), nacido, divieso (*esp. Esp*), absceso (de la piel), grano (grande); *vt* (*water*) hervir, hacer hervir; (*vegetables, meat, etc.*) cocer, hervir; *vi* hervir

boiled *adj* (*water*) hervido; (*vegetables*) cocido, hervido

boiling *adj* hirviendo; — **water** agua hirviendo

bolus *n* bolo

bomb *n* bomba; **atomic —** bomba atómica; **time —** bomba de tiempo

bond (*obst, psych, etc.*) *n* lazo afectivo, vínculo, enlace *m*; *vi* formar lazo afectivo

bonding (*obst, psych*) *n* formación *f* de un lazo afectivo

bone *adj* óseo; — **marrow** médula ósea; *n* hueso; (*of a fish*) espina

booger *n* (*vulg*) moco

booklet *n* folleto

boost *vt* (*one's immune system, etc.*) reforzar (*el sistema inmunitario, etc.*)

booster *adj* de refuerzo; — **dose** dosis *f* de refuerzo; — **shot** (*fam*) dosis *f* de refuerzo (*por inyección*); — **vaccination** revacunación *f*, vacunación de refuerzo

boot *n* bota

booze *n* (*fam*) bebida alcohólica (*incluyendo vino y cerveza*)

border *n* (*edge, margin*) borde *m*, margen *m*

borderline *adj* (*psych*) límite, borderline (*Ang*); (*leprosy*) dimorfa; (*hypertension, diabetes, etc.*) en el límite; **You have borderline hypertension (diabetes, etc.).**..Su presión arterial (azucar, etc.) está en el límite..Ud. tiene prehipertensión (prediabetes, etc.)

bore *vt* aburrir

bore *pret de* **bear**

bored (*pp de* **bore**) *adj* aburrido; **to become —** aburrirse; **He gets bored easily**..Se aburre fácilmente.

boric acid *n* ácido bórico

born (*pret de* **bear**) *adj* nacido; **to be —** nacer

borne *pp de* **bear**

botanical *adj* botánico; *n* medicina de origen botánico

botch *vt* hacer mal

bother *vt* molestar; **Is your neck bothering you?**..¿Le está molestando el cuello?

bottle *n* botella; *(for pills)* botella, frasco, pomo *(Mex, CA)*; **baby —** biberón *m*, mamadera *(Amer)*, pacha *(CA)*; **hot-water —** bolsa de agua caliente

bottom *n* fondo; *(fam, buttocks)* nalgas, trasero *(fam)*

botulinum toxin *n* toxina botulínica

botulism *n* botulismo

bound *pret & pp de* **bind**

bout *n* ataque *m*, episodio

bovine *adj* bovino

bowed *adj (curved)* arqueado

bowel *n* intestino, tripa *(fam, frec. pl)*; **large —** colon *m*; **small —** intestino delgado

bowel movement (BM) *n (act)* defecación *f (form)*, evacuación *f* (del intestino), deposición *f (Esp, SA)*; *(stool)* heces *fpl* (fecales) *(form)*, popó *(fam)*, caca *(fam or vulg)*, deposición *f (Esp, SA)*, evacuación *f*, excremento; **painful — —** defecación *or* evacuación dolorosa, dolor cuando va al baño *(fam)*; **to have a — —** defecar *(form)*, ir al baño *(euph)*, hacer del baño *(Mex)*, dar del cuerpo *(Carib)*, hacer del cuerpo *(SA)*, hacer popó *(fam)*, hacer caca *(fam or vulg)*; **When was the last time you had a bowel movement?**..¿Cuándo fue la última vez que defecó (fue al baño, etc.)?

bowlegged *adj* con las piernas arqueadas

boy *n* niño, muchacho, chico

boyfriend *n* novio, enamorado

bra *(fam) V.* **brassiere.**

brace *n* aparato ortopédico (para estabilizar una articulación); *npl* aparato (de ortodoncia), corrector *m* dental *(esp. Esp)*, brackets *mpl (fam)*, frenos *or* frenillos *(Amer, fam)*

bracelet *n* pulsera, brazalete *m*; **iden-tification (ID) —** pulsera *or* brazalete de identifición; **medic alert —** pulsera *or* brazalete de alerta médica

brachial *adj (plexus)* braquial, *(artery)* humeral

brachytherapy *n* braquiterapia

brackets *n (orthodontia)* brackets *mpl*

bradycardia *n* bradicardia

Braille *n* braille *m*, método de lectura para ciegos

brain *n* cerebro; **brain-dead** con muerte cerebral, que tiene muerte cerebral; **— death** muerte cerebral

brainstem *n* tronco del encéfalo

bran *n* salvado

branch *n* rama

brassiere *n* sostén *m*, sujetador *m*, brassiere *m (esp. Mex)*

brave *adj* valiente; **Be brave!**..¡Sé valiente!

bread *n* pan *m*

break *n (ortho)* fractura *(form)*, quebradura; *vt, vi (pret* **broke**; *pp* **broken)** *(ortho, etc.)* fracturar(se) *(form)*, quebrar(se), romper(se); **I broke my foot** *o* **My foot broke**..Me fracturé (quebré, rompí) el pie; **to — out** *(one's skin)* salir(le) (a uno) granos; **When did your skin break out?**..¿Cuándo le salieron granos?

breakdown *n* colapso, crisis *f*; **nervous —** crisis nerviosa; **skin —** deterioro de la piel *(que precede a una úlcera de decúbito)*

breakfast *n* desayuno; **to have —** desayunar(se)

breakthrough *adj* **— pain** dolor que aparece a veces a pesar del medicamento tomado diariamente para controlarlo; *n* avance *m*, adelanto

breast *n (chest)* pecho; *(female)* mama, seno, pecho

breastbone *n* esternón *m (form)*, hueso del pecho

breast-feed *vt, vi (pret & pp* **-fed)** amamantar *(form)*, dar el pecho, dar de mamar; **Are you breast-feeding him?**..¿Le está dando el pecho?

breast-feeding *n* lactancia materna

(form), (el) dar el pecho; **Breast-feeding will protect your baby against disease.**.Darle el pecho al niño le protegerá de enfermedades.

breath *n* aliento, respiración *f*; **bad** — mal aliento; — **test** prueba del aliento; **shortness of** — falta de aire, dificultad *f* para respirar; **to be short of** — faltar(le) (a uno) el aire, tener dificultad para respirar; **Do you get short of breath when you walk?**..¿Le falta el aire cuando camina?..¿Tiene dificultad para respirar cuando camina?...**How many blocks can you walk before you get short of breath?**..¿Cuántas cuadras puede caminar antes de que le falte el aire (que tenga dificultad para respirar)? **to hold one's** — contener la respiración, aguantar la respiración *(fam)*; **Hold your breath.**.Contenga (Aguante) la respiración; **to take a deep** — respirar profundo; **Take a deep breath.**. Respire profundo.

breathe *vt, vi* respirar; **Breathe quietly while I listen to your heart.**. Respire suavemente mientras le escucho el corazón; **to** — **in** inspirar *(form)*, inhalar *(form)*, respirar *(fam)*, tomar aire *(fam)*; **Breathe in.**.Inspire (Respire, Tome aire); **to** — **out** espirar *(form)*, exhalar *(form)*, sacar aire *(esp. Mex, CA; fam)*, botar aire *(esp. Carib, SA; fam)*

bridge *n (dent, etc.)* puente *m*; — **of the nose** puente nasal

bring *vt (pret & pp brought)* **to** — **on** *(pain, etc.)* provocar, causar, despertar

bristle *n (of a brush)* cerda; **soft-bristle** de cerda suave; **stiff-bristle** o **hard-bristle** de cerda dura

brittle *adj (nails, etc.)* quebradizo, frágil; *(diabetes)* difícil de controlar

broccoli *n* brécol *m*, bróculi *or* brócoli *m*

broil *adj* asar a la parrilla, asar

broke *pret de* break

broken *(pp de break) adj* quebrado, roto

bromide *n* bromuro

bromine *n* bromo

bromocriptine *n* bromocriptina

bronchi *pl de* **bronchus**

bronchial *adj* bronquial

bronchiectasis *n* bronquiectasia

bronchiole *n (pl -oles)* bronquiolo

bronchiolitis *n* bronquiolitis *f*; — **obliterans** bronquiolitis obliterante

bronchitis *n* bronquitis *f*; **chronic** — bronquitis crónica

bronchoalveolar *adj* broncoalveolar

bronchoconstriction *n* broncoconstricción *f*

bronchodilator *n* broncodilatador *m*

bronchogenic *adj* broncogénico

bronchoscope *n* broncoscopio

bronchoscopy *n (pl -pies)* broncoscopia, broncoscopía *(Amer, esp. spoken)*

bronchospasm *n* broncoespasmo

bronchus *n (pl -chi)* bronquio

broth *n* caldo

brother *n* hermano

brother-in-law *n (pl brothers-in-law)* cuñado

brought *pret & pp de* bring

brow *n (forehead)* frente *f*; *(eyebrow)* ceja

brown *adj* castaño, de color café, marrón; *(eyes)* marrón, castaño; *(hair)* castaño; *(sugar)* moreno; *(bread)* integral, moreno

brown recluse *V.* **spider.**

brucellosis *n* brucelosis *f*

bruise *n* moretón *m*, magulladura, cardenal *m (Esp)*; *vt* producir moretones (magulladuras, cardenales); *vi* salirse(le) *or* hacerse(le) (a uno) moretones (magulladuras, cardenales); **Do you bruise easily?**.. ¿Se le salen (hacen) moretones (magulladuras, cardenales) fácilmente?

bruised *adj* que tiene moretón, con moretones, magullado, que tiene cardenal *(Esp)*, con cardenales *(Esp)*

brush *n* cepillo; *vt* cepillar; **to** — **one's hair** cepillarse el pelo; **to** — **one's teeth** cepillarse los dientes

brushing *n (dent, etc.)* cepillado; **bronchial** — cepillado bronquial

bruxism *n* bruxismo

bubble *n* burbuja

bubo n (pl **buboes**) bubón m
bubonic adj bubónico
buckle n hebilla; vt abrochar(se)
bucktooth n (pl **-teeth**) diente m de conejo, diente salido
buddy tape vt fijar (un dedo) al dedo adyacente con cinta adhesiva
budesonide n budesonida, budesónida (OMS)
buffer n tampón m, amortiguador m
bug n insecto, bicho; (fam, microbe) microbio, virus m, bacteria; (fam, illness) gripe f, resfriado, enfermedad f de tipo gripal
build n contextura, físico, complexión f; vt (pret & pp **built**) **to — up** (one's strength, muscles, etc.) fortalecer; (one's resistance) aumentar (la resistencia); vi **to — up** acumularse
buildup n depósito, acumulación f
bulbar adj bulbar
bulimia n bulimia
bulimic adj bulímico
bullet n bala
bullous adj (enfisema) bulloso; (penfigoide) ampolloso
bumetanide n bumetanida
bump n nódulo (form), bola, bolita, bulto (esp. Esp), (due to trauma, esp. about the head) chichón m
bunion n juanete m
buprenorphine n buprenorfina
bupropion n bupropión m
burden n carga; **tumor —** carga tumoral
burdock n (bot) bardana, lampazo
burn n quemadura; **first (second, third) degree —** quemadura de primer (segundo, tercer) grado; vt (pret & pp **burned**) quemar; **Did you burn your hand?**..¿Se quemó la mano? **to — oneself** o **to get burned** quemarse; **Did you burn yourself?**..¿Se quemó? vi arder; **Does it burn when you urinate?**.. ¿Le arde al orinar?
burning (pain) adj quemante, ardiente; **— sensation** ardor m, sen-
sación f de quemazón; n ardor m, quemazón f, (smarting) escozor m
burnout n desgaste m profesional, burnout m (Ang)
burnt adj **burned**. V. **burn**.
burp vt (a baby) hacer eructar; **You should burp your baby after each meal**..Debe hacerle eructar a su bebé después de cada comida; vi eructar
burrow n (of scabies) túnel m (de la sarna); vi hacer un túnel
bursa n bolsa
bursitis n bursitis f; **anserine —** bursitis anserina; **olecranon —** bursitis olecraneana; **prepatellar —** bursitis prepatelar, bursitis prerrotuliana (Esp); **subacromial —** bursitis subacromial; **trochanteric —** bursitis trocantérica (Amer), bursitis trocantérea (Esp)
burst vt, vi (pret & pp **burst**) reventar(se)
buspirone n buspirona
bust n busto, pecho
busulfan n busulfán m, busulfano (OMS)
butcher n carnicero -ra mf
butt n (vulg) **buttock(s)**. V. **buttock**.
butter n mantequilla
buttock n nalga; npl trasero (fam)
button n botón m; **call —** botón de llamada; **If you need the nurse, press the call button**..Si necesita la enfermera, presione el botón de llamada; vt (también **to — up**) abotonar(se), abrochar(se)
buzzing n zumbido
bypass n bypass m (Ang), derivación f; **cardiopulmonary —** derivación cardiopulmonar; **coronary artery — graft surgery** cirugía de revascularización coronaria; **femoropopliteal —** bypass femoropoplíteo; **gastric —** bypass gástrico, derivación gástrica; **triple (quadruple, etc.) —** triple (cuádruple, etc.) bypass

C

cactus *n* (*pl* **-ti**) cactus *m*, cacto
cadaver *n* cadáver *m*
cadaveric *adj* de cadáver, cadavérico
cadmium *n* cadmio
caffeine *n* cafeína
calamine *n* calamina
calcification *n* calcificación *f*
calcify *vi* (*pret & pp* **-fied**) calcificar(se)
calcitonin *n* calcitonina
calcitriol *n* calcitriol *m*
calcium *n* calcio; — **carbonate** carbonato cálcico (*form*), carbonato de calcio; — **gluconate** gluconato cálcico (*form*), gluconato de calcio
calculus *n* (*stone, form*) cálculo (*form*), piedra; (*dent*) cálculo (*form*), sarro (dental); **renal** — cálculo renal, piedra en el riñón
calf *n* (*pl* **calves**) (*anat*) pantorrilla
calibrate *vt* calibrar
calisthenics *n* calistenia
call *n* llamada; **on** — de guardia; *vt, vi* llamar; **Call for the nurse.**. Llame a la enfermera.
callus *n* (*pl* **-luses**) callo, (*thin*) callosidad *f*
calm *adj* tranquilo; *vt* calmar; *vi* **to** — **down** tranquilizarse, calmarse
calorie *n* caloría
calves *pl de* **calf**
campaign *n* campaña; **anti-smoking** — campaña antitabaco, campaña contra el tabaco; **vaccination** — campaña de vacunación
camphor *n* alcanfor *m*
can *n* lata
canal *n* canal *m*, conducto; **auditory** — conducto auditivo; **birth** — canal del parto; **semicircular** — conducto semicircular
cancel *vt* (*pret & pp* **-celed** *o* **-celled**; *ger* **-celing** *o* **-celling**) cancelar
cancer *n* cáncer *m*; **bladder** — cáncer vesical (*form*), cáncer de vejiga; **bone** — cáncer óseo (*form*), cáncer de hueso (*fam*); **breast** — cáncer

de mama (*form*), cáncer de pecho (*fam*); **cervical** — cáncer de cuello uterino, cáncer cervical *or* de cérvix; **colon** — cáncer de colon; **colorectal** — cáncer colorrectal; **esophageal** — cáncer de esófago; **gastric** — (*form*) cáncer gástrico (*form*), cáncer de estómago; **head and neck** — cáncer de cabeza y cuello; **laryngeal** — cáncer de laringe; **liver** — cáncer de hígado; **lung** — (**non-small cell; small cell**) cáncer de pulmón (de células no pequeñas, no microcítico [*esp. Esp*]; de células pequeñas, microcítico [*esp. Esp*]); **ovarian** — cáncer de ovario; **pancreatic** — cáncer de páncreas; **prostate** — cáncer de próstata; **rectal** — cáncer de recto; **renal** (**cell**) — cáncer de riñón; **skin** — cáncer cutáneo (*form*), cáncer de piel; **stomach** — cáncer gástrico (*form*), cáncer de estómago; **thyroid** — cáncer de tiroides; **uterine** — cáncer de útero, cáncer uterino
cancer-causing *adj* cancerígeno, que causa cáncer
cancerous *adj* canceroso
candesartan *n* candesartán *m*
candidate *n* candidato -ta *mf*; **candidate for a heart transplant**..candidato a trasplante cardíaco *or* de corazón
candidiasis *n* candidiasis *f*, (tipo de) infección *f* por hongos
candy *n* (*pl* **-dies**) dulce(s) *m(pl)*, caramelo(s), golosina(s)
cane *n* bastón *m*
canker sore *n* afta, pequeña úlcera generalmente en la boca
cannabinoid *adj & n* cannabinoide *m*
cannabinol *n* cannabinol *m*
cannabis *n* cannabis *m*
cannula *n* cánula; **nasal** — cánula nasal
cap *n* (*of a bottle*) tapa; (*of a needle*)

capuchón *m*; (*dent, fam*) corona (*esp. una del color del diente*); (*head covering*) gorro; **bathing** *o* **shower** — gorro de baño; **cervical** — capuchón *m* cervical; **safety** — tapa de seguridad; **scrub** *o* **surgical** — gorro quirúrgico *or* de cirugía

capable *adj* capaz

capacity *n* (*pl* **-ties**) capacidad *f*; **forced vital** — capacidad vital forzada

capillary *adj & n* (*pl* **-ries**) capilar *m*

capitation *n* capitación *f*, sistema *m* de seguro médico en el cual los proveedores están pagados una cantidad fija por persona cubierta

capsaicin *n* capsaicina

capsule *n* cápsula

capsulitis *n* capsulitis *f*; **adhesive** — capsulitis adhesiva *or* retráctil, hombro congelado (*fam*)

captopril *n* captopril *m*

car *n* coche *m*, carro (*Amer*)

carat *n* quilate *m*; **14** — **gold** oro de 14 quilates

carb (*fam*) *V*. **carbohydrate**.

carbamazepine *n* carbamazepina *or* carbamacepina

carbamide peroxide *n* peróxido de carbamida

carbidopa *n* carbidopa

carbohydrate *n* hidrato de carbono

carbon *n* (*element*) carbono; — **dioxide** dióxido de carbono; — **monoxide** monóxido de carbono; — **tetrachloride** tetracloruro de carbono

carbonate *n* carbonato

carbonated *adj* carbonatado

carbuncle *n* ántrax *m*

carcinogen *n* carcinógeno

carcinogenic *adj* cancerígeno

carcinoid *adj* carcinoide; — **tumor** tumor carcinoide

carcinoma *n* carcinoma *m*; **basal cell** — carcinoma basocelular; **bronchogenic** — carcinoma broncogénico; **ductal** — **in situ** carcinoma ductal in situ; **hepatocellular** — carcinoma hepatocelular; **non-small cell** — carcinoma de células no pequeñas, carcinoma no microcítico (*Esp*); **renal cell** — carcinoma renal; **small cell** — carcinoma de células pequeñas, carcinoma microcítico (*Esp*); **squamous cell** — carcinoma escamoso; **transitional cell** — carcinoma de células transicionales

carcinomatosis *n* carcinomatosis *f*

card *n* (*business, insurance, etc.*) tarjeta

cardiac *adj* cardíaco *or* cardiaco

cardiogenic *adj* cardiogénico

cardiologist *n* cardiólogo -ga *mf*, médico -ca *mf* especialista en las enfermedades del corazón, especialista *mf* del corazón (*fam*)

cardiology *n* cardiología, estudio del corazón y de sus funciones y enfermedades

cardiomyopathy *n* (*pl* **-thies**) miocardiopatía, cardiopatía, cardiomiopatía; **dilated** — miocardiopatía dilatada; **hypertrophic** — miocardiopatía hipertrófica, cardiomiopatía hipertrófica (*esp. Mex*); **ischemic** — cardiopatía isquémica; **restrictive** — miocardiopatía restrictiva

cardiopulmonary *adj* cardiopulmonar

cardiorespiratory *adj* cardiorrespiratorio

cardiovascular *adj* cardiovascular

cardioversion *n* cardioversión *f*; **electrical** — cardioversión eléctrica

cardioverter *n* cardioversor *m*

carditis *n* carditis *f*

care *n* cuidado; **The care in this hospital is excellent**..El cuidado en este hospital es excelente; **day** — cuidado para niños durante el día (*esp. niños de madres que trabajan*); **foot** —, **skin** —, **wound** —, **etc**. cuidado del pie, cuidado de la piel, cuidado de la herida, etc.; **health** — *V*. health care *como artículo independiente*; **home** — atención domiciliaria; **intensive** — cuidados intensivos, terapia intensiva (*SA*); **long-term** — cuidados prolongados, cuidados de larga duración (*Esp*); **nursing** — cuidados de enfermería; **prenatal** — atención prenatal; **primary** —

atención primaria; **tertiary** — atención terciaria, atención de tercer nivel (*esp. Mex*); **tertiary** — **hospital** hospital de tercer nivel; **to take** — **of** cuidar a, atender a; **Who takes care of your mother at home?**..¿Quién cuida a su madre en casa? **to take** — **of oneself** cuidarse; **You should take care of yourself better**..Debe cuidarse mejor; *vi* **to** — **for** cuidar a, atender a

careful *adj* **to be** — tener cuidado. **Be careful with this medicine**.. Tenga cuidado con esta medicina.

caregiver *n* cuidador -ra *mf*, persona que atiende a un enfermo o discapacitado

careless *adj* descuidado

carelessness *n* descuido

caretaker *V.* **caregiver.**

caries *n* (*form*) caries *f*

carisoprodol *n* carisoprodol *m*

carnitine *n* carnitina

carotene *n* caroteno; **beta-carotene** beta-caroteno

carotid *adj* carotídeo, (*artery*) carótida

carpal *adj* carpiano

carpenter *n* carpintero -ra *mf*

carrier *n* portador -ra *mf*; **She is a hepatitis B carrier**..Ella es portadora del virus de la hepatitis B.

carrot *n* zanahoria

carry *vt* (*a gene, etc.*) tener; **He carries the gene for color blindness**..El tiene el gen del daltonismo.

carsickness *n* mareo (en vehículo)

cartilage *n* cartílago

carvedilol *n* carvedilol *m*

cascara sagrada *n* (*bot*) cáscara sagrada

case *n* caso; **in 9 out of 10 cases**..en 9 de 10 casos; — **manager** gestor -ra *mf* de caso; **just in** — por si acaso

cashew *n* anacardo

cast *n* (*ortho*) yeso; **removable** — férula

castrate *vt* castrar

castration *n* castración *f*

CAT *abbr* **computerized axial tomography**. *V.* **tomography**. (*V. también* **scan**.)

cat *n* gato

catabolic *adj* catabólico

cataract *n* catarata

catastrophe *n* catástrofe *f*

catatonia *n* catatonía

catatonic *adj* catatónico

catch *vt* (*pret & pp* **caught**) (*fam, a disease*) contraer (*form*), dar(le) (a uno), pegar(le) (a uno) (*fam*), coger (*esp. Esp*); **I caught a cold**..Me dio (pegó) un catarro..Cogí un catarro; **to** — **one's breath** recuperar el aliento; [*Note: coger may be considered offensive in many areas of Latin America.*]

catching (*fam*) *adj* contagioso

caterpillar *n* oruga

catgut *n* catgut *m*

cath (*fam*) *V.* **catheterization**.

catharsis *n* (*psych*) catarsis *f*

cathartic *adj* (*psych*) catártico; (*ant*) purgante, laxante; *n* (*ant*) purgante *m*, laxante *m*

catheter *n* (*venous, arterial*) catéter *m*, (*urinary*) sonda; **central venous** — catéter venoso central; **epidural** — catéter epidural; **Foley** — sonda Foley; **Hickman** — catéter Hickman; **implantable** — catéter implantable; **peripherally-inserted central** — (**PICC**) catéter central de inserción periférica; **pulmonary artery** *o* **Swan-Ganz** — catéter de arteria pulmonar, catéter de Swan-Ganz; **urinary** — sonda vesical

catheterization *n* cateterismo, cateterización *f*, (*of the bladder*) sondaje *m*; **cardiac** — cateterismo cardíaco

catheterize *vt* (*arterial, venous*) cateterizar (*form*), colocar *or* poner catéter, (*the bladder*) colocar *or* poner sonda, sondar (*Esp, form*)

caught *pret & pp de* **catch**

cauliflower *n* coliflor *f*

causalgia *n* causalgia

cause *n* causa; *vt* causar

caustic *adj* cáustico

cauterization *n* cauterización *f*

cauterize *vt* cauterizar

cautery *n* cauterio

cavity *n* (*pl* **-ties**) cavidad *f*; (*dent*) hueco producido por caries; **You have a cavity**..Tiene caries..Tiene un diente con caries..Una de sus muelas tiene un hueco producido por caries..**You have cavities**.. Tiene caries; [*Note: caries is a mass noun similar to the English word* decay, *therefore* una carie *is incorrect though sometimes used.*]

cc *abbr* **cubic centimeter**. *V.* **centimeter**.

CDC *V.* **Centers for Disease Control and Prevention**.

cecum *n* ciego (*del colon*)

ceftriaxone *n* ceftriaxona

celecoxib *n* celecoxib *m*

celery *n* apio

celiac *adj* celíaco

celibate *adj* que no tiene relaciones sexuales

cell *n* célula; **atypical squamous cells of undetermined significance (ASCUS)** células escamosas atípicas de significado indeterminado; **B** — célula B; **brain** — célula cerebral; **CD4** — célula CD4; **cytotoxic T** — célula T citotóxica; **helper T** — célula T colaboradora; **natural killer** — célula asesina natural; **packed red blood cells** concentrado de hematíes, paquete *m* globular (*esp. Mex*); **plasma** — célula plasmática; **red blood** — eritrocito (*form*), hematíe *m* (*esp. Esp, form*), glóbulo rojo; **stem** — célula madre; **suppressor T** — célula T supresora; **T** — célula T; **transitional** — célula transicional; **white blood** — leucocito (*form*), glóbulo blanco

cellular *adj* celular

cellulite *n* celulitis *f*, depósitos de grasa detrás de los muslos

cellulitis *n* celulitis *f*, infección *f* del tejido debajo de la piel

cement *n* (*dent, ortho*) cemento

center *n* centro; **day** — centro diurno; **day-care** — guardería infantil (*esp. para niños de madres que trabajan durante el día*); **fitness** — gimnasio; **medical** — centro médico, centro de salud, hospital *m*; **rural health** — centro de salud rural; **surgical** — *o* **surgery** — centro de cirugía, centro quirúrgico

Centers for Disease Control and Prevention (CDC) *n* Centros para Control de Enfermedades

Centigrade *adj* centígrado; **28 degrees Centigrade**..28 grados centígrados

centimeter (cm) *n* centímetro (cm); **cubic — (cc)** centímetro cúbico (cc)

centipede *n* ciempiés *m*

central *adj* central

cephalexin *n* cefalexina

cephalic *adj* cefálico

cephalosporin *n* cefalosporina

cerclage *n* cerclaje *m*

cereal *n* cereal *m*

cerebellar *adj* cerebeloso

cerebellum *n* cerebelo

cerebral *adj* cerebral; **— palsy** parálisis *f* cerebral

cerebrospinal *adj* cefalorraquídeo

cerebrovascular *adj* cerebrovascular

cerebrum *n* cerebro

certificate *n* certificado, acta, partida; **birth** — acta *or* partida de nacimiento; **death** — certificado (médico) de defunción

certified *adj* certificado, titulado

cerumen *n* cerumen *m*

cervical *adj* (*obst*) del cuello uterino, del cérvix, cervical; (*ortho*) cervical, del cuello

cervices *pl de* **cervix**

cervicitis *n* cervicitis *f*

cervix *n* (*pl* -vices *o* -vixes) cuello uterino, cérvix *m*

cesarean section *n* cesárea

cessation *n* abandono, deshabituación *f* (*esp. Esp*); **smoking** — abandono del tabaco, deshabituación tabáquica, (el) dejar de fumar

cetirizine *n* cetirizina

chafe *vt, vi* rozar

chain *n* cadena; **branched-chain** de cadena ramificada; **— of cold** cadena de frío; **— of custody** cadena de custodia; **— of survival** cadena de supervivencia; **— reaction** reacción *f* en cadena; **heavy** — cadena pesada; **light** — cadena ligera; **long-chain** de cadena larga; **medium-chain** de cadena media

chair *n* silla, sillón *m*; **dental** —

sillón dental

chalazion *n (pl -zia)* chalazión *m*

challenge *n* desafío, reto; provocación *f*; **methacholine —** provocación con metacolina

chamber *n* cámara; **decompression —** cámara de descompresión; **hyperbaric —** cámara hiperbárica

chamomile *n (bot)* manzanilla

chance *n* oportunidad *f*, posibilidad *f*; casualidad *f*; **There's maybe one chance in a hundred..**Puede haber una posibilidad en cien; **by —** por casualidad

chancre *n* chancro; **soft —** chancro blando

chancroid *n* chancroide *m*

change *n* cambio; **bandage —** cambio de vendaje; **— of life** *(ant)* menopausia; *vt, vi* cambiar

chap *vi (pret & pp* **chapped**) agrietarse, partirse, cortarse *(la piel o los labios)*

chaplain *n* capellán *m*, sacerdote *m*

chapped *adj* agrietado, partido, cortado *(la piel o los labios)*

Chap Stick *n (marca)* crema para los labios, bálsamo labial *(esp. Esp)*

characteristic *adj* característico; *n* característica, carácter *m*; **secondary sex** *or* **sexual characteristics** caracteres sexuales secundarios

charcoal *n* carbón *m*; **activated —** carbón activado

charge *n (frec. pl)* precio, costo, coste *m (Esp)*; *vt, vi* cobrar

charlie horse *(fam) n* calambre *m* muscular *(esp. de la pierna)*

chart *n (medical)* historia clínica, historial médico, expediente (clínico) *(Mex, CA)*; **eye —** tabla de Snellen, carta de letras *(para evaluar la agudeza visual)*

check *vt* chequear, revisar

checkup *n* chequeo, revisión médica

cheek *n* mejilla; *(fam, buttock)* nalga

cheekbone *n* pómulo

cheerful *adj* alegre

cheese *n* queso

cheilitis *n* queilitis *f*, boqueras *(fam)*

chelating *adj* quelante; **— agent** quelante *m*, agente *m* quelante; **iron-chelating agent** quelante del hierro

chelation *n* quelación *f*; **— therapy** tratamiento quelante

chemical *adj* químico; *n* sustancia química, producto químico

chemistry *n* química

chemo *(fam) V.* chemotherapy.

chemoprophylaxis *n* quimioprofilaxis *f*

chemotherapy *n (pl -pies)* quimioterapia; **high-dose —** quimioterapia a altas dosis; **induction —** quimioterapia de inducción; **neoadjuvant —** quimioterapia neoadyuvante

chest *n* tórax *(form)*, pecho

chew *vt, vi* masticar

chewable *adj* masticable

chewing gum *n* chicle *m*

chicken *n* pollo

chickenpox *n* varicela

chickweed *n (bot)* pamplina, alsine *m (Esp)*, capiquí *m (SA)*

chigger *n* larva roja de ciertos ácaros; *(chigoe)* nigua

chigoe *n* nigua

chilblain *n* sabañón *m*, inflamación e hinchazón producidas por exceso de frío en las extremidades y en las orejas

child *n (pl* **children**) niño -ña *mf*, hijo -ja *mf*; **foster —** *(US)* huérfano o niño abandonado criado por alguien que no es padre adoptivo y que recibe remuneración del gobierno; **only —** hijo único

childbirth *n* parto

childhood *n* niñez *f*, infancia

childproof *adj* a prueba de niños

children *pl de* **child**

chili pepper *n* chile *m*

chill *n* escalofrío

chin *n* mentón *m*, barbilla

chip *n* astilla, pedacito; *vt, vi (pret & pp* **chipped**; *ger* **chipping**) astillar(se), quebrar(se)

chiropodist *V.* podiatrist.

chiropractic *n* quiropráctica, quiropraxia

chiropractor *n* quiropráctico -ca *mf*

chlamydia *n* clamidia

chlarithromycin *n* claritromicina

chloral hydrate *n* hidrato de cloral

chlorambucil *n* clorambucilo

chloramphenicol n cloranfenicol m
chlordane n clordano
chlordiazepoxide n clordiazepóxido
chlorhexidine n clorhexidina
chloride n cloruro
chlorinated adj clorado
chlorination n cloración f
chlorine n cloro
chloroform n cloroformo
chloroquine n cloroquina
chlorpheniramine n clorfeniramina, clorfenamina (OMS)
chlorpromazine n clorpromazina
chlorpropamide n clorpropamida
chlorthalidone n clortalidona
chocolate n chocolate m
choice n elección f; **drug of** — medicamento de elección; **drug of first (second, third)** — medicamento de primera (segunda, tercera) elección
choke vt estrangular; vi (due to fumes, lack of air, etc.) asfixiarse (form), ahogarse; **to — on** (food, etc.) atragantarse con
choking n (due to fumes, lack of air, etc.) asfixia, ahogo; (on food, etc.) atragantamiento
cholangiocarcinoma n colangiocarcinoma m
cholangiogram n colangiografía (estudio imagenológico)
cholangiography n colangiografía (técnica imagenológica); **percutaneous transhepatic** — colangiografía transhepática percutánea
cholangitis n colangitis f
cholecystectomy n (pl -mies) colecistectomía
cholecystitis n colecistitis f; **acalculous** — colecistitis alitiásica
cholelithiasis n colelitiasis f
cholera n cólera m
cholestatis n colestasis; — **of pregnancy** colestasis (intrahepática) del embarazo
cholesteatoma n colesteatoma m
cholesterol n colesterol m; **LDL** —, **HDL** —, etc. colesterol LDL, colesterol HDL, etc.; **total** — colesterol total
cholestyramine n colestiramina
chondrocalcinosis n condrocalcinosis f

chondroitin sulfate n sulfato de condroitina
chondrosarcoma n condrosarcoma m
chorea n corea m&f; **Huntington's** — corea de Huntington
choriocarcinoma n coriocarcinoma m
chorioretinitis n coriorretinitis f
chromate n cromato
chromium n cromo
chromomycosis n cromomicosis f
chromosomal adj cromosómico
chromosome n cromosoma m
chronic adj crónico
chronically adv crónicamente
cidofovir n cidofovir m
cigar n puro, tabaco (esp. Carib)
cigarette n cigarrillo, cigarro (esp. Mex); **filter-tipped** — cigarrillo or cigarro con filtro
cilostazol n cilostazol m
cimetidine n cimetidina
ciprofloxacin n ciprofloxacino, ciprofloxacina (esp. Amer)
circadian adj circadiano; — **rhythm** ritmo circadiano
circle n círculo; **dark circles under one's eyes** ojeras; **vicious** — círculo vicioso
circulate vi circular
circulation n circulación f; **collateral** — circulación colateral; **extracorporeal** — circulación extracorpórea; **fetal** — circulación fetal; **pulmonary** — circulación pulmonar; **systemic** — circulación sistémica
circulatory adj circulatorio
circumcise vt circuncidar
circumcised adj circunciso
circumcision n circuncisión f
circumference n (of a body part) perímetro
cirrhosis n cirrosis f; **primary biliary** — cirrosis biliar primaria
cirrhotic adj & n cirrótico -ca mf
cisplatin n cisplatino
citalopram n citalopram m
citrate n citrato
citric adj cítrico
citrus fruit n (pl fruit o fruits) fruta(s) cítrica(s)
clammy adj pegajoso y frío
clamp n pinza; vt pinzar

clap *n* (*fam, ant*) gonorrea
clarithromycin *n* claritromicina
class *n* clase *f*
claudication *n* claudicación *f*; **inter-mittent —** claudicación intermitente
claustrophobia *n* claustrofobia
clavicle *n* clavícula
claw *n* garra; *vt* arañar
clean *adj* limpio; **— and sober** limpio y sobrio (*Ang*), sin haber tomado ningúna bebida alcohólica; *vt* limpiar
cleaning *n* (*dent, etc.*) limpieza
cleanliness *n* limpieza
cleanser *n* producto de limpieza
clear *adj* claro; *vi* **to — up** (*a rash, illness, etc.*) resolverse, quitarse; *vt* **to — one's throat** aclarar la garganta, carraspear
cleft *adj* hendido; **— lip** labio leporino; **— palate** fisura palatina
clench *vt* (*teeth, fist*) apretar (*los dientes, el puño*)
click *n* (*card*) chasquido
climacteric *n* climaterio
climate *n* clima *m*
climax *n* (*sexual*) orgasmo
clindamycin *n* clindamicina
clinic *n* clínica, consulta externa, centro ambulatorio; **free —** clínica gratuita; **urgent care —** clínica de urgencias
clinical *adj* clínico
clinician *n* clínico -ca *mf*
clip (*surg*) *n* grapa; *vt* (*pret & pp* **clipped**; *ger* **clipping**) grapar, engrapar, cerrar con grapas
clitoris *n* (*pl* **-rides**) clítoris *m*
clofazimine *n* clofazimina
clofibrate *n* clofibrato
clogged *adj* (*fam*) obstruido, tapado
clomiphene *n* clomifeno
clonazepam *n* clonazepam *m*
clone *n* clon *m*
clonic *adj* clónico
clonidine *n* clonidina
clonus *n* clonus *m*
clopidogrel *n* clopidogrel *m*
close *adj* cercano; **— friend** amigo -ga *mf* cercano; **— relative** pariente *mf* cercano; *adv* cerca de; **too close to your aorta..**demasiado cerca de su aorta

close *vt, vi* cerrar(se); **Close your eyes..**Cierre los ojos.
closed *adj* (*trauma*) cerrado
clostridium *n* clostridio
closure *n* (*psych*) conclusión *f*; (*surg*) cierre *m*
clot *n* coágulo; *vi* (*pret & pp* **clotted**; *ger* **clotting**) coagularse
clothes *npl* ropa
clothing *n* ropa
clotrimazole *n* clotrimazol *m*
clotting *n* coagulación *f*; **— factor** factor *m* de coagulación
cloudy *adj* (*comp* **-ier**; *super* **-iest**) (*vision*) nublado; (*urine, etc.*) turbio
club *n* club *m*
clubbing *n* dedos en palillo de tambor, hipocratismo digital
clubfoot *n* (*pl* **-feet**) pie zambo, malformación congénita del pie
clumsy *adj* torpe
cm. *V.* **centimeter.**
CMV *V.* **cytomegalovirus.**
CNS *abbr* **central nervous system.** *V.* **system.**
coagulate *vt, vi* coagular(se)
coagulation *n* coagulación *f*; **disseminated intravascular — (DIC)** coagulación intravascular diseminada
coagulopathy *n* coagulopatía
coal *n* carbón *m*
coal tar *n* alquitrán *m* de hulla
coarctation *n* coartación *f*
coat *n* abrigo
coating *n* (*of a tablet*) cubierta, capa
cobalamin *V.* **cyanocobalamin.**
cobalt *n* cobalto
coca *n* (*bot*) coca
cocaine *n* cocaína
coccidioidomycosis *n* coccidioidomicosis *f*
coccus *n* (*pl* **-ci**) coco
coccyx *n* (*pl* **-cyges**) coxis *m*, cóccix *m*
cochlea *n* (*pl* **-leae**) cóclea
cochlear *adj* coclear
cockroach *n* cucaracha
cocktail *n* cóctel *m*, (*of medications*) cóctel, mezcla (*de medicamentos*)
coconut *n* coco

coddle vt mimar, consentir

Code Blue n código azul (Ang), anuncio por parlante de emergencia solicitando a los médicos para realizar medidas de reanimación

codeine n codeína

codependency n codependencia

coenzyme Q n coenzima f Q

coffee n café m; — **grounds** posos de café; **ground** — café molido; **Did the vomit look as if it had coffee grounds in it?**...¿Se veía el vómito como si tuviera posos de café (café molido)?

cognitive adj cognitivo

coinfection n coinfección f

coitus n coito; — **interruptus** coitus interruptus m (form), coito interrumpido

coke (fam) n cocaína, coca (fam)

colchicine n colchicina

cold adj frío; **to be** — tener frío, (the weather) hacer frío; **Are you cold?** ...¿Tiene frío? **to feel** — sentir frío; n frío; (illness) resfriado, catarro; **chest** — resfriado (catarro) que afecta el pecho; **common** — resfriado común; **head** — resfriado (catarro) que afecta la cabeza; **to catch a** — resfriarse; **to have a** — estar resfriado

cold cream n crema limpiadora

cold sore n herpes labial (form), calentura (Esp, frec. pl), fuego, erupción en los labios (debida al herpes)

cold turkey adv (fam) bruscamente y completamente (refiriéndose a la suspensión de un hábito o de una adicción)

colectomy n (pl -mies) colectomía

colesevelam n colesevelam m

colestipol n colestipol m

colic n cólico (ped, etc; frec. pl)

coliform adj & n coliforme m

colitis n colitis f; **ischemic** — colitis isquémica; **pseudomembranous** — colitis seudomembranosa; **ulcerative** — colitis ulcerosa

collagen n colágeno

collapse n (person) desmayo, caída; (lung, etc.) colapso; vi (person) desmayarse, caerse; (lung, etc.) colapsarse

collar n (ortho) collarín m, collar m (esp. SA); **(hard, soft) cervical** — collarín or collar cervical (rígido, blando)

collarbone n clavícula

collateral adj colateral

colleague n colega mf

colloid n coloide m

colon n colon m; **ascending** — colon ascendente; **descending** — colon descendente; **left** — colon izquierdo; **right** — colon derecho; **sigmoid** — colon sigmoide or sigmoideo, sigmoides m (fam); **spastic** — (ant) síndrome de intestino irritable; **transverse** — colon transverso

colonic adj cólico, relativo al colon; n hidroterapia del colon, limpieza del colon para fines terapéuticos

colonization n colonización f

colonography n colonografía

colonoscope n colonoscopio

colonoscopy n (pl -pies) colonoscopia, colonoscopía (Amer, esp. spoken); **virtual** — colonoscopia virtual

color n color m

color-blind adj daltónico (form), que no diferencia bien ciertos colores

colorectal adj colorrectal

colorless adj incoloro

colostomy n (pl -mies) colostomía; — **bag** bolsa de or para colostomía

colostrum n calostro

colposcopy n (pl -pies) colposcopia, colposcopía (Amer, esp. spoken)

coltsfoot n (bot) fárfara, tusílago

column n columna; **spinal** o **vertebral** — columna vertebral, columna (fam)

coma n coma m

comatose adj comatoso (form), en coma

comb n peine m; vt peinar; **to** — **one's hair** peinarse

combative adj agresivo

combination n combinación f; **Smoking and diabetes are a bad combination**..Fumar y tener diabetes son una mala combinación

come vi (pret **came**; pp **come**) venir; (fam, to have an orgasm) alcanzar el orgasmo, acabar (*Amer, fam*), venirse (*fam*); **to — and go** ir y venir; **Does the pain come and go?**..El dolor, ¿va y viene? **to — down** bajar(se); **Your sugar came down**..Le bajó el azúcar; **to — down with** (*a disease*) dar(le) (a uno), pegar(le) (a uno) (*fam*), coger (*esp. Esp*); **to — on** (*to begin*) empezar, comenzar; **Did the pain come on suddenly or gradually?** ..¿Empezó el dolor de repente o poco a poco? [*Note: coger may be considered offensive in many parts of Latin America.*]

comfort *n* comodidad *f*, confort *m*; *vt* consolar

comfortable *adj* cómodo, confortable

comfrey *n* (*bot*) consuelda

comminuted *adj* conminuta

commode *n* inodoro portátil (*para enfermos y minusválidos*)

common *adj* común, frecuente; **a common problem**..un problema común *or* frecuente; **— sense** sentido común

communicable *adj* (*form*) transmisible, contagioso

communicate *vt* comunicar; *vi* comunicar(se)

communication *n* comunicación *f*

community *adj* comunitario; **— involvement** participación comunitaria; *n* (*pl* **-ties**) comunidad *f*; **community-acquired** adquirido en la comunidad

companion *n* compañero -ra *mf*, acompañante *mf*

compassion *n* compasión *f*

compassionate *adj* compasivo; **— use** (*pharm*) uso compasivo

compatible *adj* compatible

compensate *vi* compensar

competency *n* (*to make medical decisions*) capacidad *f* (*para hacer decisiones médicas*)

competent *adj* capaz, competente

complain *vi* quejarse

complaint *n* queja

complement *n* complemento

complete *adj* completo

complex *n* complejo; **Oedipus —**

complejo de Edipo

complexion *n* cutis *m*, tez *f*

compliance *n* cumplimiento; **— with treatment** cumplimiento del tratamiento

complication *n* complicación *f*

component *n* componente *m*

compound *n* compuesto

compress *n* compresa; **cool —** compresa fría; *vt* comprimir

compression *n* compresión *f*; **chest compressions** masaje cardíaco externo; **spinal cord —** compresión medular, compresión de la médula espinal

compulsion *n* compulsión *f*

compulsive *adj* compulsivo

computer *n* computadora, ordenador *m*

concave *adj* cóncavo

conceive *vi* concebir

concentrate *n* concentrado; *vt, vi* concentrar(se)

concentrated *adj* concentrado

concentration *n* concentración *f*

concentrator *n* concentrador *m*; **oxygen —** concentrador de oxígeno

conception *n* (*obst*) concepción *f*

concussion *n* conmoción *f* cerebral

condition *n* (*state*) estado, condición *f*; (*ailment*) afección *f*, condición *f*, enfermedad *f*; **critical —** estado crítico; **pre-existing —** condición preexistente

conditioned *adj* acondicionado

conditioner *n* (*for hair*) acondicionador *m*

conditioning *n* acondicionamiento; **physical —** acondicionamiento físico

condom *n* preservativo, condón *m*

conduction *n* conducción *f*

conduit *n* conducto; **ileal —** conducto ileal

cone *n* (*anat, gyn, ophthalmology, etc.*) cono

confabulation *n* confabulación *f*, (el) dar respuestas no verdaderas para llenar vacíos de la memoria

confidence *n* confianza

confidential *adj* confidencial; **What you tell me is strictly confidential**..Lo que Ud. me dice es estrictamente confidencial.

confidentiality *n* confidencialidad *f*, intimidad *f*; **doctor-patient** — secreto médico

confirm *vt* confirmar

conflict *n* conflicto

confront *vt* confrontar, enfrentar

confuse *vt* confundir

confused *adj* confundido; **to get** *o* **become** — confundirse

confusion *n* confusión *f*

congenital *adj* congénito

congested *adj* congestionado; (*nasally*) con congestión nasal, constipado, congestionado

congestion *n* congestión *f*; **nasal** — congestión nasal

congestive *adj* congestivo

congratulations *interj* (*obst., etc.*) ¡Felicidades! ¡Enhorabuena! (*Esp*)

conization *n* conización *f*

conjugated *adj* conjugado

conjunctiva *n* (*pl* -**vae**) conjuntiva

conjunctival *adj* conjuntival

conjunctivitis *n* conjuntivitis *f*

connect *vt* conectar

connection *n* conexión *f*, unión *f*

conscience *n* conciencia; **guilty** — cargo de conciencia

conscious *adj* consciente

consciousness *n* conciencia *or* consciencia, conocimiento; **collective** — conciencia colectiva; **loss of** — pérdida del conocimiento *or* de la conciencia; **to lose** — perder el conocimiento *or* la conciencia; **to regain** — volver en sí; [*Note: Although* conciencia *is the more common spelling, it also means* conscience, *whereas* consciencia *never means* conscience *and is therefore recommended by many authorities, including the Real Academia Española.*]

consent *n* consentimiento, permiso; **informed** — consentimiento informado; *vi* consentir; **to** — **to** consentir en

consequence *n* consecuencia

conservative *adj* (*measures, etc.*) conservador

conservator *n* tutor -ra *mf*, persona encargada de manejar los asuntos

de otra que es incapaz de hacerlo por discapacidad mental

conserve *vt* conservar; **breast-conserving** conservador de mama

consistency *n* (*pl* -**cies**) consistencia

console *vt* consolar

consolidation *n* consolidación *f*

constant *adj* constante, continuo

constipate *vt* estreñir

constipated *adj* estreñido

constipation *n* estreñimiento

constitution *n* constitución *f*, complexión *f*

constrict *vt* apretar

constriction *n* constricción *f*

consult *n* interconsulta (*form*), consulta (con un especialista); *vt* consultar (a un especialista)

consumption *n* consumo; (*ant*) tuberculosis *f*

contact *n* contacto; **close** — contacto cercano; **eye** — contacto visual

contagious *adj* (*disease*) contagioso; (*fam, person*) contagioso (*fam*), que puede transmitir una enfermedad, que puede infectar a los demás; [*Note: properly, both* contagious *and* contagioso *apply to diseases, not people, though both are often applied to people in colloquial speech.*]

contain *vt* contener

container *n* envase *m*, recipiente *m*

contaminate *vt* contaminar

contaminated *adj* contaminado; **to become** — contaminarse

contamination *n* contaminación *f*

content *n* (*frec. pl*) contenido

continual *adj* continuo

continuous *adj* continuo

contour *n* contorno

contraception *n* anticoncepción *f*, contracepción *f*

contraceptive *adj* & *n* anticonceptivo; **oral** — anticonceptivo oral

contract *n* contrato; *vt* (*a disease*) contraer, dar(le) (a uno), coger (*esp. Esp*); *vi* (*a muscle*) contraerse; [*Note: coger may be considered offensive in many parts of Latin America.*]

contraction *n* contracción *f*; **Braxton-Hicks contractions** contracciones de Braxton-Hicks, falsos dolores de parto; **premature atrial — (PAC)** contracción auricular prematura (CAP); **premature ventricular — (PVC)** contracción ventricular prematura (CVP)

contracture *n* contractura; **Dupuytren's —** contractura de Dupuytren

contraindicated *adj* contraindicado

contraindication *n* contraindicación *f*

contrast *n* (*fam, contrast medium*) medio de contraste, contraste *m* (*fam*)

control *n* control *m*; **birth —** anticoncepcion *f*, control de la natalidad, método anticonceptivo; **out of — ** fuera de control; **tight —** (*of blood sugars*) control estricto (*de la glucemia*); *vt* (*pret & pp* **-trolled**; *ger* **-trolling**) controlar

controversial *adj* controvertido

contusion *n* contusión *f*

convalescence *n* convalecencia

convalescent *adj* convaleciente

conventional *adj* convencional

conversion *n* conversión *f*

convex *adj* convexo

convulsion *n* convulsión *f*, ataque *m* (*fam*)

coo *vi* (*pret & pp* **cooed**) (*ped*) hacer sonidos como una paloma (*dicho de los bebés*)

cook *n* cocinero -ra *mf*; *vt, vi* cocinar

cookie *n* galleta

cool *adj* fresco

cooperate *vi* cooperar

cooperative *adj* colaborador

coordination *n* coordinación *f*

copayment *n* copago

COPD *abbr* **chronic obstructive pulmonary disease**. *V.* **disease**.

cope *vi* **to — with** afrontar, lidiar con

copper *n* cobre *m*; **— sulfate** sulfato cúprico (*form*), sulfato de cobre

coral *n* coral *m*

cord *n* cordón *m*, cuerda; **spinal —** médula espinal; **umbilical —** cordón umbilical; **vocal —** cuerda vocal

corn *n* maíz *m*; (*foot lesion*) callo (*del pie*)

cornea *n* córnea

corneal *adj* corneal

cornstarch *n* almidón *m* de maíz, maicena

coronary *adj* coronario

coroner *n* médico -ca *mf* forense, oficial *mf* del gobierno que investiga casos de muerte

corporal *adj* corporal

corpse *n* cadáver *m*

corpus luteum *n* cuerpo lúteo

correct *vt* corregir, ajustar

correction *n* corrección *f*, ajuste *m*

corrective *adj* corrector

correlation *n* correlación *f*

corrosive *adj* corrosivo

corset *n* (*ortho*) corsé *m*

cortex *n* (*pl* **-tices**) corteza

cortical *adj* cortical

cortices *pl de* **cortex**

corticosteroid *n* corticosteroide *m*

cortisol *n* cortisol *m*

cortisone *n* cortisona

cosmetic *adj & n* cosmético

cosmetologist *n* esteticista *mf*

cost *n* costo, coste *m* (*Esp*)

cost-effective *adj* rentable, costo-efectivo, coste-efectivo (*Esp*)

cost-effectiveness *n* rentabilidad *f*, costo-efectividad *m&f*, coste-efectividad *m* (*Esp*)

costochondritis *n* costocondritis *f*

cotton *n* algodón *m*; **— ball** torunda *or* bolita de algodón; **— mouth** (*fam*) sequedad *f* de boca, boca seca (*fam*)

couch *n* (*psych*) diván *m*

cough *n* tos *f*; **barking —** tos perruna; **dry —** tos seca; **hacking —** tos fuerte; *vt* **to — up** expectorar (*form*); **Are you coughing up phlegm?**..Cuando tose, ¿hay flemas?...**Try to cough up phlegm from your lungs**..Trate de toser fuerte para sacar flemas de sus pulmones...**Are you coughing up blood?**..Cuando tose, ¿hay sangre? *vi* toser; **Cough hard**..Tosa fuerte.

counseling *n* consejo, terapia con un consejero; **genetic —** consejo genético

counselor *n* consejero -ra *mf*

count *n* recuento, conteo, número;

bacterial o **bacteria** — recuento bacteriano (form), recuento or conteo de bacterias; **complete blood** — hemograma completo; **pill** — recuento de pastillas; **platelet** — recuento plaquetario (form), recuento or conteo de plaquetas; **red blood cell** — recuento de eritrocitos (form), recuento de glóbulos rojos, número de glóbulos rojos (Mex); **sperm** — recuento de espermatozoides; **white blood cell** — recuento de leucocitos (form), recuento de glóbulos blancos, número de glóbulos blancos (Mex); vt, vi contar; **Count backwards from one hundred**..Cuente al revés a partir de cien; **to** — **calories** contar calorías

counteract vt contrarrestar

counterpulsation n contrapulsación f **intraaortic balloon** — balón m de contrapulsación (intraaórtico)

country n (pl **-tries**) (rural area) campo

county n (pl **-ties**) (US) condado

couple n pareja

course n curso; **course of the disease** ..curso de la enfermedad...**He needs a course of antibiotics**..El necesita (un curso de) antibióticos.

cousin n primo -ma mf

cover vt cubrir, tapar; **Your insurance covers this**..Su seguro cubre esto...**The wound should be covered**..La herida debe de estar cubierta...**Cover your right eye**.. Cubra (Tape) su ojo derecho.

coverage n (insurance, epidemiology, etc.) cobertura

CPAP abbr **continuous positive airway pressure**. V. **pressure**.

CPR abbr **cardiopulmonary resuscitation**. V. **resuscitation**.

crab (fam) **crab louse**. V. **louse**.

crack n (bone, teeth) fisura, (skin) grieta; (cocaine) crack m, forma de cocaína para fumar; vi agrietarse, partirse

cracked adj agrietado, partido

cracker n galleta (salada)

cradle n cuna

cradle cap n costra láctea (form),

inflamación escamosa del cuero cabelludo en infantes

cramp n calambre m, (en el abdomen) cólico (frec pl); **abdominal** — cólico abdominal, retortijón m (fam); **menstrual** — cólico or dolor m menstrual; **postpartum cramps** entuertos; vi **My leg is cramping**..Tengo un calambre en la pierna.

crania pl de **cranium**

cranial adj craneal

craniopharyngioma n craneofaringioma m

craniotomy n (pl **-ties**) craneotomía

cranium n (pl **-nia**) cráneo

crank n (fam) metanfetamina

crash cart n carro de reanimación

crave vt desear mucho

craving n (obst) antojo

crawl vi (ped) gatear

crazy adj (comp **-ier**; super **-iest**) loco; **to drive** (someone) — volver loco (a alguien); **His mother drove him crazy**..Su madre lo volvió loco; **to go** — volverse loco

cream n (medicine, cosmetic) crema, pomada; (milk product) nata, crema; **hand** — crema para manos

crease n pliegue m; **palmar** — pliegue palmar

creatine n creatina

creatinine n creatinina

cretinism n cretinismo

crib n cuna

crib death n (fam) síndrome de la muerte súbita del lactante

cricothyroid adj cricotiroideo

cried pret & pp de **cry**

cries pl de **cry**

cripple (ant) n lisiado -da mf; vt lisiar

crisis n (pl **-ses**) crisis f; **blast** — crisis blástica; **identity** — crisis de identidad; **midlife** — crisis de (la) mediana edad

critical adj crítico

cromolyn sodium n cromoglicato disódico, cromoglicato de sodio (esp. Mex)

crooked adj torcido, chueco (Mex)

crop-dust vt, vi fumigar con avioneta

cross-eyed *adj* bizco

cross-match *n* prueba cruzada; *vt* hacer *or* realizar prueba(s) cruzada(s)

cross-reactivity *n* reactividad cruzada

crotch *n* (*fam*) entrepierna (*frec. pl*)

croup *n* crup *m*, ronquera y dificultad para respirar producidas por irritación de la laringe o de la tráquea

crown *n* (*anat, dent*) corona

crowning *n* (*obst*) coronación *f*

crow's feet *n* (*fam*) patas de gallo (*fam*), arrugas al lado de los ojos

cruel *adj* cruel

cruelty *n* crueldad *f*

crush *vt* (*one's finger, hand, etc.*) aplastar, machucar; (*a tablet*) triturar (*form*), moler

crushing *adj* (*pain*) opresivo, aplastante (*fam*)

crust *n* costra

crutch *n* muleta

cry *n* (*pl* **cries**) grito; — **for help** grito de auxilio; *vi* (*pret & pp* **cried**) llorar; (*to call out*) gritar

cryoconservation *n* crioconservación *f*

cryoglobulin *n* crioglobulina

cryosurgery *n* criocirugía

cryotherapy *n* crioterapia

Cryptococcus *n* criptococo

cryptorchidism *n* criptorquidia

cryptosporidiosis *n* criptosporidiosis *f*

crystal *n* cristal *m*

C-section *V.* cesarean section.

CSF *abbr* cerebrospinal fluid. *V.* fluid.

CT *abbr* computed tomography. *V.* tomography. (*V. también* scan.)

cubic *adj* cúbico

cuddle *vt* abrazar, acariciar

cue *n* (*visual, auditory, etc.*) señal (*visual, auditiva, etc.*)

cuff *n* manguito; **blood pressure —** manguito del tensiómetro *or* esfigmomanómetro; **rotator —** manguito rotador

culdocentesis *n* (*pl* -ses) culdocentesis *f*

culture *n* cultura; (*micro*) cultivo; **blood —** hemocultivo (*form*), cultivo de sangre; **stool —** coprocultivo (*form*), cultivo de heces (popó, etc.); **throat —** cultivo faríngeo (*form*), cultivo de garganta; **urine —** urocultivo (*form*), cultivo de orina; *vt* cultivar

cumulative *adj* acumulativo

cunnilingus *n* (*form*) cunnilingus *m* (*form*), sexo oral, estimulación *f* oral de la vulva y el clítoris

cup, cupful *n* (*pl* -fuls) taza

curable *adj* curable

curative *adj* curativo

curb *vt* (*appetite, desire*) suprimir (*form*), inhibir

cure *n* cura, remedio; *vt* curar

curettage *n* legrado, curetaje *m*, raspado

curette *n* cureta

current *adj* actual; **his current condition.**.su condición actual; *n* corriente *f*

curvature *n* curvatura

curve *n* curva; **growth —** curva de crecimiento; **learning —** curva de aprendizaje

cushion *n* cojín; *vt* acojinar

cuspid *n* (*diente*) canino, colmillo

custom-fitted *adj* hecho a la medida

cut *n* cortada, cortadura, herida; *vt* (*pret & pp* **cut**; *ger* **cutting**) cortar; **Did you cut your finger?.**.¿Se cortó el dedo? **to — down (on)** (*fam*) disminuir; **You need to cut down on salt.**.Tiene que disminuir la sal; **to — off** cortar, amputar; **to — oneself** cortarse; **Did you cut yourself?.**.¿Se cortó? **to — one's nails** cortarse las uñas; **to have one's hair —** cortarse el pelo

cutaneous *adj* cutáneo

cuticle *n* cutícula

cutoff point *n* punto de corte

cyanide *n* cianuro

cyanocobalamin *n* cianocobalamina, vitamina B_{12}

cyanosis *n* cianosis *f*

cyanotic *adj* cianótico, con la piel azulada

cyclamate *n* ciclamato

cycle *n* ciclo; **anovulatory —** ciclo anovulatorio; **life —** ciclo biológico *or* vital; **menstrual —** ciclo

menstrual; **reproductive** — ciclo reproductivo
cyclic, cyclical adj cíclico
cycling n (sport) ciclismo
cyclobenzaprine n ciclobenzaprina
cyclophosphamide n ciclofosfamida
cyclosporine n ciclosporina
cylinder n cilindro
cyproheptadine n ciproheptadina
cyst n quiste m; **Baker's** — quiste de Baker; **dermoid** — quiste dermoide; **epidermal inclusion** — quiste epidermoide; **ganglion** — ganglión m; **hydatid** — quiste hidatídico; **ovarian** — quiste de ovario; **pilonidal** — quiste pilonidal; **sebaceous** — quiste epidermoide, quiste sebáceo; **thyroglossal duct** — quiste del conducto tirogloso
cystectomy n (pl -**mies**) (removal of bladder) cistectomía; (removal of cyst) quistectomía

cysteine n cisteína
cystic adj quístico; (artery, duct) cístico
cysticercosis n cisticercosis f
cystic fibrosis n fibrosis quística
cystine n cistina
cystinuria n cistinuria
cystitis n cistitis f, infección f de la vejiga; **interstitial** — cistitis intersticial
cystocele n cistocele m
cystoscope n cistoscopio
cystoscopy n (pl -**pies**) cistoscopia, cistoscopía (Amer, esp. spoken)
cytology n citología, estudio microscópico de la célula
cytomegalovirus (CMV) n citomegalovirus m (CMV)
cytometry n citometría; **flow** — citometría de flujo
cytotoxic adj citotóxico

D

Dacron n Dacron m; [Note: both terms are trademarks.]
dacryocystitis n dacriocistitis f
dad papá m
daddy n (pl -**dies**) papi m, papito
daily adj diario; adv diariamente, a diario, cada día
dairy product n producto lácteo, producto de la leche
damage n daño; **brain** — daño cerebral; vt dañar, hacer daño
damiana n (bot) damiana
damp adj húmedo, mojado
dampness n humedad f
danazol n danazol m
dandelion n (bot) diente m de león

amargón
dander n caspa (de animales)
dandruff n caspa
danger n peligro
dangerous adj peligroso
dangle vt, vi colgar; **Sit with your legs dangling**..Siéntese con las piernas colgando.
dapsone n dapsona
dark adj oscuro; (complexion) oscuro, moreno
darken vt (piel, etc.) oscurecer, causar que se le oscurezca, causar que se ponga oscuro; vi ponerse oscuro
data n o npl datos, información f
date n fecha; (fruit) dátil m; — **of**

birth *o* birth — fecha de nacimiento
daub *vt* untar
daughter *n* hija
daughter-in-law *n* (*pl* **daughters-in-
law**) nuera
daunorubicin *n* daunorubicina
day *n* día *m*; **every** — todos los días;
every other — cada dos días; **the
— after** *o* **the following** — el día
siguiente; **the — after tomorrow**
pasado mañana; **the — before** el
día anterior; **the — before yesterday** anteayer
daydream *vi* (*pret & pp* **-dreamed** *o*
-dreamt) soñar despierto
daze *n* aturdimiento, mareo, estado
de confusión o desorientación sin
agitación; **in a** — aturdido, atarantado, mareado; *vt* aturdir, atarantar
dazed *adj* aturdido, atarantado, mareado; **to become** — aturdirse, ata-
rantarse
D&C *abbr* **dilation and curettage**.
V. **dilation**.
DDT V. **dichlorodiphenyltrichloroethane**.
dead *adj* muerto
deadly *adj* mortal
deaf *adj* sordo; **— and mute** sordomudo
deaf-and-dumb *adj* (*ant*) sordomudo
deaf-mute *n* sordomudo -da *mf*
deaf-mutism *n* sordomudez *f*
deafness *n* sordera
death *n* muerte *f*, (*esp. for statistics*)
fallecimiento; **brain** — muerte
cerebral; **— wish** instinto de la
muerte, deseo inconsciente de morir; **— with dignity** muerte digna;
natural — muerte natural; **sudden**
— muerte súbita
deathbed *n* lecho de muerte
debilitated *adj* debilitado
debilitating *adj* debilitante
debride *vt* desbridar
debridement *n* desbridamiento
decaffeinated *adj* descafeinado
decay *n* (*dent*) caries *f*
deceased *adj & n* difunto -ta *mf*
decibel *n* decibel *m* (*Amer*), decibelio
(*Esp*)
deciduous tooth *n* diente primario

(*form*), diente de leche (*fam*)
deciliter *n* decilitro
decision *n* decisión *f*
decline *n* deterioro, (*in something
measured*) descenso
decompression *n* descompresión *f*
deconditioned *adj* fuera de forma,
fuera de condición física
decongestant *adj & n* descongestivo,
descongestionante *m*
decontaminate *vt* descontaminar
decrease *n* disminución *f*; *vt, vi* dis-
minuir(se)
deductible *adj* deducible
deep *adj* profundo, hondo
deep-fried *adj* frito por sumergir en
aceite hirviendo
defecate *vi* defecar
defecation *n* defecación *f*
defect *n* defecto; **atrial septal —
(ASD)** comunicación *f* interauricular (CIA); **birth** — defecto congénito (*form*), defecto de nacimiento;
neural tube — defecto del tubo
neural; **ventricular septal —
(VSD)** comunicación *f* interventricular (CIV)
defense *n* defensa
defibrillate *vt* desfibrilar
defibrillation *n* desfibrilación *f*
defibrillator *n* desfibrilador *m*; **automated external — (AED)** desfibri-
lador externo automático (DEA);
**(automatic) implantable cardio-
verter — (ICD)** desfibrilador cardioversor (automático) implantable
(DCI)
deficiency *n* (*pl* **-cies**) deficiencia,
carencia, falta
deficient *adj* deficiente; **to be — in**
carecer de, faltar(le) (a uno)
deficit *n* déficit *m*, deficiencia, falta
definitive *adj* definitivo
deformed *adj* deforme
deformity *n* (*pl* **-ties**) deformidad *f*
degeneration *n* degeneración *f*
degenerative *adj* degenerativo
degradation *n* degradación *f*
degree *n* grado; **37 degrees Centigrade**...37 grados centígrados
dehumanizing *adj* deshumanizante,
deshumanizador
dehumidifier *n* deshumidificador *m*

dehumidify *vt* (*pret* & *pp* **-fied**) deshumedecer

dehydrated *adj* deshidratado

dehydration *n* deshidratación *f*

dehydroepiandrosterone (DHEA) *n* dehidroepiandrosterona (DHEA)

déjà vu, déjà vu, ya visto, sentimiento fuerte pero falso de haber vivido anteriormente una situación

delavirdine *n* delavirdina

delay *n* retraso, retardo; **developmental** — retraso mental; *vt* retrasar, retardar

delayed *adj* retardado, tardío, retrasado; **developmentally** — retrasado mental

deletion *n* deleción *f*

delicate *adj* delicado, frágil

delirious *adj* delirante; **to be** — estar delirando; **He's delirious**..Está delirando.

delirium *n* delirio(s); — **tremens** (*form*) delirium tremens *m* (*form*), delirio con temblor y alucinaciones (*debido a la suspensión del alcohol*)

deliver (*obst*) *vt* dar a luz; (*action performed by doctor or midwife*) atender (*un parto*); **Mrs. Mata delivered a baby boy at four in the morning**..La señora Mata dio a luz a un niño a las cuatro de la madrugada...**Dr. Ford delivered Mrs. Mata**..El doctor Ford atendió el parto de la señora Mata...**Dr. Ford delivered the twins**..El Dr. Ford atendió el parto de los gemelos; *vi* dar a luz

delivery *n* (*pl* **-ries**) parto; **estimated date of** — fecha probable de parto

delta *n* delta

deltoid *n* deltoides *m*

delusion *n* delirio, falsa creencia patológica; **delusions of grandeur** delirio de grandeza

dementia *n* demencia; **Alzheimer's** — demencia tipo Alzheimer; **multi-infarct** — demencia multiinfarto; **vascular** — demencia vascular

demonstrate *vt* demostrar

demyelinating *adj* desmielinizante

denatured *adj* desnaturalizado

dengue *n* dengue *m*

denial *n* negación *f*

dense *adj* denso

density *n* (*pl* **-ties**) densidad *f*; **bone mineral** — densidad mineral ósea

dental *adj* dental

dentin *n* dentina

dentist *n* dentista *mf*, odontólogo -ga *mf* (*form*)

dentistry *n* odontología

denture *n* protesis *f* dental (*form*), dentadura postiza

deodorant *adj* & *n* desodorante *m*

deoxyribonucleic acid (DNA) *n* ácido desoxirribonucleico (ADN)

department *n* departamento, unidad *f*; **Department of Motor Vehicles (DMV)** Departamento de Vehículos Motorizados; **emergency** — unidad de urgencias; **Public Health Department** Departamento de Salud Pública

dependence *n* dependencia, hábito; — **on** dependencia de *or* a; **nicotine** — hábito tabáquico

dependency *n* dependencia; **chemical** — dependencia de sustancias, drogodependencia

dependent *adj* dependiente; **You may become dependent on this medication**..Puede crear dependencia a este medicamento.

depersonalization *n* (*psych*) despersonalización *f*

depigmentation *n* despigmentación *f*

depilatory *n* (*pl* **-ries**) depilatorio, producto para quitar el vello

deplete *vt* agotar

depletion *n* agotamiento

deposit *n* depósito, sedimento; *vt* depositar

depot *adj* (*pharm*) de depósito

depressant *adj* depresor

depressed *adj* deprimido; **to get** *o* **become** — deprimirse

depression *n* depresión *f*, tristeza profunda; **postpartum** — depresión postparto *or* posparto

depressive *adj* depresivo

deprivation *n* privación *f*; **sleep** — privación de sueño

depth *n* profundidad *f*

deranged *adj* (*mentally*) trastornado, loco

derealization n (*psych*) desrealización f

derivative n derivado; **petroleum derivatives** derivados del petróleo; **purified protein — (PPD)** derivado proteico purificado, PPD *m&f*

dermabrasion n dermoabrasión f

dermatitis n dermatitis f; **atopic —** dermatitis atópica; **cercarial —** dermatitis por cercarias; **contact —** dermatitis de contacto; **— herpetiformis** dermatitis herpetiforme; **irritant —** dermatitis irritativa; **seborrheic —** dermatitis seborreica; **stasis —** dermatitis por estasis

dermatofibroma n dermatofibroma m

dermatological, dermatologic adj dermatológico

dermatologist n dermatólogo -ga *mf*, médico -ca *mf* especialista en la piel y sus enfermedades, especialista *mf* de la piel (*fam*)

dermatology n dermatología, estudio de la piel y sus enfermedades

dermatomyositis n dermatomiositis f

dermatophyte n dermatofito

dermatophytosis n dermatofitosis f

dermographism n dermografismo

DES V. diethylstilbestrol.

descendant n descendiente *mf*

descending adj descendente

describe vt describir

desensitization n desensibilización f

desensitize vt desensibilizar

designated driver n conductor -ra *mf* designado, persona de un grupo al que le ha tocado no beber para conducir

desire n deseo; vt desear

desloratadine n desloratadina

desogestrel n desogestrel m

despair n desesperación f

desperate adj desesperado; **to become —** desesperarse

desperation n desesperación f

despondent adj deprimido

dessert n postre m

destroy vt destruir

destructive adj destructivo

detached adj desprendido

detachment n desprendimiento; **reti-** nal — desprendimiento de retina

detect vt detectar

detectable adj detectable

detection n detección f

detergent adj & n detergente m

deteriorate vi (*condition of patient*) empeorar; (*substance*) deteriorarse

deterioration n deterioro

detox (*fam*) V. detoxification.

detoxification n desintoxicación f

develop vt desarrollar; **to develop your muscles**..para desarrollar los músculos; vi desarrollarse, aparecer(se), salir(se) (*fam*); **He is developing normally**..Está desarrollándose normalmente...**When did this ulcer develop?**..¿Cuándo le apareció (salió) esta úlcera?

development n desarrollo; **physical —, sexual —**, etc. desarrollo físico, desarrollo sexual, etc.; **speech —** desarrollo del lenguaje

developmental milestone n hito del desarrollo

deviated adj desviado

device n dispositivo, aparato; **intrauterine — (IUD)** dispositivo intrauterino (DIU), aparato (*fam*); **safety —** dispositivo de seguridad

DEXA V. dual-energy X-ray absorptiometry.

dexamethasone n dexametasona

dextromethorphan n dextrometorfano

dextrose n dextrosa

DHEA V. dehydroepiandrosterone.

diabetes n diabetes f; **— insipidus** diabetes insípida; **(type 1, type 2) — mellitus** diabetes mellitus (tipo 1, tipo 2); **gestational —** diabetes gestacional

diabetic adj (*caused by or having diabetes*) diabético, (*pertaining to diabetes*) diabetológico (*form*); **— education** educación diabetológica, educación sobre la diabetes; **— foot** pie diabético; n diabético -ca *mf*

diagnose vt diagnosticar

diagnosis n (*pl* -ses) diagnóstico, (*process*) diagnosis f; **differential —** diagnóstico diferencial

diagnostic adj diagnóstico

dialysis *n* diálisis *f*; **peritoneal —** diálisis peritoneal
dialyze *vt* dializar
diameter *n* diámetro
diaper *n* pañal *m*; **cloth —** pañal de tela; **disposable —** pañal desechable
diaphragm *n* (*anat, gyn*) diafragma *m*
diarrhea *n* diarrea; **traveler's —** diarrea del viajero
diarrheal *adj* diarreico
diastolic *adj* diastólico
diathermy *n* diatermia, empleo de corrientes eléctricas para elevar la temperatura en tejidos profundos del cuerpo con fines terapéuticos
diazepam *n* diazepam *m*
DIC *abbr* **disseminated intravascular coagulation.** *V.* **coagulation.**
dichlorodiphenyltrichloroethane (DDT) *n* diclorodifeniltricloroetano (DDT)
dick *n* (*vulg, penis*) pene *m*
diclofenac *n* diclofenaco
dicloxacillin *n* dicloxacilina
didanosine *n* didanosina
die *vi* (*pret & pp* **died**; *ger* **dying**) morir(se), fallecer
dieldrin *n* dieldrin *m*
diet *n* dieta, régimen *m*, alimentación *f*; **balanced —** alimentación equilibrada (*form*), dieta equilibrada, dieta balanceada (*esp. Mex*); **diabetic —** dieta para diabéticos; **high-fiber —** dieta rica en fibra; **low-fat —** dieta baja en grasas; **Mediterranean —** dieta mediterránea; **weight loss —** dieta para bajar de peso, dieta de adelgazamiento (*esp. Esp*); *vi* (*también* **to be on a —**) estar a dieta, seguir un régimen
dietary *adj* dietético, alimenticio, alimentario, de la dieta
dietetic *adj* dietético; *npl* dietética
diethylstilbestrol (DES) *n* dietilestilbestrol *m* (DES)
dietitian, dietician *n* dietista *mf*, especialista *mf* en nutrición
differentiated *adj* diferenciado; **partially —** parcialmente diferenciado; **poorly —** pobremente *or* poco diferenciado; **well —** bien diferen-

ciado
difficulty *n* dificultad *f*
diffuse *adj* difuso
diffusion *n* difusión *f*
digest *vt* digerir
digestible *adj* digerible, digestible
digestion *n* digestión *f*
digestive *adj* digestivo
digit *n* (*finger, toe*) dedo
digital *adj* digital
digitalis *n* (*pharm*) digital *f*
dignity *n* dignidad *f*
digoxin *n* digoxina
dilate *vt, vi* dilatar(se)
dilation *n* dilatación *f*; **— and curettage (D&C)** dilatación y curetaje, dilatación y legrado
dilator *n* dilatador *m*
dildo *n* (*pl* **-dos**) consolador *m*, pene erecto artificial empleado para satisfacción sexual
diloxanide *n* diloxanida
diltiazem *n* diltiazem *m*
dilute *adj* diluido; *vt* diluir
dilution *n* dilución *f*
dilutional *adj* dilucional
dim *adj* (*comp* **dimmer**; *super* **dimmest**) oscuro, indistinto
dimension *n* dimensión *f*
dimethyl sulfoxide (DMSO) *n* dimetil sulfóxido
dimethyltryptamine (DMT) *n* dimetiltriptamina (DMT)
diminish *vi* disminuir
dimple *n* hoyuelo
dinner *n* cena
dioxide *n* dióxido
dioxin *n* dioxina
diphenhydramine *n* difenhidramina
diphenoxylate *n* difenoxilato
diphtheria *n* difteria
diplococcus *n* (*pl* **-ci**) diplococo
dipstick *n* tira reactiva (*para orina*)
direction *n* dirección *f*
dirt *n* suciedad *f*
dirty *adj* (*comp* **-ier**; *super* **-iest**) sucio; **to get —** ensuciarse; **to get (something) —** ensuciar
disability *n* (*pl* **-ties**) discapacidad *f*, (*esp. partial*) minusvalía, (*esp. with respect to work, possibly temporary*) incapacidad *f*, invalidez *f*, (*disorder*) trastorno; **cognitive —**

discapacidad intelectual; **learning** — trastorno de(l) aprendizaje; **physical** — discapacidad física

disabled *adj* discapacitado, *(esp. partially)* minusválido, *(unable to work, esp. temporarily)* incapacitado; **developmentally** — retrasado mental; **physically** — discapacitado físico

disabling *adj* incapacitante, discapacitante, invalidante

disappear *vi* desaparecer(se)

disaster *n* desastre *m*

disc *n* disco; **herniated** — hernia de disco; **intervertebral** — disco intervertebral; **optic** — disco óptico

discectomy *n* (*pl* **-mies**) discectomía

discharge *n* secreción *f*, *(vaginal)* flujo; *(from the hospital)* alta; *vt* dar de alta; **We are going to discharge you tomorrow**..Vamos a darlo de alta mañana.

discipline *n* disciplina; *vt* disciplinar

discography *n* discografía

discoid *adj* discoide

discomfort *n* molestia, incomodidad; **You're going to feel a little discomfort**..Va a sentir un poco de molestia.

discontinue *vt* suspender, *(a catheter, etc.)* retirar

discouraged *adj* desalentado, desanimado; **to get** — desalentarse, desanimarse

disease *n* enfermedad *f*, mal *m*; **Addison's** — enfermedad de Addison; **Alzheimer's** — enfermedad de Alzheimer; **benign breast** — enfermedad mamaria benigna; **cat-scratch** — enfermedad por arañazo de gato; **celiac** — enfermedad celíaca; **Chagas'** — enfermedad de Chagas; **chronic obstructive pulmonary** — (COPD) enfermedad pulmonar obstructiva crónica (EPOC); **connective tissue** — enfermedad del tejido conectivo *or* conjuntivo, conectivopatía *(Esp)*; **coronary artery** — enfermedad coronaria; **Crohn's** — enfermedad de Crohn; **Cushing's** — enfermedad de Cushing; **degenerative joint** — osteoartritis *f*; **diverticular**

— enfermedad diverticular; **fibrocystic** — of the breast enfermedad fibroquística de la mama; **fifth** — eritema infeccioso, quinta enfermedad; **gastroesophageal reflux** — **(GERD)** enfermedad por reflujo gastroesofágico (ERGE); **Gaucher's** — enfermedad de Gaucher; **graft-versus-host** — enfermedad del injerto contra el huésped; **Graves'** — enfermedad de Graves; **hand-foot-and-mouth** — enfermedad de manos, pies y boca; **Hansen's** — enfermedad de Hansen, lepra; **heart** — enfermedad cardíaca *(form)*, enfermedad del corazón; **Hirschsprung's** — enfermedad de Hirschsprung; **Hodgkin's** — enfermedad de Hodgkin; **Huntington's** — enfermedad de Huntington; **hyaline membrane** — enfermedad de membrana hialina; **infectious** — enfermedad infecciosa; **inflammatory bowel** — enfermedad inflamatoria intestinal; **interstitial lung** — enfermedad intersticial pulmonar; **Kawasaki's** — enfermedad de Kawasaki; **kidney** — enfermedad renal *(form)*, enfermedad de los riñones; **Legionnaire's** — legionelosis *f*; **liver** — enfermedad hepática *(form)*, enfermedad del hígado; **Lyme** — enfermedad de Lyme; **mad cow** — encefalopatía espongiforme bovina *(form)*, enfermedad de las vacas locas; **minimal change** — síndrome nefrótico de cambios mínimos; **mixed connective tissue** — enfermedad mixta del tejido conectivo; **motor neuron** — enfermedad de neurona motora; **Osgood-Schlatter** — enfermedad de Osgood-Schlatter; **Paget's** — enfermedad de Paget, *(of bone)* enfermedad ósea de Paget; **Parkinson's** — enfermedad de Parkinson; **pelvic inflammatory** — **(PID)** enfermedad inflamatoria pélvica; **peripheral vascular** — enfermedad vascular periférica; **polycystic kidney** — poliquistosis *f* renal; **Pott's** — mal *m* de Pott; **Raynaud's** — enfermedad de Raynaud; **rheu-**

matic heart — cardiopatía reumática; **sexually transmitted — (STD)** enfermedad de transmisión sexual (ETS), infección *f* de transmisión sexual (ITS); **sickle cell —** anemia falciforme, drepanocitosis *f*; **venereal — (VD)** (*ant*) infección *f* de transmisión sexual, enfermedad venérea (*ant*); **von Willebrand's** — enfermedad de von Willebrand; **Whipple's** — enfermedad de Whipple; **Wilson's** — enfermedad de Wilson

disinfect *vt* desinfectar

disinfectant *adj & n* desinfectante *m*

disk *V.* **disc.**

diskectomy *V.* **discectomy.**

dislocate *vt* dislocar(se); **How did he dislocate his shoulder?**..¿Cómo se dislocó el hombro?

dislocation *n* luxación *f* (*form*), dislocación *f*

disopyramide *n* disopiramida

disorder *n* trastorno; **anxiety** — trastorno de ansiedad; **attention deficit-hyperactivity — (ADHD)** trastorno por déficit de atención con hiperactividad (TDAH); **behavioral** — trastorno de comportamiento; **bipolar** — trastorno bipolar; **body dysmorphic** — trastorno dismórfico corporal; **borderline personality** — trastorno límite de la personalidad; **eating** — trastorno de alimentación; **female sexual arousal** — trastorno de la excitación sexual en la mujer; **obsessive-compulsive** — trastorno obsesivo-compulsivo; **panic** — trastorno de pánico; **personality** — trastorno de la personalidad; **posttraumatic stress** — trastorno por estrés postraumático; **sleep** — trastorno del sueño; **somatoform** — trastorno de somatización, trastorno somatomorfo *or* somatoforme; **speech** — trastorno del lenguaje

disoriented *adj* desorientado

dispense *vt* (*pharm*) dispensar

dispenser *n* dosificador *m*

displaced *adj* desplazado

disposable *adj* desechable

dissection *n* disección *f*; **aortic —**

disección aórtica

disseminate *vi* diseminarse

disseminated *adj* diseminado

dissemination *n* diseminación *f*, extensión *f*

dissociation *n* (*psych*) disociación *f*

dissolve *vt, vi* disolver(se)

distal *adj* distal

distend *vt* distender; **to become distended** distender(se)

distention, distension *n* distensión *f*

distilled *adj* destilado

distinguish *vt* distinguir

distress *n* distrés *m*, aflicción *f*; **respiratory** — distrés respiratorio

district *n* distrito, área

disturbance *n* trastorno, alteración *f*

disulfiram *n* disulfiram *m*

diuresis *n* diuresis *f*

diuretic *adj & n* diurético

diversion *n* derivación *f*; **urinary** — derivación urinaria

diverticulitis *n* diverticulitis *f*

diverticulosis *n* diverticulosis *f*

diverticulum *n* (*pl* **-la**) divertículo; **Meckel's** — divertículo de Meckel

divide *vt* dividir

diving *n* (*sport*) buceo

divorce *n* divorcio; *vt* divorciarse de; **She divorced him**..Se divorció de él; *vi* divorciarse

dizziness *n* mareo

dizzy *adj* (*comp* **-zier**; *super* **-ziest**) mareado; **to make** — dar mareo

DMSO *V.* **dimethyl sulfoxide.**

DMT *V.* **dimethlytryptamine.**

DMV *abbr* **Department of Motor Vehicles.** *V.* **department.**

DNA *V.* **deoxyribonucleic acid.**

DNR *abbr* **Do Not Resuscitate.** *V.* **resuscitate.**

doc *V.* **doctor.**

doctor *n* médico -ca *mf*, doctor -ra *mf*; **— on call** (*también* **on-call —**) médico de guardia; **family** — médico de cabecera, médico de la familia; **primary care** — médico de atención primaria, médico de cabecera; **private** — médico privado (*V. también* **physician.**)

Doctor of Medicine (MD, M.D.) *n* médico, licenciado -da *mf* en medicina

dog *n* perro; **guide —, seeing eye —**
(*ant*) perro guía
dominant *adj* dominante; **— hand**
mano dominante
donate *vt* donar
donation *n* donación *f*; **blood —** donación de sangre; **organ —** donación de órganos
donor *adj* de donante; **— semen** semen *m* de donante; *n* donante *mf*;
living — donante vivo; **universal**
— donante universal
dopamine *n* dopamina
dope *n* (*vulg*) narcótico(s), droga(s)
dopey *adj* drogado
doping *n* dopaje *m*
Doppler *n* (*imaging study*) Doppler
m
dorsal *adj* dorsal
dosage *n* dosis *f*, cantidad *f* de medicina; dosificación *f*
dose *n* dosis *f*; **When did you take**
the first dose?..¿Cuándo tomó la
primera dosis?
dosing *n* dosificación *f*
double *adj* doble; **— chin** papada; **—**
vision visión *f* doble; *adv* **to see —**
ver doble; *vt* doblar
double-jointed *adj* (*person*) que tiene hipermovilidad articular (*form*),
que tiene articulaciones hiperex-
tensibles, que puede doblar las coyunturas mucho más de lo normal;
(*joint*) hiperextensible, que se doble
mucho más de lo normal
douche *n* lavado vaginal, ducha (*vag-*
inal)
down *adj* (*depressed*) triste, deprimido; **Are you feeling down?**..¿Se
siente triste? *adv* hacia abajo; **Look**
down..Mire hacia abajo.
downer *n* (*fam*) sedante *m*, calmante
m
doxazocin *n* doxazocina
doxepin *n* doxepina
doxorubicin *n* doxorubicina
doxycycline *n* doxiciclina
doze *vi* dormitar
drain *vt* drenar; **We need to drain**
the abscess..Tenemos que drenar
el absceso; *vi* drenar, salir; **Is the**
wound still draining pus?..¿Todavía le sale pus de la herida?

drainage *n* (*of a wound, etc.*) drenaje
m, escurrimiento (*esp. Mex*); (*ma-*
terial drained) drenaje, secreciones
fpl
drank *pret de* **drink**
drape *n* paño; **surgical —** paño quirúrgico
draw *n* extracción *f* de sangre; **You**
need to go to the laboratory for a
blood draw..Tiene que ir al laboratorio para que le saquen sangre; *vt*
(*pret* **drew**; *pp* **drawn**) **to — blood**
extraer sangre (*form*), sacar sangre
dream *n* sueño; *vt*, *vi* (*pret & pp*
dreamed *o* **dreamt**) soñar; **to — of**
o **about** soñar con
dress *n* vestido; *vt* vestir; (*a wound*)
vendar; *vi* (*también* **to get dress-**
ed) vestirse
dressing *n* vendaje *m*, apósito, cura;
occlusive — vendaje oclusivo, cura
oclusiva; **pressure —** vendaje
compresivo
drew *pret de* **draw**
dried *pret & pp de* **dry**
drill (*dent*) *n* taladro; *vt* taladrar
drink *n* bebida; *vt*, *vi* (*pret* **drank**; *pp*
drunk) beber, tomar; **Do you**
drink alcohol much?..¿Toma Ud.
alcohol con frecuencia?
drinker *n* (*alcohol*) bebedor -ra *mf*,
tomador -ra *mf* (*Amer*)
drip *n* goteo; **postnasal —** goteo posnasal; *vi* (*pret & pp* **dripped**; *ger*
dripping) gotear
drive *n* impulso; **sex —** impulso
sexual; *vt*, *vi* (*pret* **drove**; *pp* **driv-**
en) (*a vehicle*) conducir, manejar
drool *n* baba; *vi* babear
drooling *n* babeo
droop *vi* (*eyelids, etc.*) caerse (*los*
párpados, etc.)
drop *n* gota; (*in level of something*
being measured) disminución *f*,
baja (*fam*); **cough —** pastilla para
la tos; **ear drops** gotas óticas, gotas
para los oídos; **eye drops** colirio,
gotas oftálmicas, gotas para los
ojos; **foot —** pie caído; **hand —**
mano péndula; *vi* (*pret & pp* **drop-**
ped; *ger* **dropping**) bajar(se); **His**
sugar dropped..Su azúcar bajó..Se
le bajó el azúcar.

drop-in *n* (*fam*) visita no programada

droplet *n* gota, gota chica de esputo que puede flotar en el aire y transmitir infección

dropper *n* gotero (*Amer*), cuentagotas *m*

drove *pret de* **drive**

drown *vt, vi* ahogar(se)

drowsy *adj* (*comp* -**sier**; *super* -**siest**) somnoliento; **to be —** tener sueño

drug *n* droga, medicamento; **designer —** droga de diseño; **hard —** droga dura; **nonsteroidal antiinflammatory — (NSAID)** antiinflamatorio no esteroideo (AINE); **soft —** droga blanda; *vt* (*pret & pp* **drugged**; *ger* **drugging**) drogar

druggist *n* (*ant*) farmacéutico -ca *mf*, boticario -ria *mf*

drugstore *n* farmacia, botica

drunk (*pp de* **drink**) *adj* borracho; **to get —** emborracharse; *n* (*person*) borracho -cha *mf*

drunkenness *n* borrachera, embriaguez *f*

dry *adj* seco; **— heaves** (*fam*) arcadas (*form*), vómito sin nada que expulsar; **— mouth** sequedad *f* de boca, boca seca (*fam*); *vt* (*pret & pp* **dried**) secar; *vi* (*también* **to get — o to — out**) secarse

drying *adj* secante

dryness *n* sequedad *f*, resequedad *f* (*esp. Mex*)

d.t.'s, the (*fam*) *V.* **delirium tremens**.

dual-energy X-ray absorptiometry (DEXA) *n* absorciometría de rayos X de doble energía

duct *n* conducto, vía; **bile —** conducto biliar; **common bile —** conducto biliar común, conducto colédoco; **cystic —** conducto cístico; **hepatic —** conducto hepático; **lacrimal —** vía *or* conducto lagrimal; **pancreatic —** conducto pancreático; **tear —** (*fam*) vía *or* conducto lagrimal

ductal *adj* ductal

ductus arteriosus *n* conducto arterioso; **patent — —** conducto arterioso persistente

due *adj* **— date** (*obst*) fecha probable de parto; **to be —** esperar dar a luz; **When are you due?**..¿Cuándo espera dar a luz?..¿Cuál es la fecha del parto? *prep* **— to** debido a; **ascites due to liver failure**..ascitis debida a insuficiencia hepática

dull *adj* romo; (*pain*) sordo; *vt* (*pain*) calmar

duloxetine *n* duloxetina

dumb *adj* (*ant, mute*) mudo

duodenal *adj* duodenal

duodenitis *n* duodenitis *f*

duodenum *n* duodeno

durable *adj* duradero

duration *n* duración *f*

dust *n* polvo; **house —** polvo de casa

DVT *abbr* **deep venous thrombosis**. *V.* **thrombosis**.

dwarf *n* enano -na *mf*

dwarfism *n* enanismo

dye *n* colorante *m*

dying *ger de* **die**

dyscrasia *n* discrasia

dysentery *n* disentería

dysfunction *n* disfunción *f*; **erectile —** disfunción eréctil; **temporomandibular joint —** disfunción de la articulación temporomandibular, disfunción temporomandibular

dysfunctional *adj* disfuncional

dyskinesia *n* discinesia; **tardive —** discinesia tardía

dyslexia *n* dislexia

dyspepsia *n* dispepsia, indigestión *f* (*fam*)

dysphasia *n* disfasia, dificultad *f* para hablar debida a un problema del cerebro

dysplasia *n* displasia, desorden *f* de crecimiento en un tejido

dysplastic *adj* displásico

dystrophy *n* distrofia; **reflex sympathetic —** distrofia simpática refleja

E

ear *n* oreja, (*organ of hearing*) oído; **external** — oído externo; **glue** — (*fam*) otitis media serosa; **inner** — oído interno; **middle** — oído medio; **outer** — oído externo; **swimmer's** — (*fam*) otitis externa

earache *n* dolor *m* de oídos, dolor de oído

eardrum *n* tímpano

earlobe *n* lóbulo de la oreja

early *adj* (*development, etc.*) temprano, precoz; *adv* temprano

earmuffs *n* orejeras

ear, nose and throat (ENT) *n* otorrinolaringología (*form*); oídos, nariz y garganta

earplugs *n* tapones auditivos (*form*), tapones para los oídos

earring *n* arete *m*

earthquake *n* terremoto, (*light*) temblor *m* (de tierra)

earwax *n* cerumen *m* (*form*), cera de los oídos

eat *vt, vi* (*pret* **ate**; *pp* **eaten**) comer

EBV *abbr* **Epstein-Barr virus.** *V.* **virus.**

ECG *V.* **electrocardiogram.**

Echinacea (*bot*) Echinacea

echinococcosis *n* equinococosis *f*

Echinococcus *n* equinococo

echo (*fam*) *V.* **echocardiogram.**

echocardiogram *n* ecocardiograma *m*

echocardiography *n* ecocardiografía; **stress** — ecocardiografía de esfuerzo; **transesophageal** — ecocardiografía transesofágica; **transthoracic** — ecocardiografía transtorácica

eclampsia *n* eclampsia

ecstasy *n* (*fam*) metilendioximetanfetamina (MDMA), éxtasis *m* (*fam*); **liquid** — (*fam*) gammahidroxibutirato, éxtasis líquido (*fam*)

ECT *abbr* **electroconvulsive therapy.** *V.* **therapy.**

ecthyma *n* ectima *m*

ectopic *adj* ectópico

ectropion *n* ectropión *m*, inversión *f* hacia fuera del párpado inferior

eczema *n* eccema *or* eczema *m*

edema *n* (*form*) edema *m* (*form*), hinchazón *f*; **pulmonary** — edema pulmonar

edge *n* borde *m*, margen *m*; **to be on** — (*fam*) estar nervioso, estar irritable; **to take the** — **off** (*fam*) calmar un poco (*dolor, ansiedad, etc.*)

educate *vt* educar

education *n* educación *f*; **diabetic** — educación diabetológica (*form*), educación para diabéticos; **health** — educación sanitaria (*form*), educación para la salud; **sex** — educación sexual

EEG *V.* **electroencephalogram.**

efavirenz *n* efavirenz *m*, efavirenzo (*OMS*)

effect *n* efecto; **adverse** — efecto adverso; **cumulative** — efecto acumulativo; **side** — efecto secundario; **to take** — hacer efecto

effective *adj* eficaz, efectivo

effectiveness *n* eficacia, efectividad *f*

effeminate *adj* afeminado

efficacy *n* eficacia

effort *n* esfuerzo

effusion *n* derrame *m*; **pericardial** — derrame pericárdico; **pleural** — derrame pleural

EGD *V.* **esophagogastroduodenoscopy.**

egg *n* huevo; (*fam, ovum*) óvulo, huevo (*fam*); — **white** clara de huevo; — **yolk** yema de huevo

ego *n* (*pl* **egos**) (*psych*) (el) yo; (*lay sense*) ego *m*

egocentric *adj* egocéntrico

egoism *n* egoísmo

egoistic *adj* egoísta

egotism *n* egotismo

egotist *n* egotista *mf*

egotistic *adj* egotista

ejaculate *n* eyaculado, semen *m*; *vi* eyacular

ejaculation *n* eyaculación *f*; **prema-ture** — eyaculación precoz
EKG *V.* **electrocardiogram**.
elastic *adj* elástico
elbow *n* codo
elderly *adj* anciano, de edad avanza-da
elective *adj* (*surg*) programado, elec-tivo
electric, electrical *adj* eléctrico
electrocardiogram (ECG) *n* electro-cardiograma *m* (ECG)
electrocardiography *n* electrocardio-grafía
electrocute *vt* electrocutar
electrocution *n* electrocución *f*
electrode *n* electrodo
electroencephalogram (EEG) *n* electroencefalograma *m* (EEG)
electroencephalography *n* electro-encefalografía
electrolyte *adj* electrolítico; *n* elec-trolito
electromyography (EMG) *n* electro-miografía (EMG)
electrophoresis *n* electroforesis *f*
electrophysiological, electrophysio-logic *adj* electrofisiológico
electrophysiology *n* electrofisiología; — **study (EPS)** estudio electrofi-siológico
element *n* elemento; **trace** — oligo-elemento, elemento traza (*frec. pl*); [*Note: the plural of* elemento traza *is* elementos traza.]
elephantiasis *n* elefantiasis *f*
eletriptan *n* eletriptán *m*
elevate *vt* elevar; **Try to keep your legs elevated as much as possi-ble**..Trate de mantener las piernas elevadas lo más posible.
elevation *n* elevación *f*
eliminate *vt* eliminar
elimination *n* eliminación *f*
elixir *n* elixir *m*
elute *vt* liberar; **drug-eluting** libera-dor de fármacos
emaciated *adj* severamente enflaque-cido, demacrado
emasculate *vt* emascular
embarrass *vt* **Don't feel embarrass-ed**..No tenga pena..No se apene..No tenga vergüenza.

embarrassment *n* vergüenza, pena
embolectomy *n* (*pl* -**mies**) embolec-tomía
embolism *n* embolia; **pulmonary** — embolia pulmonar
embolization *n* embolización *f*; **uter-ine artery** — embolización de las arterias uterinas
embolus *n* (*pl* -**li**) émbolo
embrace *n* abrazo; *vt* abrazar
embryo *n* (*pl* -**os**) embrión *m*
embryology *n* embriología
embryonal *adj* embrionario
emergency *adj* de urgencia, urgente (*esp. Esp*); — **C-section** cesarea de urgencia, cesarea urgente; — **ser-vices** servicio(s) de urgencias; *n* (*pl* -**cies**) urgencia, (*esp. non-medical*) emergencia
emerging *adj* emergente; — **disease** enfermedad *f* emergente
emery board *n* lima para uñas
emesis *n* emesis *f*
emetic *adj* & *n* emético, vomitivo
EMG *V.* **electromyography**.
emollient *adj* & *n* emoliente *m*
emotion *n* emoción *f*
emotional *adj* emocional, afectivo; (*person*) emotivo
empathy *n* empatía
emphysema *n* enfisema *m*
employ *vt* emplear
employer *n* empleador -ra *mf*, patrón -na *mf*
employment *n* empleo
empower *vt* (*psych*) apoyar, dar con-fianza
empty *adj* vacío; **on an** — **stomach** en ayunas; *vt* (*pret & pp* -**tied**) va-ciar; **You need to empty your bladder**..Necesita vaciar la vejiga.
emptying *n* vaciamiento
empyema *n* empiema *m*
emtricitabine *n* emtricitabina
enalapril *n* enalapril *m*
enamel *n* esmalte *m*
encephalitis *n* encefalitis *f*
encephalomyelitis *n* encefalomielitis *f*
encephalopathy *n* encefalopatía; **bo-vine spongiform** — encefalopatía espongiforme bovina, enfermedad de las vacas locas (*fam*); **hepatic** —

encefalopatía hepática; **Wernicke's** — encefalopatía de Wernicke

end *n* fin *m*; **end-stage** en fase terminal

endarterectomy *n* (*pl* **-mies**) endarterectomía; **carotid** — endarterectomía carotídea

endemic *adj* endémico

endocarditis *n* endocarditis *f*; **infectious** — endocarditis infecciosa

endocardium *n* (*pl* **-dia**) endocardio

endocervical *adj* endocervical

endocervix *n* endocérvix *m*

endocrine *adj* endocrino

endocrinologist *n* endocrinólogo -ga *mf*, médico -ca *mf* especialista en las hormonas y sus funciones

endocrinology *n* endocrinología, estudio de las hormonas y sus funciones

endometriosis *n* endometriosis *f*

endometritis *n* endometritis *f*

endometrium *n* endometrio

endorphin *n* endorfina

endoscope *n* endoscopio

endoscopic *adj* endoscópico; — **retrograde cholangiopancreatography (ERCP)** colangiopancreatografía retrógrada endoscópica (CPRE)

endoscopy *n* (*pl* **-pies**) endoscopia, endoscopía (*Amer, esp. spoken*); **capsule** — cápsula endoscópica; **upper** — endoscopia digestiva alta

endotracheal *adj* endotraqueal

endure *vt* aguantar, tolerar

enema *n* enema *m*, lavativa (*fam*); **barium** — enema de bario, enema opaco (*Esp*); **retention** — enema de retención

energetic *adj* activo, con mucha energía

energy *n* energía

enfuvirtide *n* enfuvirtida

engineering *n* ingeniería; **genetic** — ingeniería genética

enlarge *vt, vi* agrandar(se), aumentar de tamaño

enlargement *n* aumento de tamaño, dilatación *f*, hipertrofia (*form*), (*thickening*) engrosamiento

enrich *vt* enriquecer

ENT *V.* **ear, nose, and throat**.

enteral *adj* enteral

enteric *adj* entérico; **enteric-coated** con cubierta entérica, con capa entérica (*esp. Mex*)

enteritis *n* enteritis *f*; **eosinophilic** — enteritis eosinofílica; **regional** — enfermedad *f* de Crohn, enteritis regional

enterococcus *n* (*pl* **-ci**) enterococo

enterocolitis *n* enterocolitis *f*

enteropathy *n* (*pl* **-thies**) enteropatía; **protein-losing** — enteropatía perdedora de proteínas, enteropatía pierde-proteínas (*Esp*)

enterotoxin *n* enterotoxina

entrance *n* entrada

entrapment *n* compresión *f*, atrapamiento; **entrapment of the median (sciatic, etc.) nerve**..compresión *or* atrapamiento del nervio mediano (ciático, etc.); **peripheral nerve** — compresión *or* atrapamiento de un nervio periférico

entropion *n* entropión *m*, inversión *f* hacia dentro del párpado inferior

entry *n* entrada; **portal of** — puerta de entrada

enuresis *n* enuresis *f*, (el) mojar la cama

envenomation *n* envenenamiento (*de origen animal*)

environment *n* (*in general*) medio ambiente; (*immediate surroundings*) ambiente *m*, entorno

environmental *adj* (*in general*) ambiental, del medio ambiente; (*immediate surroundings*) ambiental

enzyme *n* enzima *m&f*; **angiotensin converting** — enzima de conversión de la angiotensina

eosinophil *n* eosinófilo

eosinophilia *n* eosinofilia

ephedra *n* (*bot*) efedra, belcho

ephedrine *n* efedrina

epicondyle *n* (*of elbow*) (*lateral*) epicóndilo; (*medial*) epitróclea

epicondylitis *n* (*lateral*) epicondilitis *f*; (*medial*) epitrocleítis *f*

epidemic *adj* epidémico; *n* epidemia

epidemiology *n* epidemiología

epididymis *n* (*pl* **-mides**) epidídimo

epididymitis *n* epididimitis *f*

epidural *adj* epidural

epigastric *adj* epigástrico

epiglottis *n* epiglotis *f*
epiglottitis *n* epiglotitis *f*
epilepsy *n* epilepsia
epileptic *adj & n* epiléptico -ca *mf*
epinephrine *n* epinefrina
epiphyseal *adj* epifisario
epiphysis *n* epífisis *f*
episiotomy *n* (*pl* -mies) episiotomía
episode *n* episodio
epispadias *n* epispadias *m*
epoetin alfa *n* epoetina alfa, eritropoyetina
EPS *abbr* **electrophysiology study.** *V.* **electrophysiology.**
epulis *n* épulis *m*
equilibrium *n* equilibrio
equipment *n* equipo, material *m*, instrumental *m*
equivalent *adj & n* equivalente *m*
ER *abbr* **emergency room.** *V.* **room.**
eradicate *vt* erradicar
eradication *n* erradicación *f*
ERCP *V.* **endoscopic retrograde cholangiopancreatography.**
erect *adj* erecto
erectile *adj* eréctil
erection *n* erección *f*
ergocalciferol *n* ergocalciferol *m*
ergonomic *adj* ergonómico -ca
ergonomics *n* ergonomía
ergotamine *n* ergotamina
erode *vt* erosionar
erogenous *adj* erógeno
erosion *n* erosión *f*
erosive *adj* erosivo
erotic *adj* erótico
error *n* error *m*; **inborn — of metabolism** error congénito del metabolismo; **laboratory —** error de laboratorio; **medication —** error de medicación
eruption *n* erupción *f*; **fixed drug —** erupción fija (medicamentosa); **polymorphous light —** erupción polimorfa lumínica
erysipelas *n* erisipela
erythema *n* eritema *m*; **— chronicum migrans** eritema crónico migratorio; **— infectiosum** eritema infeccioso; **— marginatum** eritema marginado; **— multiforme** eritema multiforme; **— nodosum** eritema nodoso *or* nudoso

erythrocyte *n* eritrocito; **— sedimentation rate (ESR)** velocidad *f* de sedimentación globular (VSG)
erythromycin *n* eritromicina
erythropoetin *n* eritropoyetina
eschar *n* (*form*) escara (*form*), costra
escitalopram *n* escitalopram *m*
esomeprazole *n* esomeprazol *m*
esophageal *adj* esofágico
esophagitis *n* esofagitis *f*; **erosive —** esofagitis erosiva; **reflux —** esofagitis por reflujo
esophagogastroduodenoscopy (EGD) *n* endoscopia digestiva alta
esophagus *n* (*pl* -gi) esófago; **Barrett's —** esófago de Barrett
ESR *abbr* **erythrocyte sedimentation rate.** *V.* **erythrocyte.**
essential *adj* esencial
esthetic *adj* estético
estradiol *n* estradiol *m*
estriol *n* estriol *m*
estrogen *n* estrógeno; **conjugated estrogens** estrógenos conjugados
eszopiclone *n* eszopiclona
etanercept *n* etanercept *m*
ethambutol *n* etambutol *m*
ethanol *n* etanol *m*
ether *n* éter *m*
ethical *adj* ético
ethinylestradiol *n* etinilestradiol *m*
ethionamide *n* etionamida
ethmoid *adj* etmoidal
ethnic *adj* étnico
ethosuximide *n* etosuximida
ethyl alcohol *n* etanol *m*, alcohol etílico
ethylene glycol *n* etilenglicol *m*
etretinate *n* etretinato
eucalyptus *n* (*bot*) eucalipto
eunuch *n* eunuco
euphoria *n* euforia
Eustachian tube *n* trompa de Eustaquio
euthanasia *n* eutanasia
evacuate *vt* evacuar
evacuation *n* evacuación *f*
evaluate *vt* valorar, evaluar
evaluation *n* valoración *f*, evaluación *f*
evaporate *vi* evaporarse
evaporation *n* evaporación *f*
evening *n* (*early*) tarde *f*, (*after dark*)

noche f

event recorder n monitor portátil transtelefónico del ritmo cardíaco

eventually adv con el tiempo

evidence n evidencia; **There's no evidence of tumor**..No hay evidencia de tumor; **evidence-based** basado en la evidencia; **scientific** — evidencia científica

evil eye n mal m de ojo

evolution n evolución f

evolve vi evolucionar, desarrollarse

ex- pref ex; **ex-husband** ex marido; **ex-smoker** ex fumador -ra mf; **ex-wife** ex esposa

exacerbation n exacerbación f, agudización f

exact adj exacto

exam (fam) V. **examination**.

examination n exploración f (form), reconocimiento (form), examen m, tacto, revisión f (fam); **breast** — examen mamario (form), examen de mamas or senos; **breast self-examination** (form) autoexploración mamaria (form), autoexamen de los senos, examen de los proprios senos (fam); **eye** — examen oftalmológico (form), examen de los ojos, examen de la vista; **pelvic** — examen pélvico, examen de las partes (íntimas) (fam); **physical** — exploración física (form), examen físico; **rectal** — tacto rectal

examine vt explorar (form), reconocer (form), examinar, revisar (fam); **May I examine your leg?**..¿Puedo examinarle la pierna?

examiner n examinador -ra mf

exanthem subitum n exantema súbito

excess n exceso

excessive adj excesivo

exchange n intercambio

excipient n excipiente m

excise vt resecar, extirpar, sacar (fam)

excision n escisión or excisión f, resección f

excisional adj escisional or excisional

excoriate vt excoriar

excoriation n excoriación f

excrement n excremento

excrete vt excretar

excretory adj excretor

excuse n excusa; **work** — justificante médico, excusa médica para no trabajar

exercise n ejercicio; **Kegel exercises** ejercicios de Kegel; **regular physical** — ejercicio físico regular; **stretching exercises** ejercicios de estiramiento; **warmup exercises** ejercicios de calentamiento; vi hacer ejercicio

exert vt **to** — **oneself** esforzarse

exertion n esfuerzo; **physical** — esfuerzo físico, ejercicio

exfoliation n exfoliación f

exfoliative adj exfoliativo

exhale vt, vi exhalar

exhaust n (gas) gas m de escape; vt agotar

exhausted adj exhausto, agotado; **to become** — agotarse

exhaustion n agotamiento

exit n salida

expand vt, vi expandir, dilatar(se)

expectant adj (obst, fam) embarazada, esperando (fam)

expectorant adj & n expectorante m

experiment n experimento; vi experimentar

experimental adj experimental

expert adj & n experto -ta mf, especialista mf; — **opinion** opinión f de expertos

expiration n (of a drug) caducidad f, vencimiento; (breathing out) espiración f; — **date** fecha de caducidad or vencimiento

expiratory adj espiratorio

expire vi (to die) fallecer, morir

exploratory adj (surg) explorador

expose vt exponer

exposed adj expuesto, (uncovered) descubierto; **sun-exposed** áreas expuestas al sol...**Have you been exposed to tuberculosis?**..¿Ha estado expuesto a la tuberculosis?

exposure n exposición f, contacto

express vt (thoughts, ideas, etc.) expresar; (pus) exprimir; **to** — **oneself** expresarse

expulsion n expulsión f

extend *vt, vi* extender(se)
extension *n* extensión *f*
extensive *adj* extenso
extensor *adj & n* extensor *m*
exterior *adj & n* exterior *m*
external *adj* externo
extra *adj* extra
extract *n* (*pharm*) extracto; *vt* (*to remove, take out*) extraer, sacar
extraction *n* (*dent, etc.*) extracción *f*
extreme unction *n* extremaunción *f*
extremity *n* (*pl* **-ties**) extremidad *f*
extrovert *n* extrovertido -da *mf*
extroverted *adj* extrovertido
extubate *vt* extubar
extubation *n* extubación *f*
eye *n* ojo; **angle** *o* **corner of the —** ángulo del ojo; **— shadow** sombras de *o* para ojos; **with the naked —** a simple vista
eyeball *n* globo ocular (*form*), globo

del ojo
eyebright *n* (*bot*) eufrasia
eyebrow *n* ceja; **Raise your eyebrows..**Levante las cejas.
eyedropper *n* gotero (*Amer*), cuentagotas *m*
eyeglasses *npl* lentes *mpl*, anteojos (*esp. Amer*), espejuelos (*esp. Carib*), gafas (*V. también* **glasses**.)
eyeground *n* fondo de ojo
eyelash *n* pestaña
eyelid *n* párpado
eyesight *n* visión *f*, vista
eyestrain *n* fatiga *or* cansancio visual
eyewash *n* colirio, gotas para los ojos
eyewear *n* gafas, lentes *mpl*, anteojos (*esp. Amer*), espejuelos (*esp. Carib*); **protective —** gafas protectoras, gafas de seguridad, lentes protectores (*esp. Mex*)
ezetimibe *n* ezetimiba

F

face *n* cara, rostro; *vt* (*to confront*) enfrentar; (*to turn facing*) voltearse; **Face the wall please..**Voltéese hacia la pared por favor.
facedown *adj* boca abajo
facelift *n* ritidectomía (*form*), estiramiento facial, cirugía plástica para eliminar las arrugas de la cara
face mask *n* (*for oxygen*) mascarilla, máscara
face shield *n* escudo facial
faceup *adj* boca arriba
facial *adj* facial; *n* tratamiento facial, masaje *m* facial
facility *n* (*pl* **-ties**) centro, hospital, asilo, residencia (*esp Esp*); **skilled nursing —** asilo *or* residencia de

ancianos; asilo *or* residencia para ancianos, enfermos, u otros descapacitados donde se ofrecen servicios de enfermería
factitious *adj* facticio, simulado, fingido
factor *n* factor *m*; **clotting —** factor de coagulación; **— V Leiden** factor V de Leiden; **intrinsic —** factor intrínseco; **Rh —** factor Rh; **rheumatoid —** factor reumatoide, factor reumatoideo (*SA*); **risk —** factor de riesgo; **sun protection — (SPF)** factor de protección solar (FPS)
facts of life *npl* (*ped, fam*) como se hacen los bebés

faculty *n* (*pl* **-ties**) facultad *f*
Fahrenheit *adj* Fahrenheit
fail *vi* fracasar, fallar
failure *n* insuficiencia, fallo, falla (*Amer*); (*treatment*) fracaso; **acute renal** — insuficiencia renal aguda; **adrenal** — insuficiencia suprarrenal; **chronic renal** — insuficiencia renal crónica; **congestive heart** — insuficiencia cardíaca congestiva; — **to thrive** fallo de medro (*Esp, form*), detención *f* del desarrollo, bajo peso para la edad; **heart** — insuficiencia cardíaca; **liver** — insuficiencia hepática; **multi-system organ** — fallo multiorgánico, falla orgánica múltiple (*esp. Mex*); **respiratory** — insuficiencia respiratoria; **treatment** — fracaso terapéutico, fracaso del tratamiento
faint *adj* **to feel** — sentir que se va a desmayar, estar mareado; **Do you feel faint?**..¿Siente que se va a desmayar? *n* desmayo; *vi* desmayarse
fair *adj* (*complexion*) blanco, güero (*Mex*)
fall *n* caída; (*in level of something being measured*) descenso (*form*), baja (*fam*); (*season*) otoño; *vi* (*pret* **fell**; *pp* **fallen**) caerse; bajar(se); **to** — **down** caerse
fallen *pp de* **fall**
fallout *n* lluvia radiactiva
false *adj* falso, (*tooth, eye, etc.*) postizo; — **teeth** dentadura postiza, dientes postizos
famciclovir *n* famciclovir *m*
familial *adj* familiar
family *adj* familiar; — **member** familiar *m*; — **planning** planificación *f* familiar; — **practice** medicina familiar; *n* (*pl* **-lies**) familia; **dysfunctional** — familia disfuncional; **extended** — familia extendida
famotidine *n* famotidina
fan *n* (*electric*) ventilador *m*
fang *n* colmillo
fantasy *n* (*pl* **-sies**) fantasía
farmer *n* agricultor -ra *mf*, granjero -ra *mf*
farsighted *adj* hipermétrope (*form*), que tiene dificultad para ver los objetos cercanos
farsightedness *n* hipermetropía (*form*), dificultad *f* para ver los objetos cercanos
fart (*vulg*) *n* flato (*form*), ventosidad *f*, pedo (*vulg*); *vi* expulsar gases, ventosear, tirarse pedos, (*vulg*) tirarse un pedo (*vulg*)
fascia *n* (*pl* **-ciae**) fascia
fasciitis *n* fascitis *f*; **necrotizing** — fascitis necrotizante *or* necrosante
fascioliasis *n* fascioliasis *f*
fasciotomy *n* (*pl* **-mies**) fasciotomía
fast *adj* rápido
fast *n* ayuno; *vi* ayunar, no comer nada
fasting *adj* en ayunas; — **glucose** glucemia en ayunas (*form*), glucosa en ayunas; *n* ayuno, (el) ayunar; **Fasting for a day won't do you any harm**..Ayunar por un día no le hará ningún daño.
fat *adj* (*comp* **fatter**; *super* **fattest**) gordo; **to get** — engordar(se); *n* grasa; **animal** — grasa animal; **milk** — grasa de leche; **saturated** — grasa saturada
fatal *adj* mortal, fatal
fat burner *n* quemador *m* de grasa
father *n* padre *m*
fatherhood *n* paternidad *f*
father-in-law *n* (*pl* **fathers-in-law**) suegro
fatigue *n* fatiga, cansancio
fatty *adj* (*comp* **-tier**; *super* **-tiest**) adiposo (*form*), graso; — **tissue** tejido adiposo
fatty acid *n* ácido graso; **essential** — — ácido graso esencial; **monounsaturated** — — ácido graso monoinsaturado; **omega-3** — — ácido graso omega-3; **polyunsaturated** — — ácido graso poliinsaturado; **saturated** — — ácido graso saturado; **trans** — — ácido graso trans; **unsaturated** — — ácido graso insaturado
favorable *adj* favorable
FDA *abbr* **Food and Drug Administration**. *V.* **administration**.
fear *n* miedo, temor *m*; **fear of needles**..miedo a las agujas
features *npl* facciones *fpl*, rasgos

febrile *adj* febril
fecal *adj* fecal
feces *npl* heces *fpl* (fecales)
fed *pret & pp de* **feed**
fee *n* honorarios
feeble *adj* débil
feed *vt* (*pret & pp* **fed**) alimentar (*form*), dar de comer
feedback *n* retroalimentación *f*
feeding *n* alimentación *f*; **tube** — alimentación por sonda
feel *vt* (*pret & pp* **felt**) sentir; **Can you feel this?**..¿Puede sentir esto? ...**Do you feel any pain?**..¿Siente algún dolor? *vi* sentirse; **How do you feel?**..¿Cómo se siente?...**Do you feel sick?**..¿Se siente enfermo?
feeling *n* (*sensation*) sensación *f*; (*emotion*) sentimiento, emoción *f*; (*sense of touch*) sensibilidad *f*; **feeling of warmth**..sensación de calor...**strong feelings** sentimientos fuertes...**Have you lost feeling in your feet?**..¿Ha perdido la sensibilidad en los pies?
feet *pl de* **foot**
fell *pret de* **fall**
fellatio *n* (*form*) felación *f* (*form*), sexo oral, estimulación *f* oral del pene
felodipine *n* felodipino, felodipina (*esp. SA*)
felon *n* panadizo (herpético), infección de la piel detrás de la uña (*producida por el herpes en la mayoría de los casos*)
felt *pret & pp de* **feel**
female *adj* femenino; *n* mujer *f*, niña, chica
feminine *adj* femenino
feminization *n* feminización *f*
femoral *adj* femoral
femur *n* fémur *m*
fenofibrate *n* fenofibrato
fenoprofen *n* fenoprofeno
fentanyl *n* fentanilo
ferric *adj* férrico
ferritin *n* ferritina
ferrous *adj* ferroso; — **sulfate** sulfato ferroso
fertile *adj* fértil
fertilization *n* fecundación *f*, fertilización *f*; **in vitro** — **(IVF)** fecundación *or* fertilización in vitro **(FIV)**
fertilize *vt* fecundar, fertilizar
fetal *adj* fetal
fetish *n* fetiche *m*
fetus *n* feto
fever *n* fiebre *f*, calentura; **hay** — fiebre del heno, alergia al polen; **hemorrhagic** — fiebre hemorrágica; **Mediterranean spotted** — fiebre botonosa mediterránea; **Q** — fiebre Q; **relapsing** — borreliosis; **rheumatic** — fiebre reumática; **Rocky Mountain spotted** — fiebre maculosa de las Montañas Rocosas; **scarlet** — escarlatina; **typhoid** — fiebre tifoidea; **valley** — (*fam*) coccidioidomicosis *f*; **yellow** — fiebre amarilla
fever blister *n* herpes labial (*form*), calentura (*Esp, frec. pl*), fuego, erupción en los labios (*debida al herpes*)
feverfew *n* (*bot*) matricaria
feverish *adj* con fiebre *or* calentura
few *adj* (*comp* less; *super* least) poco
fexofenadine *n* fexofenadina
fiancé *n* novio, prometido
fiancée *n* novia, prometida
fiber *n* fibra; **dietary** — fibra dietética; **insoluble** — fibra insoluble; **muscle** — fibra muscular; **nerve** — fibra nerviosa; **soluble** — fibra soluble
fiberoptic *adj* de fibra óptica
fibrillation *n* fibrilación *f*; **atrial** — fibrilación auricular; **ventricular** — fibrilación ventricular
fibrin *n* fibrina
fibrinogen *n* fibrinógeno
fibrinolysis *n* fibrinólisis *f*
fibrinolytic *adj* fibrinolítico
fibroadenoma *n* fibroadenoma *m*
fibrocystic *adj* fibroquístico
fibroid *n* (*of the uterus*) mioma *or* leiomioma uterino, tumor benigno del útero
fibroma *n* fibroma *m*
fibromyalgia *n* fibromialgia, dolor crónico en todo el cuerpo
fibrosis *n* fibrosis *f*; **idiopathic pulmonary** — fibrosis pulmonar idiopática

fibrotic *adj* fibrótico
fibula *n* peroné *m*
fidget *vi* moverse (*con impaciencia o nerviosismo*), hacer movimientos inconscientes (*debido a impaciencia o nerviosismo*)
field *adj* de campaña; — **hospital** hospital *m* de campaña; *n* campo; **visual** — campo visual
figure *n* (*of a person*) figura, línea
filariasis *n* filariasis *f*
file *n* (*patient chart*) historia clínica, historial médico, expediente (clínico) (*Mex, CA*); **nail** — lima de uñas; *vt* **to** — **one's nails** limarse las uñas
filgrastim *n* filgrastim *m*
fill *vt* llenar; (*a prescription, by a pharmacist*) surtir, surtir medicamento de acuerdo con (*una receta*); (*a prescription, by a patient*) presentar (*una receta*) para obtener medicamento; (*dent*) empastar, rellenar (*Amer*), tapar (*fam*); **Any pharmacist can fill this prescription for you.**.Cualquier farmacéutico puede surtirle medicamento de acuerdo con esta receta...**You can fill this prescription at any pharmacy.**.Ud. puede presentar esta receta en cualquier farmácia para obtener el medicamento.
filling *n* (*dent*) empaste *m*, relleno (*Amer*)
film *n* (*X-ray*) radiografía, placa (*fam*)
filter *n* filtro; *vt, vi* filtrar(se)
filtration *n* filtración *f*
finasteride *n* finasterida
finding *n* hallazgo
finger *n* dedo (de la mano); **index** — dedo índice; **little** — dedo meñique; **middle** — dedo medio, dedo del corazón; **ring** — dedo anular
fingernail *n* uña (de la mano)
finger-stick *n* punción *f* digital (*form*), pinchazo en el dedo, piquete *m* en el dedo (*esp. Mex*); **finger-stick glucose** glucemia capilar (*form*), medición *f* del azúcar a través de un pinchazo (piquete) en el dedo
fingertip *n* punta del dedo

fire *n* fuego, incendio; — **department** cuerpo de bomberos; — **extinguisher** extintor *m* de incendios, extinguidor *m* de incendios (*Amer*); — **retardant** retardante *m* de fuego
fire ant *n* hormiga de fuego, tipo de hormiga cuya picadura es muy dolorosa
firearm *n* arma de fuego
firefighter *n* bombero -ra *mf*
firm *adj* firme
first *adj* primero; — **aid** primeros auxilios
fish *n* (*pl* **fish** *o* **fishes**) pez *m*; (*after being caught, as food*) pescado
fishbone *n* espina
fisherman *n* (*pl* **-men**) pescador *m*
fisherwoman *n* (*pl* **-women**) pescadora
fishhook *n* anzuelo
fissure *n* fisura; **anal** — fisura anal
fist *n* puño; **Make a fist**..Cierre el puño.
fistula *n* (*pl* **-las** *o* **-lae**) fístula; **anal** — fístula anal *or* de ano; **arteriovenous** — fístula arteriovenosa
fit *adj* (*comp* **fitter**; *super* **fittest**) en forma, en buen estado físico; *n* (*attack*) ataque *m*, acceso; *vt* (*pret & pp* **fitted**; *ger* **fitting**) (*glasses, etc.*) ajustar; *vt, vi* (*shoes, clothing*) quedar (bien); **You need shoes that fit you better**..Necesita zapatos que le queden mejor.
fitness *n* condición física, acondicionamiento físico, aptitud física
fix *vt* arreglar, reparar
fixation *n* fijación *f*
fixed *adj* fijo
flab *n* rollos (de grasa)
flabby *adj* (*comp* **-bier**; *super* **-biest**) flácido, flojo
flaccid *adj* flácido
flake (*skin*) *n* escama; *vi* descamarse (*form*), caerse en escamas
flaky *adj* (*comp* **-ier**; *super* **-iest**) escamoso
flame *n* llama; — **retardant** retardante *m* de fuego
flammable *adj* inflamable
flank *n* flanco, costado entre las costillas y la cadera
flap *n* colgajo

flare n reagudización f (form), empeoramiento nuevo y súbito; vi (también **to — up**) reagudizarse (form), recrudecer(se) (form), volver(se) a agravar

flashback n recurrencia de alucinaciones producidas por una droga tomada en el pasado; recuerdo vivo hasta con alucinaciones de una experiencia traumática en el pasado

flat adj (comp **flatter**; super **flattest**) plano; **Do you get short of breath when you sleep flat in bed?**..¿Le falta el aire al acostarse sin almohadas?

flatfoot n (pl **-feet**) pie plano

flatline n asistolia, ausencia de actividad eléctrica (indicada por monitor cardíaco)

flatulence n flatulencia

flatulent adj flatulento

flatworm n platelminto (form), gusano plano

flavonoid n flavonoide m

flavor n sabor m, gusto; **cherry-flavored, banana-flavored, etc.** con sabor a cereza, con sabor a plátano, etc.

flea n pulga

fleeting adj (pain, etc.) pasajero

flesh n carne f; **flesh-eating** necrosante (form), devorador de carne; **raw —** carne viva

fleshy adj carnoso

flex vt flexionar (form), doblar

flexible adj flexible

flexor adj & n flexor m

flies pl de **fly**

flip vt (pret & pp **flipped**; ger **flipping**) **to — out** (fam) volverse loco

floater n (in the eye) mosca volante, puntos o hilos flotando en el campo visual

flood n inundación f

floor n piso, suelo (Esp); **— of the mouth** piso or suelo de la boca; **pelvic —** piso or suelo pélvico

flora n flora, microflora

floss n (también **dental —**) hilo dental; vt, vi limpiar (los dientes) con hilo dental

flour n harina

flow n flujo; **blood —** flujo sanguíneo (form), circulación f (de la sangre); **peak —** (spirometry) flujo espiratorio máximo; vi fluir, circular

flu n gripe f, influenza; **Asian —** gripe asiática; **avian** o **bird —** gripe aviar; **stomach —** (fam) gastroenteritis f; **swine —** influenza porcina

fluconazole n fluconazol m

fluctuate vi fluctuar, oscilar, variar

fludrocortisone n fludrocortisona

fluid n líquido, fluido; **amniotic —** líquido amniótico; **body —** fluido corporal; **cerebrospinal — (CSF)** líquido cefalorraquídeo (LCR); **pleural —** líquido pleural; **seminal —** líquido seminal; **synovial —** líquido sinovial

fluke n trematodo, (tipo de) gusano plano parasítico

flumetasone n flumetasona

flunisolide n flunisolida

fluorescent adj fluorescente

fluoridation n fluoración f

fluoride n fluoruro

fluorine n flúor m

fluoroscopy n (pl **-pies**) fluoroscopia, fluoroscopía (Amer, esp. spoken)

fluorouracil n fluorouracilo

fluoxetine n fluoxetina

fluphenazine n flufenazina

flurazepam n flurazepam m

flush (physio) n enrojecimiento (de la piel), rubefacción f (form), rubor m; (due to menopause) rubor m, sofoco, bochorno; vi ruborizarse, sonrojarse

flushing n enrojecimiento (de la piel), rubefacción f (form), rubor m

fluticasone n fluticasona

flutter n aleteo, flúter m (Ang); **atrial —** aleteo or flúter auricular

fluvastatin n fluvastatina

fly n (pl **flies**) mosca

foam rubber n goma espuma, hule m espuma (esp. Mex, CA)

foamy adj (comp **-ier**; super **-iest**) espumoso

focal adj focal

focus n (pl **foci** o **focuses**) foco; vt (pret & pp **focused** o **focussed**; ger **focusing** o **focussing**) enfocar

fold n pliegue m; **nail —** pliegue ungueal; **skin** — pliegue cutáneo; *vt* **to** — **one's arms** cruzar los brazos; **Fold your arms while I listen to your lungs**..Cruce los brazos mientras le escucho los pulmones.

folic acid *n* ácido fólico

follicle *n* folículo; **hair** — folículo piloso; **ovarian** — folículo ovárico

folliculitis *n* foliculitis *f*

follow *vt (medically)* estar tratando; **Who follows you for your diabetes?**..¿Quién lo está tratando para su diabetes?

follow-up *n* seguimiento, consulta subsecuente (*Mex*), atención médica subsecuente

fondle *vt* acariciar, molestar

fontanelle, fontanel *n* fontanela, mollera

food *n* comida, alimento *(frec. pl)*; **baby** — alimentos infantiles, comida para bebés; **canned** — alimentos enlatados, comida enlatada; **fast** — comida rápida; — **coloring** colorante *m*, colorante vegetal, colorante alimentario; — **handler** manipulador -ra *mf* de alimentos; — **poisoning** intoxicación alimentaria, intoxicación por productos bacterianos en la comida; — **value** valor nutritivo; **health** *o* **natural** — alimentos naturales; **health** — **store** *o* **natural** — **store** tienda de productos naturales, tienda naturista (*Mex*); **junk** — comida chatarra, comida basura (*esp. Esp*); **processed** — alimentos procesados

foodborne *adj* de transmisión alimentaria *(form)*, transmitido por los alimentos

foot *n (pl* **feet***)* pie *m; (unit of measure)* 0,3048 metros; **diabetic** — pie diabético

football *n* fútbol (americano)

footrest *n* reposapiés *m*

footwear *n* calzado *(zapatos, botas)*

foramen ovale *n* foramen *m* oval; **patent** — — foramen oval permeable

force *n* fuerza; **shear** — fuerza de cizallamiento *or* cizalla

forceps *n (pl* **-ceps***) (obst)* fórceps *m*

forearm *n* antebrazo

forefinger *n* dedo índice

forefoot *n* antepié *m*, parte *f* anterior del pie

forehead *n* frente *f*

foreign *adj* extraño; **Your body recognizes foreign proteins**..Su organismo reconoce las proteínas extrañas; — **body** cuerpo extraño

forensic *adj* forense

foreplay *n* caricias eróticas que preceden al acto sexual

foreskin *n* prepucio

forget *vt, vi (pret* **-got***; pp* **-gotten***; ger* **-getting***)* olvidar

forgetful *adj* olvidadizo

forgetfulness *n* dificultad *f* para recordar, falta de memoria

form *n* forma; *(paper to fill out)* formulario; *vt, vi* formar(se)

formaldehyde *n* formaldehído

formalin *n* formol *m*

formation *n* formación *f*

former *adj* ex; — **smoker** ex fumador -ra *mf*

formoterol *n* formoterol *m*

formula *n (pharm, math)* fórmula; *(ped)* fórmula, leche *f* artificial para lactantes

formulary *n (pl* **-ries***)* formulario, lista de medicamentos disponibles

fortify *vt (pret & pp* **-fied***)* enriquecer, fortificar

forward *adv* adelante, hacia adelante; **Lean forward**..Inclínese hacia adelante.

fosamprenavir *n* fosamprenavir *m*

fosinopril *n* fosinopril *m*

fossa *n* fosa

foster care *n (US)* crianza de huérfanos o niños abandonados por alguien que no es padre adoptivo y que recibe remuneración del gobierno

foul-smelling *adj* que tiene mal olor, que huele mal

fourth *n* cuarta parte, cuarto; **a fourth of the patients**..una cuarta parte de los pacientes

fowl *n* aves *fpl* de corral

fox *n* zorro -ra *mf*

fraction *n* fracción *f*; **ejection** — **fracción** de eyección

fracture *n* fractura; **closed** — fractura cerrada; **comminuted** — fractura conminuta; **compound** — fractura abierta; **cranial** — fractura craneal; **hairline** — fisura, fractura pequeña, grieta; **open** — fractura abierta; **skull** — fractura de cráneo; **spiral** — fractura espiroidea; **stress** — fractura de estrés; **vertebral compression** — (fractura por) aplastamiento vertebral, fractura vertebral (debida a la osteoporosis); *vt, vi* fracturar(se), quebrar(se); **He fractured his femur** ..Se fracturó el fémur...**The bullet fractured his femur**..La bala le fracturó el fémur.

fragile *adj* frágil, delicado, quebradizo

fragment *n* fragmento

frail *adj* frágil, débil

frames *npl* (*for eyeglasses*) armazón *m&f*, montura (*Esp*)

fraternal *adj* fraterno

freak *n* (*vulg*) monstruo; *vi* **to** — **out** enloquecerse, perder el control, tener pánico

freckle *n* peca

free *adj* libre, suelto; **fat-free, sugar-free, etc**. sin grasa, sin azúcar, etc.; — **of pain** (*también* **pain-free**) (*person*) sin dolor, (*method, procedure*) que no duele; *vt* soltar

freebase *n* (*cocaine*) base *f* libre (*cocaína*)

freeze *vt, vi* (*pret* **froze**; *pp* **frozen**) congelar(se)

freeze-dried *adj* liofilizado

frequency *n* (*pl* **-cies**) frecuencia

frequent *adj* frecuente

frequently *adv* frecuentemente, a menudo

fresh *adj* fresco

friction *n* fricción *f*

fried (*pret & pp de* **fry**) *adj* frito

friend *n* amigo -ga *mf*

friendly *adj* amable

friendship *n* amistad *f*

fright *n* susto

frighten *vt* asustar

frigid *adj* (*ant*) frígida, que tiene deseo sexual disminuido (*dicho de una mujer*)

frigidity *n* (*ant*) frigidez *f*, disminución *f* del apetito sexual en la mujer

frontal *adj* frontal

frostbite *n* congelamiento, daño a los tejidos producido por exposición al frío

frovatriptan *n* frovatriptán *m*

frown *vi* fruncir el ceño *or* entrecejo

froze *pret de* **freeze**

frozen *pp de* **freeze**

fructose *n* fructosa

fruit *n* (*pl* **fruit** *o* **fruits**) fruta; **citric** — fruta cítrica

fry *vt* (*pret & pp* **fried**) freír

FSH *abbr* **follicle-stimulating hormone**. *V.* **hormone**.

Fucus *n* (*bot*) Fucus

full *adj* lleno; **I feel full**..Me siento lleno.

fullness *n* saciedad *f* (*form*), plenitud *f* (*form*), sensación *f* de llenado (*fam*)

fulminant *adj* fulminante

fumes *npl* humo

fumigate *vt* fumigar

function *n* función *f*; *vi* funcionar

funeral home *n* funeraria

fungal *adj* fúngico, micótico

fungus *n* (*pl* **-gi**) hongo

funny *adj* (*fam, unusual*) extraño, raro; *adv* de una manera extraña *or* rara; **She walks funny**..Camina de una manera extraña (rara).

funny bone *n* (*fam*) codo

furosemide *n* furosemida

furuncle *n* forúnculo

fuse *vt, vi* (*ortho*) fusionar(se)

fusion *n* fusión *f*

G

gabapentin *n* gabapentina
gadolinium *n* gadolinio
gag *vt* (*pret & pp* **gagged**; *ger* **gagging**) (*también* **to make** —) provocar náuseas; **It gagged him..It made him gag**..Le provocó náuseas; *vi* sentir náuseas; **She gagged**.. Sintió náuseas.
gain *n* ganancia, aumento; **weight** — ganancia de peso; *vt* **to** — **weight** subir de peso, ganar peso
gait *n* marcha (*form*), forma de andar
galactose *n* galactosa
galactosemia *n* galactosemia
gallbladder *n* vesícula (biliar)
gallium *n* galio
gallop *n* (*card*) galope *m*
gallstone *n* cálculo biliar (*form*), piedra de *or* en la vesícula
gamma *n* gamma
gamma-hydroxybutyrate (GHB) *n* gammahidroxibutirato, éxtasis líquido (*fam*)
gammopathy *n* gammapatía; **monoclonal** — **of undetermined significance** gammapatía monoclonal de significado incierto
gancyclovir *n* ganciclovir *m*
gang *n* pandilla
ganglion *n* (*pl* **-glia**) (*neural*) ganglio; (*cyst*) ganglión *m*
ganglioneuroma *n* ganglioneuroma *m*
gangrene *n* gangrena; **dry** — gangrena seca; **gas** — gangrena gaseosa
gap *n* espacio
gardener *n* jardinero -ra *mf*
gargle *vi* hacer gárgaras
garlic *n* ajo
gas *n* gas *m*; (*US, fam*) gasolina; **natural** — gas natural; **tear** — gas lacrimógeno; **to have** — tener distensión *f* abdominal (*form*), tener gases; **to pass** — expulsar gases, ventosear; **Are you passing gas yet?**..¿Ya está expulsando gases?
gash *n* herida, herida grande (*produ-*

cida por un objeto cortante)
gasoline *n* (*US*) gasolina
gasp *vi* hacer esfuerzos para respirar, hacer esfuerzo marcado con cada respiración, boquear
gastrectomy *n* (*pl* **-mies**) gastrectomía
gastric *adj* gástrico
gastrin *n* gastrina
gastrinoma *n* gastrinoma *m*
gastritis *n* gastritis *f*
gastrocnemius *n* gastrocnemio, músculo gemelo
gastroenteritis *n* gastroenteritis *f*
gastroenterologist *n* gastroenterólogo -ga *mf*, médico -ca *mf* especialista en el aparato digestivo y sus enfermedades, médico del estómago (*fam*)
gastroenterology *n* gastroenterología, estudio del aparato digestivo y sus enfermedades
gastroesophageal *adj* gastroesofágico
gastrointestinal (GI) *adj* gastrointestinal, digestivo
gastroparesis *n* gastroparesia
gastrostomy *n* (*pl* **-mies**) gastrostomía; **percutaneous endoscopic** — **(PEG)** gastrostomía endoscópica percutánea
gauge *n* calibre *m*; **21** — **needle** aguja de calibre 21
gauze *n* gasa
gave *pret de* **give**
gay *adj* gay, homosexual; — **man** gay *m*, homosexual *m*; — **woman** lesbiana
gaze *n* mirada (*acto de mantener fija la vista en una dirección determinada*)
gel *n* gel *m*
gelatin *n* gelatina
gemfibrozil *n* gemfibrozilo
gender *n* género, sexo; — **identity** identidad *f* de género
gene *n* gen *m*

general *adj* general
generalized *adj* generalizado
generation *n* generación *f*; **first —, second —,** etc. primera generación, segunda generación, etc.
generator *n* (*of a pacemaker, etc.*) generador *m*
generic *adj & n* (*pharm*) genérico
genetic *adj* genético
geneticist *n* genetista *mf*
genetics *n* genética
genital *adj* genital; *npl* genitales *mpl*
genius *n* genio
genome *n* genoma *m*; **human —** genoma humano
genotype *n* genotipo
gentamicin *n* gentamicina
Gentian violet *n* violeta de genciana
gentle *adj* suave, ligero
genu valgum *adj* genu valgo
genu varum *adj* genu varo, piernas arqueadas (*fam*)
geranium oil *n* (*bot*) aceite *m* de geranio
GERD *abbr* **gastroesophageal reflux disease.** *V.* **disease.**
geriatric *adj* geriátrico
geriatrician *n* geriatra *mf*
geriatrics *n* geriatría
germ *n* germen *m*, microbio; (*of a seed*) germen *m*; **wheat —** germen de trigo
germander *n* (*bot*) camedrio
German measles *n* (*fam*) rubéola
germinoma *n* germinoma *m*
gerontologist *n* gerontólogo -ga *mf*, médico -ca *mf* especialista en la vejez y sus enfermedades
gerontology *n* gerontología, estudio de la vejez y sus enfermedades
gestation *n* gestación *f*
gestational *adj* gestacional
get *vt* (*pret* **got**; *pp* **gotten**; *ger* **getting**) (*a disease*) dar(le) (a uno), pegar(le) (a uno), coger (*esp. Esp*); **I got the flu..**Me dio (pegó) la gripe..Cogí la gripe; **to — over** (*an illness, etc.*) recuperarse; **to — up** levantarse; [*Note:* coger *may be considered offensive in many parts of Latin America.*]
GH *abbr* **growth hormone.** *V.* **hormone.**

GHB *V.* **gamma-hydroxybutyrate.**
GI *adj* (*fam*) *V.* **gastrointestinal.**
giant *adj* gigante
giardiasis *n* giardiasis *f*
giddy *adj* (*comp* **-dier**; *super* **-diest**) mareado
GIFT *abbr* **gamete intrafallopian transfer.** *V.* **transfer.**
gifted *adj* superdotado
gigantism *n* gigantismo
Gila monster *n* monstruo de Gila
ginger *n* (*bot*) jengibre *m*
gingiva *n* (*pl* **-vae**) encía
gingivitis *n* gingivitis *f*; **acute necrotizing ulcerative —** angina de Vincent, gingivitis úlceronecrotizante aguda
ginkgo biloba *n* (*bot*) ginkgo biloba *m*
ginseng *n* (*bot*) ginseng *m*, mandrágora
girdle *n* cintura; **pelvic —** cintura pélvica *or* pelviana; **shoulder —** cintura escapular
girl *n* niña, muchacha, chica
girlfriend *n* (*romantic*) novia, enamorada
girth *n* perímetro
give *vt* (*pret* **gave**; *pp* **given**) dar; (*a disease*) contagiar (*form*), pegar, dar, pasar; **Don't give me your cold..**No me contagie (pegue, etc.) su resfriado; **to — out** (*knee, etc.*) fallar(le), no dar más; **Your knee gave out?..**¿Le falló la rodilla?.. ¿Su rodilla no dio más? **to — up** (*smoking, etc.*) dejar de; **You have to give up smoking..**Tiene que dejar de fumar; **to — up on** (*diet, treatment, etc.*) abandonar
gland *n* glándula; (*fam, lymph node*) ganglio linfático; **adrenal —** glándula suprarrenal, suprarrenal *f* (*fam*); **endocrine —** glándula endocrina; **lacrimal —** glándula lagrimal; **mammary —** glándula mamaria; **parathyroid —** glándula paratiroides, paratiroides *f* (*fam*); **parotid —** glándula parótida, parótida (*fam*); **pineal —** glándula pineal; **pituitary —** hipófisis *f*; **prostate —** glándula prostática, próstata (*fam*); **salivary —** glándu-

la salival; **sweat** — glándula sudorípara; **thyroid** — glándula tiroides, tiroides *m&f (fam)*

glans *n* glande *m*

glass *n (material)* vidrio; *(tumbler)* vaso; **a glass of milk**..un vaso de leche

glasses *npl* lentes *mpl*, anteojos *(esp. Amer)*, espejuelos *(esp. Carib)*, gafas; **bifocal** — lentes (anteojos, etc.) bifocales, bifocales *mpl (fam)*; **reading** — lentes *or* anteojos de lectura, gafas de lectura *(Esp)*; **safety** — gafas protectoras *or* de seguridad, lentes protectores *(esp. Mex)*

glaucoma *n* glaucoma *m*

glimepiride *n* glimepirida

glioblastoma *n* glioblastoma *m*; **glioblastoma multiforme** glioblastoma multiforme

glioma *n* glioma *m*

glipizide *n* glipizida

global *adj* global

globulin *n* globulina; **gamma** — gammaglobulina; **immune** — inmunoglobulina *(exógena)*

glomerulonephritis *n* glomerulonefritis *f*

glossitis *n* glositis *f*

glottis *n* glotis *f*

glove *n* guante *m*

glucagon *n* glucagón *m*

glucagonoma *n* glucagonoma *m*

glucocorticoid *adj & n* glucocorticoide *m*

Glucometer *n (marca)* **(blood) glucose meter** *o* **monitor**. *V.* **meter** *o* **monitor**.

glucosamine *n* glucosamina

glucose *n* glucosa

glue *n (as drug of abuse)* pegamento

glutamic acid *n* ácido glutámico

glutamine *n* glutamina

glutaraldehyde *n* glutaraldehído

gluteal *adj* glúteo

gluten *n* gluten *m*

gluteus *n* glúteo

glyburide *n* glibenclamida

glycerol, glycerin *n* glicerol *m*, glicerina

glycine *n* glicina

GMO *abbr* **genetically modified organism**. *V.* **organism**.

gnash *vt (one's teeth)* rechinar *(los dientes)*

gnat *n (type that bite)* jején *m*, insecto pequeño parecido al mosquito

gnawing *adj (pain)* sordo y persistente

GnRH *abbr* **gonadotropin-releasing hormone**. *V.* **hormone**.

go *vi (pret* **went**; *pp* **gone**) ir; **to be going around** *(a virus, etc.)* estar circulando, estar dando(se); **The flu virus is going around now**..El virus de la gripe está circulando (se está dando) ahora; **to — away** *(pain, etc.)* quitarse, pasarse; **The pain should go away in a few days**..El dolor debe quitarse (pasarse) dentro de unos días; **to — down** *(temperature, blood glucose, etc.)* bajar(se); **to — to the doctor** ir *or* acudir al médico; **to — up** subir(se)

goal *n* meta

goggles *npl* gafas, gogles *mpl (Mex)*; **safety** — gafas protectoras *or* de seguridad, lentes protectores *(esp. Mex)*; **swimming** — gafas de natación *or* para nadar

goiter *n* bocio; **toxic multinodular** — bocio multinodular tóxico

gold *n* oro

goldenseal *n (bot)* botón *m* de oro

gold standard *n* patrón *m* oro

golf *n* golf *m*

golfer's elbow *n* epitrocleítis *f (form)*, codo de golfista

gonad *n* gónada

gonadorelin *n* gonadorelina

gonadotropin *n* gonadotropina, gonadotrofina *(OMS)*; **human chorionic** — **(HCG)** gonadotropina coriónica humana, *(esp. pharm)* gonadotrofina coriónica humana

gonococcus *n (pl* **-ci)** gonococo

gonorrhea *n* gonorrea

good *adj (comp* **better**; *super* **best)** bueno; *n* bien *m*; **for your own** — por su propio bien

good-looking *adj* bien parecido, guapo *(fam)*

goosebumps *n* piel *f or* carne *f* de ga-

llina
goserelin *n* goserelina
got *pret de* get
gotten *pp de* get
gout *n* gota
gouty *adj* gotoso
gown *n* bata
grade *n* (*degree*) grado; **low-grade**
(*fever, infection*) leve, (*tumor*) de
bajo grado; **high-grade** (*tumor*) de
alto grado
gradual *adj* gradual
gradually *adv* gradualmente
graduated *adj* graduado
graft *n* injerto; **bone** — injerto
óseo; **coronary artery bypass** — injerto
coronario, cirugía de revascularización
coronaria; **skin** — injerto
cutáneo; *vt* injertar, colocar un injerto
grain *n* (*pharm*) unidad *f* de peso
equivalente a 0,0648 gramos;
(*food*) grano, cereal *m*
gram *n* gramo
Gram-negative *adj* Gram negativo
Gram-positive *adj* Gram positivo
grandchild *n* (*pl* -children) nieto -ta
mf
granddaughter *n* nieta
grandfather *n* abuelo
grandiose *adj* grandioso
grandmother *n* abuela
grandparent *n* abuelo -la *mf*; *npl*
abuelos
grandson *n* nieto
granulation *n* granulación *f*
granule *n* gránulo
granulocyte *n* granulocito
granuloma *n* granuloma *m*; **pyogenic**
— granuloma piógeno
grapefruit *n* toronja, pomelo (*esp.
Esp*)
graph *n* gráfica *or* gráfico
grasp *vt* agarrar
grass *n* hierba; (*fam*) marihuana, mariguana
(*Mex*), hierba (*fam*), mota
(*Mex, CA; fam*)
gratification *n* gratificación *f*
grave *adj* grave
gray *adj* gris; *n* (*radiology*) gray *m*
grayish *adj* grisáceo
graze *vt* rozar
grease *n* grasa

greasy *adj* (*comp* -ier; *super* -iest)
graso, grasoso, grasiento (*Esp*)
great-grandchild *n* (*pl* -children)
bisnieto -ta *mf*
great-granddaughter *n* bisnieta
great-grandfather *n* bisabuelo
great-grandmother *n* bisabuela
great-grandparent *n* bisabuelo -la
mf; *npl* bisabuelos
great-grandson *n* bisnieto
green *adj* verde; (*fruit*) verde, no maduro
greenish *adj* verdoso
greens *npl* verduras
grew *pret de* grow
grief *n* duelo, pena, lamento, dolor *m*
emocional por una pérdida, (*due to
death*) luto
grill *vt* asar a la parrilla, asar
grind *vt* (*pret & pp* ground) (*a pill,
etc.*) triturar (*form*), moler; (*one's
teeth*) rechinar (*los dientes*)
grip *n* prensión *f*; — **strength** fuerza
de prensión; *vt* (*pret & pp* **gripped**;
ger **gripping**) agarrar, apretar
griseofulvin *n* griseofulvina
groan *n* gemido; *vi* gemir
groggy *adj* mareado, débil (*debido a
una droga, falta de sueño, etc.*)
groin *n* ingle *f*
group *adj* de grupo, grupal; *n* grupo;
age — grupo de edad; **peer** — grupo
de iguales, grupo de pares, personas
de la misma edad y aproximadamente
el mismo estatus social
que comparten los mismos intereses
y creencias y que influyen uno en el
otro; **support** — grupo de apoyo
grow *vi* (*pret* grew; *pp* grown) crecer;
to — **old** envejecer(se); **to** —
out of (a habit) quitarse(le) (a uno)
con el tiempo, perder con la edad;
She will grow out of it..Se le quitará
con el tiempo..Lo perderá con
la edad; **to** — **up** crecer; **when you
grow up**..cuando crezcas...**when
you are grown up**..cuando seas
grande
growl *vi* (*one's stomach*) gruñir, rugir
grown *pp de* grow
grown-up (*fam*) *adj* adulto
grownup (*fam*) *n* adulto -ta *mf*

growth n crecimiento; (*on body*) lesión f, sobrecrecimiento de la piel; — **spurt** estirón m

grunt n gruñido; vi gruñir

G-tube (*fam*) **gastrostomy tube**. *V.* **tube**.

guaifenesin n guaifenesina

guard n protector m; **mouth** — protector bucal; **shin** — espinillera, canillera (*CA, SA*)

guardian n (*legal*) tutor -ra mf

guidance n orientación f, guía, consejo

guideline n pauta, norma, guía

guilt n culpa; **feelings of** — sentimientos de culpa

guinea pig n cobayo or cobaya m

gum n goma; (*anat*) encía; **chewing** — chicle m, goma de mascar

gumma n goma m

gun n pistola; (*rifle*) fusil m

gurgle n gorgoteo

gurney n camilla

gut n intestino, tripa (*fam, frec. pl*)

gymnasium n gimnasio

gymnastics n gimnasia

gynecologic, gynecological adj ginecológico

gynecologist n ginecólogo -ga mf, médico -ca mf especialista en el aparato reproductor femenino

gynecology n ginecología, estudio del aparato reproductor femenino

H

HAART abbr **highly active antiretroviral therapy**. *V.* **therapy**.

habit n hábito, costumbre f; **bad** — vicio, mal hábito; **eating habits** hábitos alimenticios, hábitos de comer (*fam*)

habit-forming adj que crea hábito

habitual adj habitual

habituation n habituación f

had pret & pp de **have**

hair n pelo, (*head*) cabello, (*body*) vello; **axillary** — vello axilar; **body** — vello corporal, vello; **facial** — vello facial; **gray** — cana; — **remover** depilatorio (*form*), crema o aerosol m para quitar el vello (*esp. de las piernas*); **ingrown** — pelo encarnado; **pubic** — vello púbico

hairbrush n cepillo (para el pelo)

haircut n corte m de pelo; **to get a** — cortarse el pelo

haircutter n peluquero -ra mf, barbero

hairline n (línea de) nacimiento del pelo, perfil m del cuero cabelludo; **receding** — retroceso de la línea de nacimiento del pelo, entradas (*fam*)

hairspray n laca (*para el cabello, en aerosol*)

hairy adj peludo

half adj medio; **Take a half pill every morning**..Tome media pastilla todas las mañanas; — **brother** medio hermano; — **sister** media hermana; adv medio; **half asleep**..medio dormido; n (*pl* **halves**) mitad f

half-life n vida media, semivida

halfway house n (*US*) casa de rehabilitación (*esp. para drogadictos y*

alcohólicos después de tratamiento y antes de volver a la sociedad)
halitosis *n* halitosis *f*, mal aliento
hallucination *n* alucinación *f*
hallucinogen *n* alucinógeno
hallux valgus *n* hallux valgus *m*
hallux varus *n* hallux varus *m*
hallway *n* pasillo, corredor *m*
halo *n* halo *m*
haloperidol *n* haloperidol *m*
halves *pl de* **half**
ham *n* jamón *m*; (*muscle*) corva
hamartoma *n* hamartoma *m*
hammertoe *n* dedo (del pie) en martillo
hamstring *n* tendón *m* de la corva
hand *n* mano *f*
handgun *n* pistola
handheld *adj* manual, de mano
handicap *n* (*ant*) *V*. **disability**.
handicapped *adj* (*ant*) *V*. **disabled**.
handkerchief *n* pañuelo
hand lens *n* lupa, lente *m&f* de aumento
handout *n* folleto (con consejos médicos)
hand sanitizer *n* gel antiséptico para manos
handwriting *n* escritura, letra
hang *vt* (*pret & pp* **hanged** *o* **hung**) (*by the neck*) ahorcar; **to — oneself** ahorcarse; *vi* colgar
hangnail *n* padrastro (*en el dedo*)
hangover *n* resaca, cruda (*Mex*), goma (*CA*); **to have a —** tener una resaca *or* cruda, estar crudo (*Mex*), estar de goma
hantavirus *n* hantavirus *m*
happiness *n* felicidad *f*
happy *adj* feliz, contento
harassment acoso; **sexual —** acoso sexual
hard *adj* duro; **— of hearing** duro de oído, que no oye bien
harden *vt, vi* endurecer(se); **hardened arteries** (*fam*) arterias ateroscleróticas, arterias cuyas paredes han sido endurecidas por el colesterol elevado y otros factores
hardening *n* endurecimiento; **— of the arteries** aterosclerosis *f* (*form*), endurecimiento de las arterias
hard hat *n* casco de seguridad

harelip *n* (*vulg*) labio leporino
harm *n* daño; *vt* dañar, hacer daño
harmful *adj* nocivo, dañino
harmless *adj* inofensivo, que no hace daño
harsh *adj* áspero
hashish *n* hachís *m*
hat *n* sombrero
hate *n* odio; *vt* odiar
have *vt* (*pret & pp* **had**) tener; **You have herpes**..Ud. tiene herpes.
hawk *vi* **to — up** (*fam*) expectorar (*form*), desgarrar (*fam*)
hawthorn *n* (*bot*) espino
hay fever *n* fiebre *f* del heno, alergia al polen
hazard *n* peligro, riesgo
hazardous *adj* peligroso, riesgoso
HBV *abbr* **hepatitis B virus**. *V*. **virus**.
HCG *abbr* **human chorionic gonadotropin**. *V*. **gonadotropin**.
HCV *abbr* **hepatitis C virus**. *V*. **virus**.
HDL *abbr* **high density lipoprotein**. *V*. **lipoprotein**.
head *n* cabeza; (*of an abscess*) parte blanca donde hay pus; (*of a bed*) cabecera; (*of a family*) jefe -fa *mf*, cabeza (*de una familia*); **to come to a —** (*an abscess*) madurar (*un absceso*)
headache *n* cefalea (*form*), dolor *m* de cabeza; **cluster —** cefalea en racimos; **migraine —** migraña, jaqueca; **tension —** cefalea de tensión *or* tensional; **vascular —** cefalea vascular
headgear *n* sombrero, prenda que sirve para cubrir o proteger la cabeza; (*orthodontics*) aparato extraoral
headrest *n* reposacabezas *m*
heal *vt, vi* curar(se), sanar; **The wound is healed**..La herida está curada..La herida ha sanado.
healer *n* persona que cura, curandero -ra *mf*, sanador -ra *mf*; **faith —** curandero, sanador; **folk** o **traditional —** curandero, sanador
healing *n* curación *f*, (el) curar; (*wound*) cicatrización *f*; **the art of healing**..el arte de curar..**Steroids can retard healing**..Los esteroides

pueden retardar la cicatrización; **faith** — curanderismo; **folk** — *o* **traditional** — medicina popular *or* tradicional, curanderismo

health *n* salud *f*, sanidad *f* (*esp. Esp*); — **care** *V.* **health care**; — **club** gimnasio, club *m* de salud (*Ang*); — **enthusiast** naturista; — **resort** balneario, spa *m*; **mental** — salud mental; **occupational** — salud laboral *or* ocupacional; **women's** — salud de la mujer

health care *n* cuidado médico, atención médica, asistencia médica, asistencia sanitaria (*esp. Esp, SA*); **You should get more involved in your own health care**..Debería participar más en su propio cuidado médico; **access to** — — acceso a la atención médica (asistencia sanitaria); — — **delivery** prestación *f* de asistencia médica (asistencia sanitaria); **home** — — atención domiciliaria; **quality** — — atención médica de calidad

healthful *adj* saludable

healthy *adj* (*comp* -**ier**; *super* -**iest**) sano, saludable

hear *vt, vi* (*pret & pp* **heard**) oír

hearing *n* (*sense*) audición *f* (*form*), oído; **How's your hearing?**..¿Cómo está escuchando?..¿Cómo está oyendo? — **aid** audífono

heart *n* corazón *m*

heartbeat *n* latido del corazón

heartburn *n* acidez *f* (estomacal), agruras (*esp. Mex*), ardor *m* del estómago (que se siente en el pecho)

heart-healthy *adj* cardiosaludable

heat *n* calor *m*; **body** — calor corporal; *vt* (*también* **to** — **up**) calentar

heater *n* calefactor *m*

heating *n* calefacción *f*

heating pad *n* almohadilla eléctrica, cojín eléctrico (*esp. Mex*)

heat rash *n* sudamina, sarpullido, salpullido (*esp. Mex*), erupción *f* por calor, erupción por sudar en exceso durante tiempos de calor

heatstroke *n* insolación *f*, golpe *m* de calor

heat wave *n* ola de calor

heaviness *n* pesadez *f*

heavy *adj* (*comp* -**ier**; *super* -**iest**) pesado; — **drinker** persona que bebe mucho; — **smoker** persona que fuma mucho

heavyset *adj* robusto

heel *n* talón *m*; (*of the hand*) talón (de la mano); (*of the sole of a shoe*) tacón *m*; **high-heeled** de tacón alto; **low-heeled** de tacón bajo

height *n* altura; (*of a person*) estatura, altura, talla

held *pret & pp de* **hold**

helical *adj* helicoidal

helium *n* helio

helix *n* hélice *f*; **double** — doble hélice

hellebore *n* (*bot*) eléboro

helmet *n* casco

help *interj* ¡Auxilio!, ¡Socorro!; *n* ayuda, auxilio; *vt, vi* ayudar

hemangioma *n* hemangioma *m*; **cavernous** — hemangioma cavernoso

hematocele *n* hematocele *m*

hematocrit *n* hematocrito

hematologist *n* hematólogo -ga *mf*, médico -ca *mf* especialista en la sangre y sus enfermedades, especialista *mf* de la sangre (*fam*)

hematology *n* hematología, estudio de la sangre y sus enfermedades

hematoma *n* hematoma *m*; **subdural** — hematoma subdural

hemiplegia *n* hemiplejía *o* hemiplejia

hemisphere *n* hemisferio

hemlock *n* (*bot*) cicuta

hemochromatosis *n* hemocromatosis *f*

hemodialysis *n* hemodiálisis *f*

hemoglobin *n* hemoglobina; **glycosylated** — hemoglobina glucosilada *or* glicosilada

hemoglobinuria *n* hemoglobinuria; **paroxysmal nocturnal** — hemoglobinuria paroxística nocturna

hemolysis *n* hemólisis *f*

hemolytic *adj* hemolítico; **beta-hemolytic** beta-hemolítico

hemophilia *n* hemofilia

hemophiliac *n* hemofílico -ca *mf*

hemorrhage *n* hemorragia, sangrado (*fam*); **subarachnoid** — hemorragia subaracnoidea

hemorrhagic *adj* hemorrágico

hemorrhoid *n* hemorroide *f*, almorrana

hemorrhoidectomy *n* (*pl* -mies) hemorroidectomía

hemosiderosis *n* hemosiderosis *f*

henna *n* (*bot*) henna, alheña (*Esp*)

heparin *n* heparina; **low-molecular-weight** — heparina de bajo peso molecular

hepatic *adj* hepático

hepatitis *n* hepatitis *f*; — **A (B, C, etc.)** hepatitis A (B, C, etc.)

hepatologist *n* hepatólogo -ga *mf*, médico -ca *mf* especialista en el hígado y sus enfermedades, especialista *mf* del hígado (*fam*)

hepatology *n* hepatología, estudio del hígado y sus enfermedades

hepatoma *n* hepatoma *m*

hepatorenal *adj* hepatorrenal

herb *n* (*medical*) planta medicinal, hierba

herbal *adj* herbario, herbal

herbalism *n* herbolaria, fitoterapia

herbalist *n* herbolista *mf*, yerbero -ra *mf*, herbolario -ria *mf*, persona que utiliza hierbas para curar

herbicide *n* herbicida *m*

hereditary *adj* hereditario

heredity *n* herencia

heritable *adj* hereditario

hermaphrodite *adj & n* hermafrodita *mf*

hermaphroditism *n* hermafroditismo

hernia *n* hernia; **femoral** — hernia crural; **hiatal** — hernia hiatal; **incarcerated** — hernia incarcerada; **incisional** — eventración *f*, hernia incisional; **inguinal** — hernia inguinal; **reducible** — hernia reductible, hernia reducible (*esp. Esp*); **strangulated** — hernia estrangulada; **umbilical** — hernia umbilical

herniorrhaphy *n* (*pl* -phies) herniorrafia

heroin *n* heroína

herpangina *n* herpangina

herpes *n* herpes *m*; — **simplex** herpes simple; — **zoster** herpes zoster, culebrilla (*fam*), zona *m* (*fam*); **labial** — herpes labial, calentura (*Esp,*

frec. pl), fuego, erupción en los labios (*debida al herpes*)

herpesvirus *n* (*pl* -ruses) herpesvirus *m*; **human** — **6, human** — **8, etc.** herpesvirus humano 6, herpesvirus humano 8, etc.

herpetic *adj* herpético

heterosexual *adj & n* heterosexual *mf*

hiccup *n* hipo; **to have the hiccups** tener hipo; *vi* (*pret & pp* -cuped *o* -cupped; *ger* -cuping *o* -cupping) hipar, tener hipo

hickey *n* chupón *m*, chupete *m*, chupetón *m*, marca roja en la piel producida por un beso fuerte

hidradenitis suppurativa *n* hidradenitis supurativa (*form*), golondrino, inflamación *f* de las glándulas sudoríparas de la axila

high *adj* alto, elevado; (*fam, on drugs*) drogado; **Your cholesterol is high.**.Su colesterol está alto (elevado).

high-dose *adj* a altas dosis

higher (*comp de* high) *adj* (*physically*) más alto, más arriba; (*numerically*) superior a (*form*), por encima de, arriba de (*Amer*); **higher on my back**..más arriba en mi espalda; **higher than 100**..superior a 100.. por encima de 100..arriba de 100

high-pitched *adj* agudo, de tono alto

hike *n* caminata

hiking *n* senderismo

hip *n* cadera

hipbone *n* hueso de la cadera

Hippocratic Oath *n* Juramento Hipocrático

hirsute *adj* hirsuto, velludo, peludo (*fam*)

hirsutism *n* hirsutismo

histamine *n* histamina

histidine *n* histidina

histiocytosis *n* histiocitosis *f*; — **X** histiocitosis X

histology *n* histología

histoplasmosis *n* histoplasmosis *f*

history *n* (*pl* -ries) (*medical*) historia, historia clínica, información médica obtenida al entrevistar al paciente y al revisar los antecedentes médicos; antecedentes *mpl*; **family** — antecedentes familiares;

health — historia de salud; — **and physical** historia clínica, historia clínica y examen físico; — **of** (*cancer, trauma, etc.*) antecedentes de (*cáncer, traumatismo, etc.*); **natural** — (*of a disease*) evolución *f* natural; **past medical** — antecedentes médicos

histrionic *adj* histriónico

hit *vt* (*pret & pp* hit; *ger* hitting) golpear, pegar

HIV *abbr* **human immunodeficiency virus.** *V.* **virus.**

hive *n* roncha, habón *m*; *npl* urticaria (*form*), ronchas

HLTV *abbr* **human T-lymphotrophic virus.** *V.* **virus.**

HMO *abbr* **health maintenance organization.** *V.* **organization.**

hoarse *adj* ronco; **to be** — tener la voz ronca

hoarseness *n* ronquera

hobby *n* (*pl* -bies) pasatiempo

hold *vt* (*pret & pp* held) **to** — **one's breath** contener la respiración, aguantar la respiración (*fam*)

hole *n* perforación *f*, hueco, agujero

holistic *adj* holístico, integral

hollow *adj & n* hueco; — **of the hand** hueco de la mano

Holter monitor *n* Holter *m*, monitor ambulatorio del ritmo cardíaco

home *adj* domiciliario, casero; — **care** atención domiciliaria; — **remedy** remedio casero; *n* casa, hogar, domicilio; **You can go home**.. Puede regresar a la casa; **at** — en casa; **convalescent** — casa de reposo, residencia que ofrece cuidado de convalecencia; **rest** — casa de reposo, asilo *or* residencia de ancianos

homebound *adj* incapaz de abandonar la casa

homeless *adj* sin hogar

homemaker *n* ama de casa

homeopath *n* homeópata *mf*

homeopathic *adj* homeopático

homeopathy *n* homeopatía, sistema curativo en que se administra dosis pequeñas de sustancias que en dosis más grandes podrían causar o agravar la misma enfermedad que

se pretende de curar

homesick *adj* nostálgico; **to be** — sentir nostalgia (del hogar), tener morriña (*Esp*)

homesickness *n* nostalgia (del hogar), morriña (*Esp*)

homophobia *n* homofobia

homophobic *adj* homofóbico

homosexual *adj & n* homosexual *mf*

honey *n* miel *f* (de abeja)

hooked *adj* (*fam, on drugs*) adicto

hookworm *n* anquilostoma *m*

hop *n* salto; *vi* (*pret & pp* hopped; *ger* hopping) saltar; **Hop on one foot**..Salte en un pie.

hope *n* esperanza; **to lose** — perder la esperanza, desesperarse; *vt, vi* esperar; **to** — **for** esperar, tener esperanzas de

hopeless *adj* desesperado, sin esperanza

hops *n* (*bot*) lúpulo

horizontal *adj* horizontal

hormonal *adj* hormonal

hormone *n* hormona; **adrenocorticotropic** — **(ACTH)** corticotropina *or* corticotrofina; **antidiuretic** — vasopresina, hormona antidiurética; **bovine growth** — hormona de(l) crecimiento bovina; **follicle-stimulating** — **(FSH)** hormona folículo estimulante, folitropina; **gonadotropin-releasing** — **(GnRH)** hormona liberadora de gonadotropinas; **growth** — **(GH)** hormona de(l) crecimiento, somatotropina; **luteinizing** — **(LH)** hormona luteinizante; **parathyroid** — **(PTH)** hormona paratiroidea; **thyroid** — hormona tiroidea; **thyroid-stimulating** — **(TSH)** tirotropina *or* tirotrofina, hormona estimulante de la tiroides

hornet *n* avispón *m*

horsefly *n* (*pl* -flies) tábano

horsetail *n* (*bot*) cola de caballo

hose *n* (*tube*) manguera

hose *npl* (*stockings*) medias; **support** — medias elásticas, medias de compresión *or* compresivas

hospice *n* atención domiciliaria para pacientes terminales

hospital *adj* hospitalario; *n* hospital

m; **community** — hospital comunitario; **county** — (*US*) hospital del condado; **general** — hospital general; **mental** — hospital psiquiátrico; **private** — hospital privado; **public** — hospital público; **teaching** — hospital de enseñanza; **Veteran's Administration (VA)** — (*US*) hospital de veteranos

hospitalist *n* médico -ca *mf* especializado en atender pacientes hospitalizados

hospitalization *n* hospitalización *f*

hospitalize *vt* hospitalizar, internar (en un hospital); **Have you ever been hospitalized before?**..¿Ha sido hospitalizado alguna vez?

hostile *adj* hostil

hostility *n* hostilidad *f*

hot *adj* (*comp* **hotter**; *super* **hottest**) caliente; (*to the taste*) picante; **to be** — tener calor; (*the weather*) hacer calor; **to feel** — sentir calor; **Do you feel hot all the time?**..¿Siente calor todo el tiempo?

hot flash *n* sofoco, bochorno (*esp. Mex*), sensación repentina de calor que suelen sufrir las mujeres durante la menopausia

hot flush (*form*) *V.* **hot flash**.

hot sauce *n* salsa picante

hot springs *npl* aguas termales

hot tub *n* baño de agua caliente (*grande, frecuentemente al aire libre, con fines recreativos o terapéuticos*)

hot-water bottle *n* bolsa de agua caliente

hour *n* hora; **office hours** horario de consulta; **visiting hours** horario de visita

housebound *adj* incapaz de abandonar la casa

house call *n* visita domiciliaria, visita a domicilio

housecleaner *n* persona que limpia casas

housefly *n* (*pl* **-flies**) mosca doméstica

housewife *n* (*pl* **-wives**) ama de casa

HPV *abbr* **human papillomavirus**. *V.* **papillomavirus**.

HSV *abbr* **herpes simplex virus**. *V.*

virus.

hug *n* abrazo; *vt* (*pret & pp* **hugged**; *ger* **hugging**) abrazar

hum *n* (*buzz or ringing*) zumbido; *vt, vi* (*pret & pp* **hummed**; *ger* **humming**) (*a tune, etc.*) canturrear

human *adj* humano; — **being** ser humano; *n* humano

humanitarian *adj* humanitario

humerus *n* (*pl* **-ri**) húmero

humid *adj* húmedo

humidifier *n* humidificador *m*, aparato para aumentar la humedad del aire

humidify *vt* (*pret & pp* **-fied**) humidificar, humedecer

humidity *n* humedad *f*

humor *n* (*anat., etc.*) humor *m*; **aqueous** — humor acuoso; **sense of** — sentido del humor; **vitreous** — humor vítreo

hump *n* (*on the back*) joroba

humpback *n* joroba

humpbacked *adj* jorobado

hunchback *n* (*person*) jorobado -da *mf*; (*hump*) joroba

hung *pret & pp de* **hang**

hunger *n* hambre *f*

hungover *adj* **to be** — tener una resaca, tener una cruda (*Mex*), estar crudo (*Mex*), estar de goma (*CA*)

hungry *adj* **to be** — tener hambre; **Are you hungry?**..¿Tiene hambre?

hurricane *n* huracán *m*

hurt *vt* (*pret & pp* **hurt**) (*to cause pain*) doler, causar dolor; (*to injure*) lastimar, herir; (*to harm*) hacer daño; **This won't hurt you**.. Esto no le va a doler...**I'm not going to hurt you**..No voy a causarle dolor...**Did you hurt your finger?** ..¿Se lastimó el dedo?...**Eating oranges won't hurt you**..Comer naranjas no le hará daño; **to** — **oneself** *o* **to get** — lastimarse; **Did you hurt yourself?**..¿Se lastimó? *vi* doler, sentir dolor; **Where does it hurt?**..¿Dónde le duele?...**Do you hurt all over?**..¿Le duele todo?...**Tell me if it hurts**..Dígame si le duele..Dígame si siente dolor.

husband *n* esposo, marido

hyaluronic acid *n* ácido hialurónico

hydatid *adj* hidatídico
hydatidiform *adj (obst)* hidatiforme
hydralazine *n* hidralazina
hydrangea *n (bot)* hortensia
hydrate *n* hidrato; *vt* hidratar
hydrocarbon *n* hidrocarburo
hydrocele *n* hidrocele *m*
hydrocephalus *n* hidrocefalia; **normal pressure —** hidrocefalia normotensiva
hydrochloric acid *n* ácido clorhídrico
hydrochloride *n* clorhidrato
hydrochlorothiazide *n* hidroclorotiazida
hydrocodone *n* hidrocodona
hydrocolloid *n* hidrocoloide *m*
hydrocortisone *n* hidrocortisona
hydrogel *n* hidrogel *m*
hydrogenated *adj* hidrogenado
hydrogen peroxide *n* peróxido de hidrógeno *(form)*, agua oxigenada
hydronephrosis *n* hidronefrosis *f*
hydrophobia *n* hidrofobia, terror *m* al agua *(esp. en rabiosos)*
hydroquinone *n* hidroquinona
hydrotherapy *n* hidroterapia, método curativo por medio del agua
hydroxide *n* hidróxido
hydroxychloroquine *n* hidroxicloroquina
hydroxyurea *n* hidroxiurea
hydroxyzine *n* hidroxicina, hidroxizina *(OMS)*
hygiene *n* higiene *f (form)*, aseo; **oral —** higiene *or* aseo bucal
hygienic *adj* higiénico
hygienist *n* higienista *mf*; **dental —** higienista dental
hymen *n* himen *m*; **imperforate —** himen imperforado, imperforación *f* de himen
hyoid bone *n* hioides *m*
hyper *(fam)* hiperactivo, acelerado *(fam)*
hyperactive *adj* hiperactivo
hyperactivity *n* hiperactividad *f*
hyperalimentation *n* hiperalimentación *f*
hyperbaric *adj* hiperbárico
hypercalcemia *n* hipercalcemia
hyperemesis gravidarum *n (obst)* hiperemesis gravídica, estado grave de náuseas y vómitos que aparece en etapas tempranas del embarazo
hyperglycemia *n* hiperglucemia
hyperhidrosis *n* hiperhidrosis *f*, sudoración excesiva principalmente de las manos y de los pies
hyperlipidemia *n* hiperlipemia, hiperlipidemia
hypermobile *adj* hipermóvil
hypernatremia *n* hipernatremia
hyperosmolar *adj* hiperosmolar
hyperparathyroid *adj* hiperparatiroideo
hyperparathyroidism *n* hiperparatiroidismo
hyperpigmentation *n* hiperpigmentación *f*
hyperplasia *n* hiperplasia; **benign prostatic —** hiperplasia prostática benigna; **congenital adrenal —** hiperplasia suprarrenal congénita
hyperprolactinemia *n* hiperprolactinemia
hypersensitive *adj* hipersensible
hypersensitivity *n* hipersensibilidad *f*
hypertension *n* hipertensión *f* arterial *(form)*, hipertensión, presión alta *(fam)*; **benign intracranial —** hipertensión intracraneal benigna; **essential —** hipertensión (arterial) esencial; **malignant —** hipertensión (arterial) maligna; **portal —** hipertensión portal; **pulmonary —** hipertensión pulmonar; **renovascular —** hipertensión renovascular; **white-coat —** hipertensión de bata blanca
hyperthermia *n* hipertermia
hyperthyroid *adj* hipertiroideo
hyperthyroidism *n* hipertiroidismo
hypertrophic *adj* hipertrófico
hypertrophy *n* hipertrofia
hyperuricemia *n* hiperuricemia
hyperventilate *vi* hiperventilar, respirar demasiado rápido
hyperventilation *n* hiperventilación *f*
hyphema *n* hipema *m*
hypnosis *n* hipnosis *f*
hypnotic *adj & n* hipnótico
hypnotism *n* hipnotismo
hypnotist *n* hipnotizador -ra *mf*

hypnotize vt hipnotizar
hypoallergenic adj hipoalergénico
hypocalcemia n hipocalcemia
hypochondriac n (ant) hipocondríaco -ca mf
hypochondriasis n (ant) hipocondría
hypodermic adj hipodérmico; n (ant, fam) inyección f
hypoglycemia n hipoglucemia
hypoglycemic adj (pertaining to hypoglycemia) hipoglucémico, (causing hypoglycemia) hipoglucemiante; — episode episodio de hipoglucemia; oral — agent hipoglucemiante m oral
hypokalemia n hipopotasemia
hyponatremia n hiponatremia
hypoparathyroid adj hipoparatiroideo
hypoparathyroidism n hipoparatiroidismo
hypopigmentation n hipopigmentación f
hypopituitarism n hipopituitarismo
hypospadias n hipospadias m
hypotension n hipotensión f; orthostatic — hipotensión ortostática
hypotensive adj hipotensor, hipotensivo
hypothalamus n hipotálamo
hypothermia n hipotermia
hypothyroid adj hipotiroideo
hypothyroidism n hipotiroidismo
hypovolemic adj hipovolémico
hysterectomy n (pl -mies) histerectomía; total abdominal — histerectomía total abdominal; vaginal — histerectomía vaginal
hysteria n (ant) histeria, crisis f de ansiedad, ansiedad severa
hysterical adj (ant) histérico, severamente ansioso, relativo a la ansiedad

I

ibandronate n ibandronato
ibuprofen n ibuprofeno, ibuprofen m
ICD abbr implantable cardioverter defibrillator. V. defibrillator.
ID V. identification.
ice n hielo; (fam, methamphetamine) metanfetamina; — chips pedacitos or trocitos de hielo; — pack bolsa de hielo; vt (an injury) aplicar hielo (a una herida)
ice cream n helado
ichthyosis n ictiosis f
ICU abbr intensive care unit. V. unit.
id n (psych) ello m, fuente f inconsciente de toda energía psíquica
I&D abbr incision and drainage. V. incision.
ideal adj ideal
identical adj idéntico
identification (ID) n identificación f
identify vt (pret & pp -fied) identificar; vi to — with (psych) identificarse con
identity n (pl -ties) identidad f; — crisis crisis f de identidad
idiopathic adj idiopático, sin causa conocida
ileal adj ileal
ileitis n ileítis f

ileostomy *n* (*pl* **-mies**) ileostomía
ileum *n* íleon *m*
ileus *n* íleo
iliac *adj* ilíaco, iliaco (*esp. Mex*)
ilium *n* ilion *m*, hueso ilíaco, hueso iliaco (*esp. Mex*), hueso de la cadera (*fam*)
ill *adj* enfermo
illiteracy *n* analfabetismo
illiterate *adj* analfabeto
illness *n* enfermedad *f*, mal *m*; **mental** — enfermedad mental; **occupational** — enfermedad profesional; **present** — enfermedad actual
IM *V.* intramuscular.
image *n* imagen *f*; **body** — imagen corporal, esquema corporal
imaging *n* imagenología, uso de técnicas radiológicas para obtener imágenes del interior del cuerpo; **diagnostic** — diagnóstico por imagen; **— study** estudio por imagen, estudio radiológico; **magnetic resonance — (MRI)** resonancia magnética nuclear (RMN), resonancia magnética (*fam*); **open MRI** resonancia magnética abierta
imbalance *n* desequilibrio; **chemical** — desequilibrio químico
imipenem *n* imipenem *m*
imipramine *n* imipramina
imiquimod *n* imiquimod *m*
immature *adj* inmaduro
immaturity *n* inmadurez *f*
immediate *adj* inmediato
immediately *adv* inmediatamente
immersion *n* inmersión *f*
immobile *adj* inmóvil
immobilization *n* inmovilización *f*
immobilize *vt* inmovilizar
immobilizer *n* inmovilizador *m*; **shoulder** — inmovilizador de hombro
immune *adj* inmune, inmunitario, inmunológico; **immune to..**inmune a; **— reconstitution** reconstitución inmunológica
immunity *n* inmunidad *f*; **immunity to..**inmunidad frente a, inmunidad contra (*esp. Amer*); **herd** — inmunidad colectiva, inmunidad de grupo *or* rebaño
immunization *n* inmunización *f*;

(*vaccination*) vacunación *f*
immunize *vt* inmunizar, (*vaccinate*) vacunar
immunizing *adj* inmunizante, inmunizador
immunocompetent *adj* inmunocompetente
immunocompromised *adj* inmunocomprometido, inmunodeprimido
immunodeficiency *n* inmunodeficiencia; **common variable** — inmunodeficiencia variable común
immunodeficient *adj* inmunodeficiente
immunodepressed *adj* inmunodeprimido
immunodepression *n* inmunodepresión *f*
immunodepressive *adj* inmunodepresor
immunoglobulin *n* inmunoglobulina (*endógena*)
immunologic, immunological *adj* inmunológico
immunologist *n* inmunólogo -ga *mf*, médico -ca *mf* especialista en el sistema inmune y sus enfermedades
immunology *n* inmunología, estudio del sistema inmune y sus enfermedades
immunosuppressant *n* inmunosupresor *m*
immunosuppressed *adj* inmunosuprimido
immunosuppression *n* inmunosupresión *f*
immunosuppressive *adj* inmunosupresor
immunotherapy *n* inmunoterapia
impact *n* impacto; **low** — bajo impacto
impacted *adj* (*dent*) retenido, impactado, incluido (*Esp*), que no ha podido salir porque no tiene espacio
impaction *n* impactación *f*; **cerumen** — tapón de cerumen; **dental** — diente retenido *or* impactado, inclusión dentaria (*Esp*), diente que no ha podido salir porque no tiene espacio; **fecal** — impactación fecal
impair *vt* dañar, perjudicar
impairment *n* trastorno, deficiencia, pérdida; **hearing** — pérdida de la

audición

impediment *n* **speech** — (*ant*) trastorno del lenguaje

imperforate *adj* imperforado

impetigo *n* impétigo

impingement *n* pinzamiento

implant *n* implante *m*; **breast** — prótesis mamaria, implante mamario; **silicone** — implante de silicona; *vt* implantar

implantation *n* implantación *f*

impossible *adj* imposible

impotence *n* (*ant, sexual*) disfunción *f* eréctil, impotencia (sexual)

impotent *adj* (*ant*) impotente, con disfunción eréctil

impression *n* (*dent, etc.*) impresión *f*

improve *vt* mejorar; *vi* mejorarse, (*patient*) recuperarse

improvement *n* mejoría

impulse *n* impulso

impulsive *adj* impulsivo

impurity *n* (*pl* -**ties**) impureza

inability *n* incapacidad *f*

inactive *adj* inactivo

inactivity *n* inactividad *f*

inadequate *adj* (*not suited*) inadecuado, (*insufficient*) insuficiente

inappropriate *adj* inadecuado, inapropiado, indebido

inbred *adj* procreado por uniones entre la misma familia extendida

incapable *adj* incapaz

incapacitating *adj* incapacitante

incarcerated *adj* incarcerado

incest *n* incesto

incestuous *adj* incestuoso

inch *n* pulgada, 2,54 centímetros

incidence *n* incidencia

incidentaloma *n* incidentaloma *m* (*Ang*)

incision *n* incisión *f*, herida; — **and drainage (I&D)** incisión y drenaje

incisor *n* incisivo

incoherent *adj* incoherente

incompatible *adj* incompatible

incompetence *n* incompetencia, insuficiencia; **cervical** — incompetencia *or* insuficiencia cervical

incompetent *adj* incompetente

incomplete *adj* incompleto

incontinence *n* incontinencia; **fecal** — incontinencia fecal, incapacidad

f para retener las heces; **overflow** — incontinencia por rebosamiento; **stress** — incontinencia de esfuerzo; **urge** — incontinencia (urinaria) de urgencia; **urinary** — incontinencia urinaria, incapacidad *f* para retener la orina

incontinent *adj* incontinente, (*of urine*) incapaz de retener la orina, (*of stool*) incapaz de retener las heces

increase *n* aumento; *vt* aumentar, incrementar (*form*); **I'm going to increase your furosemide**..Voy a aumentar la dosis de su furosemida; *vi* aumentar(se)

incubator *n* (*ped*) incubadora

incurable *adj* incurable

independent *adj* independiente; **to become** — independizarse

index *n* (*pl* **indexes** *o* **indices**) índice *m*; **body mass** — **(BMI)** índice de masa corporal (IMC)

indication *n* indicación *f*

indices *pl de* index

indifference *n* indiferencia

indigestion *n* indigestión *f*

indinavir *n* indinavir *m*

indistinct *adj* indistinto

individual *n* individuo (*inv*)

indomethacin *n* indometacina

induce *vt* inducir, provocar

induced *adj* inducido; **exercise-induced** inducido por (el) ejercicio

induction *n* inducción *f*

ineffective *adj* ineficaz

inert *adj* inerte

infancy *n* primer período de la vida, lactancia

infant *n* lactante *mf* (*form*), bebé *mf*, recién nacido -da *mf*, nene -na *mf* (*fam*)

infantile *adj* infantil, relativo a los bebés

infarct *n* infarto

infarction *n* infarto, acción *f* y efecto de un infarto; **acute myocardial** — infarto agudo de miocardio

infect *vt* infectar

infected *adj* infectado; — **with** infectado por *or* con; **to become infected** infectarse

infection *n* infección *f*; **fungal** —

infección fúngica (*form*), infección micótica (*form*), infección por hongos; **upper respiratory tract** — infección respiratoria alta; **urinary tract** — **(UTI)** infección urinaria, infección del tracto urinario (ITU), infección de orina (*fam*); **yeast** — infección por levaduras (*form*), infección por hongos (*fam*)

infectious *adj* infeccioso

inferior *adj* (*anat*) inferior

infertile *adj* infértil, estéril

infertility *n* infertilidad *f*, esterilidad *f*

infest *vt* infestar

infestation *n* infestación *f*

infested *adj* infestado; — **with** infestado de; **to get o become** — **with** infestarse con *or* de

infiltrate *vt, vi* infiltrar(se)

infiltrating *adj* infiltrante

infiltration *n* infiltración *f*

infirmary *n* (*pl* **-ries**) (*ant*) enfermería, local *m or* dependencia para enfermos

inflame *vt* inflamar; **to become inflamed** inflamarse

inflammable *adj* inflamable

inflammation *n* inflamación *f*

inflammatory *adj* inflamatorio

infliximab *n* infliximab *m*

influenza *n* gripe *f*, influenza; **Asian** — gripe asiática; **avian** — gripe aviar; **swine** — influenza porcina

information *n* información *f*

infraorbital *adj* infraorbitario

infrared *adj* & *n* infrarrojo

infuse *vt* infundir

infusion *n* infusión *f*

ingest *vt* ingerir

ingestion *n* ingestión *f*

ingredient *n* ingrediente *m*; **active** — principio activo

ingrown *adj* encarnada, enterrada (*Mex, CA, Carib*)

inguinal *adj* inguinal

INH *V.* **isoniazid.**

inhalation *n* inhalación *f*; **smoke** — inhalación de humo

inhale *vt, vi* inhalar; **inhaled steroids** esteroides inhalados

inhaler *n* inhalador *m*, aerosol *m*; **dry powder** — inhalador de polvo seco; **metered dose** — inhalador *or* aerosol dosificador; **nasal** — inhalador nasal

inherit *vt* heredar

inhibit *vt* inhibir

inhibited *adj* inhibido, cohibido

inhibition *n* inhibición *f*, cohibición *f*

inhibitor *n* inhibidor *m*; **angiotensin converting enzyme** — inhibidor de la enzima convertidora de la angiotensina, inhibidor de conversión de la angiotensina; **cholinesterase** — inhibidor de la colinesterasa; **fusion** — inhibidor de fusión; **integrase** — inhibidor de la integrasa; **mono-amine oxidase** — inhibidor de la monoaminooxidasa; **non-nucleoside reverse transcriptase** — inhibidor no nucleósido de la transcriptasa inversa, inhibidor no nucleósido de la transcriptasa reversa (*esp. Amer*); **nucleoside reverse transcriptase** — inhibidor nucleósido de la transcriptasa inversa, inhibidor nucleósido de la transcriptasa reversa (*esp. Amer*); **protease** — inhibidor de la proteasa; **proton pump** — inhibidor de la bomba de protones; **selective serotonin reuptake** — inhibidor selectivo de la recaptación de serotonina

initial *adj* inicial; *npl* iniciales *fpl*; *vi* poner iniciales; **Initial here please** ..Ponga sus iniciales aquí por favor.

inject *vt* inyectar, (*oneself*) inyectarse

injectable *adj* inyectable

injection *n* inyección *f*; **The nurse will give you an injection**..La enfermera le va a poner una inyección.

injure *vt* herir, lastimar, lesionar

injury *n* (*pl* **-ries**) herida, lesión *f*, traumatismo; **spinal cord** — lesión de la médula espinal; **sports** — lesión deportiva

inlay *n* (*dent*) incrustación *f*

innards *npl* (*fam*) vísceras, tripas (*fam*), entrañas

inner *adj* interno, interior

inoculate *vt* inocular

inoculation *n* inoculación *f*

inoperable *adj* inoperable

inorganic *adj* inorgánico
inpatient *n* paciente hospitalizado
INR *abbr* **international normalized ratio**. *V.* **ratio**.
insane *adj* loco
insanity *n* locura
insect *n* insecto
insecticide *n* insecticida *m*
insecure *adj* inseguro
insecurity *n* inseguridad *f*
inseminate *vt* inseminar
insemination *n* inseminación *f*; **artificial** — inseminación artificial
insert *vt* introducir, insertar
inside *adj* interior, interno; *adv* dentro, adentro; *n* interior *m*, parte *f* de adentro; *prep* dentro de; **inside your body**..dentro de su cuerpo
insight *n* (*psych*) autoconocimiento, conocimiento de uno mismo
in situ, in situ, localizado
insole *n* plantilla (*del zapato*)
insoluble *adj* insoluble
insomnia *n* insomnio
instep *n* empeine *m* (*del pie*)
instinct *n* instinto
institution *n* asilo; residencia; hospital *m*; establecimiento que ofrece cuidados prolongados (*esp. para pacientes psiquiátricos*); **mental** — hospital psiquiátrico
instrument *n* instrumento
insufficiency *n* insuficiencia; **adrenal** —, **aortic** —, **venous** —, etc. insuficiencia suprarrenal, insuficiencia aórtica, insuficiencia venosa, etc.
insufficient *adj* insuficiente
insulin *n* insulina; **human** — insulina humana; — **aspart** insulina aspart, insulina asparta (*OMS*); — **glargine** insulina glargina; — **lispro** insulina lispro; **intermediate-acting** — insulina de acción intermedia; **lente** — insulina lenta, forma de insulina de acción intermedia; **long-acting** — insulina de acción prolongada; **NPH** — insulina NPH; **rapid-acting** — insulina de acción rápida; **rapid-acting** — **analog** análogo de insulina de acción rápida, insulina ultrarrápida; **recombinant** — insulina recombi-

nante; **regular** — insulina regular; **to take** — ponerse insulina; **ultralente** — insulina ultralenta, forma de insulina de acción prolongada
insulinoma *n* insulinoma *m*
insurance *n* seguro; **health care** *o* **medical** — seguro médico; **private** — seguro privado
insured *adj* asegurado, con seguro (médico)
intact *adj* intacto
intake *n* consumo, ingesta; **tolerable daily** — ingesta diaria admisible
intellectual *adj* intelectual
intellectualize *vi* intelectualizar
intelligence *n* inteligencia; — **quotient (IQ)** cociente *m or* coeficiente *m* intelectual (CI)
intelligent *adj* inteligente
intense *adj* intenso, fuerte
intensify *vt* (*pret & pp* **-fied**) intensificar
intensity *n* (*pl* **-ties**) intensidad *f*
intensive *adj* intensivo
intensivist *n* intensivista *mf*
interact *vi* interactuar
interaction *n* interacción *f*; **drug** — interacción de drogas
intercostal *adj* intercostal
intercourse *n* coito (*form*), relaciones sexuales, relaciones (*fam*), (el) acto sexual; **When was the last time you had intercourse?**...¿Cuándo fue la última vez que tuvo relaciones (sexuales)?...**during intercourse**..durante el acto sexual..durante las relaciones sexuales
interfere *vi* interferir
interferon *n* interferón *m*; **alpha** —, **beta** —, etc. interferón alfa, interferón beta, etc.; **pegylated** — interferón pegilado
interior *adj & n* interior *m*
intermediate *adj* intermedio
intermittent *adj* intermitente
intern *n* interno -na *mf*
internal *adj* interno
internalize *vt* interiorizar
internet *n* internet *m&f*; **on the** — en internet
internist *n* internista *mf*
interpersonal *adj* interpersonal
interpret *vt, vi* interpretar

interpreter *n* intérprete *mf*
interrogate *vt* (*a pacemaker*) interrogar (*un marcapasos*)
interruption *n* interrupción *f*
interstitial *adj* intersticial
intertrochanteric *adj* intertrocantéreo, intertrocantérico (*esp. Amer*)
interval *n* intervalo
intervention *n* intervención *f*
interventional *adj* intervencionista
interventricular *adj* interventricular
intervertebral *adj* intervertebral
intestinal *adj* intestinal
intestine *n* intestino, tripa (*fam, frec. pl*); **large** — intestino grueso; **small** — intestino delgado
intimacy *n* intimidad *f*
intimate *adj* íntimo
intolerance *n* intolerancia; **lactose** — intolerancia a la lactosa
intolerant *adj* intolerante; — **of** *o* **to** intolerante a
intoxication *n* intoxicación *f*
intraabdominal *adj* intraabdominal
intraarticular *adj* intraarticular
intracranial *adj* intracraneal, intracraneano
intractable *adj* resistente al tratamiento
intradermal *adj* intradérmico
intramuscular (IM) *adj* intramuscular (IM)
intranasal *adj* intranasal
intraocular *adj* intraocular
intraoperative *adj* intraoperatorio
intrauterine *adj* intrauterino
intravenous (IV) *adj* intravenoso (IV)
intrinsic *adj* intrínseco
introspection *n* introspección *f*
introvert *n* introvertido -da *mf*
introverted *adj* introvertido
intubate *vt* intubar
intubation *n* intubación *f*
intussusception *n* invaginación *f* intestinal
in utero, en el útero
invade *vt* invadir
invalid *n* (*ant*) **disabled person.** *V.* **person.**
invasive *adj* (*procedure, surgery*) invasivo, (*disease*) invasor; **minimally** — mínimamente invasivo

investigational *adj* (*medication, etc.*) en investigación
invisible *adj* invisible
in vitro, in vitro, en el laboratorio
involuntary *adj* involuntario
involvement *n* participación *f*; (*path*) afección *f*; **lymph node** — afección ganglionar
iodide *n* yoduro
iodine *n* yodo
iodized *adj* yodado
ion *n* ion *m*
iontophoresis *n* iontoforesis *f*
ipecac *n* ipecacuana; **syrup of** — jarabe *m* de ipecacuana
ipratropium bromide *n* bromuro de ipratropio
IQ *abbr* **intelligence quotient.** *V.* **intelligence.**
irbesartan *n* irbesartán *m*
iris *n* (*pl* **irides** *o* **irises**) iris *m*
iritis *n* iritis *f*
iron *n* hierro
irradiate *vt* irradiar, tratar con radiación
irradiation *n* irradiación *f*; **food** — irradiación de alimentos
irregular *adj* irregular
irreversible *adj* irreversible
irrigate *vt* irrigar
irrigation *n* irrigación *f*
irritability *n* irritabilidad *f*
irritable *adj* irritable
irritant *n* irritante *m*, agente *m* irritante
irritate *vt* irritar; **to become irritated** irritarse
irritating *adj* (*person, event, etc.*) molesto; (*substance*) irritante
irritation *n* irritación *f*
ischemia *n* isquemia
ischemic *adj* isquémico
islet *n* islote *m*; **pancreatic islets** islotes pancreáticos
isolate *vt* aislar
isolation *n* aislamiento; **protective** — aislamiento protector; **respiratory** — aislamiento respiratorio; **reverse** — aislamiento inverso
isoleucine *n* isoleucina
isometric *adj* isométrico
isoniazid (INH) *n* isoniazida *or* isoniacida

isopropyl alcohol *n* alcohol isopropílico

isosorbide *n* isosorbida

isotope *n* isótopo

isotretinoin *n* isotretinoína

isradipine *n* isradipino, isradipina (*esp. SA*)

itch *n* comezón *f*, picazón *f*; *vi* picar, sentir *or* tener comezón (picazón); **Where does it itch?**..¿Dónde le pica?...**Does your arm itch?**..¿Le pica el brazo?...**Do you itch?**.. ¿Siente comezón (picazón)?..¿Tiene comezón (picazón)?

itching, itchiness *n* comezón *f*, picazón *f*

ITP *abbr* **idiopathic thrombocytopenic purpura**. *V.* **purpura**.

itraconazole *n* itraconazol *m*

IUD *abbr* **intrauterine device**. *V.* **device**.

IV *V.* **intravenous**.

ivermectin *n* ivermectina

IVF *abbr* **in vitro fertilization**. *V.* **fertilization**.

IVP *abbr* **intravenous pyelogram**. *V.* **pyelogram**.

J

jabbing *adj* (*pain*) punzante

jack *vi* **to — off** (*vulg*) masturbarse, hacerse la paja (*vulg*), hacerse una paja (*Esp, vulg*)

jacket *n* chaqueta, chamarra (*esp. Mex*)

jaundice *n* ictericia (*form*), coloración amarilla de la piel y los ojos

jaw *n* mandíbula, quijada (*fam*); **lower — ** maxilar *m* inferior (*form*), mandíbula (*fam*); **upper — ** maxilar *m* superior (*form*)

jawbone *n* mandíbula (*form*), quijada

Jehovah's Witness *npl* Testigo de Jehová

jejunal *adj* yeyunal

jejunum *n* yeyuno

jellyfish *n* (*pl* **-fish** *o* **-fishes**) medusa, aguamala

jet lag *n* jet lag *m* (*Ang*), desequilibrio del ritmo circadiano producido por viajar en avión a través de los husos horarios

jigger *n* nigua

job *n* trabajo, empleo

jock itch *n* (*fam*) tiña inguinal *or* crural

jockstrap *n* (*fam*) suspensorio

jog *vi* (*pret & pp* **jogged**; *ger* **jogging**) trotar

jogging *n* (el) trotar, jogging (*Ang*)

join (*two objects*) *vt* juntar; *vi* unirse

joint *adj* articular; **— pain** dolor *m* articular, dolor en la coyuntura; *n* articulación *f*, coyuntura (*fam*); (*fam, marijuana cigarette*) cigarrillo de marihuana, porro (*fam*); **knee —, ankle —,** etc. articulación de la rodilla, articulación del tobillo, etc.

judo *n* judo

jugular *adj* yugular

juice *n* jugo, zumo; **fruit — ** jugo de fruta; **orange — ** jugo de naranja

junction *n* unión *f*; **atrioventricular — ** unión auriculoventricular

junk food *n* comida chatarra, comida

basura (*esp. Esp*)
junkie *n* (*fam*) adicto -ta *mf* a la heroína

just in case, por si acaso
juvenile *adj* juvenil

K

karate *n* karate *m*
karyotype *n* cariotipo
kava *n* (*bot*) kava *m&f*
keloid *n* queloide *m*
kelp *n* tipo de alga marina
keratectomy *n* (*pl* **-mies**) queratectomía; **photorefractive —** (**PRK**); queratectomía fotorrefractiva
keratin *n* queratina
keratitis *n* queratitis *f*
keratomileusis *n* queratomileusis *f*; **laser-assisted in situ —** (**LASIK**) queratomileusis in situ asistida con láser
keratosis *n* queratosis *f*; **actinic —** queratosis actínica; **seborrheic —** queratosis seborreica
keratotomy *n* (*pl* **-mies**) queratotomía; **radial —** queratotomía radial
kernicterus *n* kernicterus *m*
ketamine *n* ketamina
ketoacidosis *n* cetoacidosis *f*
ketoconazole *n* ketoconazol *m*
ketone *n* cetona
ketoprofen *n* ketoprofeno
ketorolac *n* ketorolaco
ketotic *adj* cetónico
kick *n* patada; *vt, vi* dar una patada, dar patadas, patear; (*fam, a habit*) dejar (*un vicio*); **Can you feel your baby kicking?**..¿Siente que le patea su bebé?..¿Siente las patadas de su bebé?

kid *n* (*fam*) niño -ña *mf*
kidney *n* riñón *m*
kill *vt* matar
kilo (*fam*) *V.* **kilogram.**
kilocalorie *n* kilocaloría
kilogram *n* kilogramo, kilo (*fam*)
kin *n* parientes *mf*, familia; **next of —** parientes más cercanos
kind *adj* amable
kinesiology *n* cinesiología
kinetic *adj* cinético
kiss *n* beso; *vt* besar
kissing bug *n* chinche hocicona *or* besucona (*Mex*), chinche (*fam*), vinchuca (*esp. SA*)
kit *n* botiquín *m*; **first-aid —** botiquín de primeros auxilios
knee *n* rodilla; **back of the —** corva
knee bend *n* sentadilla
kneecap *n* rótula
kneepad *n* rodillera
knife *n* (*pl* **knives**) cuchillo
knife-like *adj* (*pain*) punzante
knit *vi* (*pret & pp* **knitted**); *ger* **knitting**) (*ortho*) soldar
knives *pl de* **knife**
knock-kneed *adj* con las rodillas hacia adentro,
knot *n* nudo
knuckle *n* nudillo
kwashiorkor *n* kwashiorkor *m*
kyphoscoliosis *n* cifoescoliosis *f*
kyphosis *n* cifosis *f*

L

lab (*fam*) *V.* **laboratory**.
label *n* etiqueta
labetolol *n* labetolol *m*
labia *pl de* **labium**
labial *adj* labial
labium *n* (*pl* **labia**) labio (genital)
labor *n* trabajo de parto; **Labor and Delivery** sala de partos; — **pain** dolor *m* del parto; **to be in** — estar en trabajo de parto, estar de parto (*esp. Esp*); **to go into** — entrar en trabajo de parto, ponerse de parto (*Esp*)
laboratory *n* (*pl* **-ries**) laboratorio; **catheterization** — laboratorio de cateterismo
labyrinth *n* (*anat*) laberinto
labyrinthitis *n* laberintitis *f*
laced with, adulterado con
lacerate *vt* lacerar, desgarrar
laceration *n* laceración *f*, desgarro
lachrymal *V.* **lacrimal**.
lack *n* falta, carencia; *vt* faltar(le) (a uno), carecer de
lacrimal *adj* lagrimal
lactase *n* lactasa
lactate *n* lactato; *vi* producir y secretar leche
lactation *n* producción *f* y secreción *f* de leche; (*period of milk production*) lactancia
lactic *adj* láctico; — **acid** ácido láctico; — **dehydrogenase** deshidrogenasa láctica
lactobacillus *n* lactobacilo
lactose *n* lactosa; — **intolerance** intolerancia a la lactosa
lactulose *n* lactulosa
lag *n* retraso, intervalo; *vi* (*pret & pp* **lagged**; *ger* **lagging**) retrasarse
laid up, (*fam*) incapacitado temporalmente
lain *pp de* **lie**
Lamaze method, Lamaze technique *n* método Lamaze
lamb *n* (*meat*) carne *f* de cordero, cordero; **lamb's wool** *n* lana de oveja
lame *adj* cojo
laminaria *n* laminaria
laminectomy *n* (*pl* **-mies**) laminectomía
lamivudine *n* lamivudina
lamotrigine *n* lamotrigina
lamp *n* lámpara; **heat** — lámpara de calor; **Wood's** — lámpara de Wood
lance *vt* abrir con bisturí (*un absceso*)
lancet *n* lanceta; **diabetic** — lanceta para diabéticos
language *n* (*referring to structure and development*) lenguaje *m*; **body** — lenguaje corporal
lanolin *n* lanolina
lansoprazole *n* lansoprazol *m*
lanugo *n* lanugo, vello de los bebés
lap *n* (*of a person*) regazo
laparoscope *n* laparoscopio
laparoscopic *adj* laparoscópico
laparoscopy *n* (*pl* **-pies**) laparoscopia, laparoscopía (*Amer, esp. spoken*)
laparotomy *n* (*pl* **-mies**) laparotomía; **exploratory** — laparotomía exploradora
lard *n* manteca de cerdo
large *adj* grande
larva migrans *n* larva migrans *f*; **cutaneous** — — larva migrans cutánea; **visceral** — — larva migrans visceral
laryngeal *adj* laríngeo
laryngectomy *n* (*pl* **-mies**) laringectomía
larynges *pl de* **larynx**
laryngitis *n* laringitis *f*
laryngoplasty *n* (*pl* **-ties**) laringoplastia
laryngoscope *n* laringoscopio
laryngoscopy *n* (*pl* **-pies**) laringoscopia, laringoscopía (*Amer, esp. spoken*)
larynx *n* (*pl* **larynges** *o* **larynxes**) laringe *f*

laser *n* láser *m*

LASIK *abbr* **laser-assisted in situ keratomileusis.** *V.* **keratomileusis.**

last *adj* último; **your last period**..su último período menstrual..su última regla; *vi* durar; **How long did the pain last?**..¿Cuánto tiempo le duró el dolor?...**These pills should last a month**..Estas pastillas deben durar un mes.

last rites *npl* extremaunción *f*, santos óleos

latanoprost *n* latanoprost *m*

late *adj* (*development, etc.*) tardío; *adv* tarde

latent *adj* latente

lateral *adj* (*anat*) lateral, externo

latex *n* látex *m*

latrine *n* letrina

laugh *n* risa; *vi* reír(se)

laughing gas *n* gas *m* hilarante

lavage *n* lavado; **bronchoalveolar —** lavado broncoalveolar; **gastric —** lavado gástrico; **peritoneal —** lavado peritoneal

lawsuit *n* demanda, pleito (legal)

lax *adj* laxo, flojo

laxative *adj* & *n* laxante *m*; **bulk —** laxante incrementador del bolo intestinal, laxante que aumenta el volumen de las heces

lay *adj* lego (*form*), no profesional; **— opinion** opinión lega (no profesional)

lay *pret de* **lie**

layer *n* capa; **layers of the skin**..capas de la piel

lazy eye *n* ambliopía (*form*), ojo vago, debilidad *f* de la vista sin lesión orgánica del ojo

lb *V.* **pound.**

L-carnitine *n* L-carnitina

LDL *abbr* **low density lipoprotein.** *V.* **lipoprotein.**

lead *n* (*ECG*) derivación *f*

lead *n* (*metal*) plomo

lean *adj* (*person*) flaco, delgado; (*meat*) magro, sin grasa; *vi* inclinarse; **Lean forward**..Inclínese hacia adelante.

learn *vt, vi* aprender; **to learn to read**..aprender a leer

learning *n* aprendizaje *m*

least (*super de* **little** *and* **few**) *adj* menor; **the least harm**..el menor daño; *adv* menor; **the least invasive option**..la opción menos invasiva

lecithin *n* lecitina

leech *n* sanguijuela

LEEP *abbr* **loop electrosurgical excision procedure.** *V.* **procedure.**

left *adj* izquierdo; *n* (*left-hand side*) izquierda

left-handed *adj* zurdo

leg *n* pierna

legume *n* legumbre *f*

leiomyoma *n* leiomioma *m*; **uterine — leiomioma uterino**

leiomyosarcoma *n* leiomiosarcoma *m*

leishmaniasis *n* leishmaniasis *f*; **cutaneous —** leishmaniasis cutánea; **mucocutaneous —** leishmaniasis mucocutánea, espundia; **visceral — leishmaniasis visceral**

leisure *n* ocio

lemon *n* limón *m*

lemon eucalyptus oil *n* aceite *m* de eucalipto limón

lemon flower *n* (*bot*) azahar *m*

length *n* longitud *f*, largo

lens *n* lente *m&f*; (*of the eye*) cristalino; **bifocal —** lente bifocal; **(hard, soft) contact —** lente de contacto (rígido, blando); **progressive —** lente progresivo; **trifocal —** lente trifocal

lentigo *n* lentigo

lepromatous *adj* lepromatoso

leprosy *n* lepra, enfermedad *f* de Hansen; **borderline —** lepra dimorfa; **lepromatous —** lepra lepromatosa; **tuberculoid —** lepra tuberculoide

leptospirosis *n* leptospirosis *f*

lesbian *adj* lesbiana; *n* lesbiana, mujer *f* homosexual

lesion *n* lesión *f*

less (*comp de* **little** *or* **few**) *adj* menos; **less pills**..menos pastillas; **— than** menos de; **less than there was before**..menos de lo que había antes; *adv* menos; **— than** menos que; **less than usual**..menos que de costumbre

letdown *n* (*obst*) reflejo de eyección

de la leche (*form*), bajada de la leche
lethal *adj* letal
lethargic *adj* letárgico
lethargy *n* letargo, somnolencia
leucine *n* leucina
leukemia *n* leucemia; **acute lymphoblastic** *o* **lymphocytic** — leucemia linfoblástica *or* linfocítica aguda; **acute myeloid** *o* **myelogenous** — leucemia mieloide *or* mielógena aguda; **chronic lymphocytic** — leucemia linfocítica *or* linfática crónica; **chronic myelogenous** *o* **myeloid** — leucemia mieloide crónica
leukocyte *n* leucocito, glóbulo blanco
leukoencephalopathy *n* leucoencefalopatía; **progressive multifocal** — leucoencefalopatía multifocal progresiva
leukoplakia *n* leucoplasia, manchas blancas en la boca o lengua
leuprolide *n* leuprorelina
levamisol *n* levamisol *m*
level *adj* plano; **How far can you walk on level ground before you get short of breath?**..¿Qué distancia puede caminar en superficie plana antes de que le falte el aire? *n* nivel *m*, concentración *f*; **blood sugar** — nivel *or* concentración de azúcar en la sangre; — **of consciousness** nivel de conciencia *or* consciencia; **socioeconomic** — nivel socioeconómico; **therapeutic** — nivel terapéutico
levodopa *n* levodopa
levofloxacin *n* levofloxacino, levofloxacina (*esp. Amer*)
levonorgestrel *n* levonorgestrel *m*
levothyroxine *n* levotiroxina
LGV *V.* **lymphogranuloma venereum.**
LH *abbr* **luteinizing hormone.** *V.* **hormone.**
libido *n* libido *f*, deseo sexual
lice *pl de* **louse**
lichen planus *n* liquen plano
lick *vt* lamer
licorice *n* regaliz *m*
lid *V.* **eyelid.**
lidocaine *n* lidocaína

lie *vi* (*pret* **lay;** *pp* **lain;** *ger* **lying**) **to** — **down** acostarse; **Lie down please**..Acuéstese por favor.
life *n* vida; **for** — de por vida; **for the rest of your** — por el resto de su vida; — **expectancy** expectativa *or* esperanza de vida; **life-saving** que salva vidas, que puede salvar la vida; **life-threatening** que amenaza la vida, potencialmente mortal; **sex** — vida sexual; **social** — vida social
lifelong *adj* de por vida
lifestyle *n* estilo de vida
lifetime *n* vida, toda una vida, período de tiempo vivido
lift *n* **heel** — cojín *m* que se coloca en el calzado para levantar el talón; *vt* levantar; **to** — **weights** levantar pesas
ligament *n* ligamento
ligation *n* ligadura; **tubal** — ligadura de trompas
light *adj* (*case of disease*) leve; (*touch*) suave, ligero; (*weight*) ligero, liviano; — **sleeper** persona que tiene un sueño ligero, persona de sueño ligero; *n* luz *f*
lightening *n* (*obst*) descenso del feto al final del embarazo
lightheaded *adj* mareado; **to be** *o* **feel** — sentir que se va a desmayar, estar mareado
lightheadedness *n* sensación *f* de desmayo, mareo
lightning *n* relámpago
limb *n* extremidad *f* (*form*), miembro
limber *adj* ágil
lime *n* (*fruit*) lima
limit *n* límite *m*; **Your potassium is below normal limits**..Su potasio está por debajo de los límites normales; **lower** — **of normal** límite inferior normal; **upper** — **of normal** límite superior normal; **Your sugar is over twice the upper limit of normal**..Su azúcar está dos veces por encima del límite superior normal; **within normal limits** dentro de límites normales; *vt* limitar
limp *adj* flácido, relajado; *n* cojera; **She has a limp**..Cojea..Ella está

cojeando; *vi* cojear
lindane *n* lindano
linden *n* (*bot*) tila
line *n* línea; (*catheter*) catéter; **arterial** — catéter arterial; **central** — catéter (venoso) central; **first** —, **second** —, etc. de primera línea, de segunda línea, etc.; **gum** — (*dent*) linea de la(s) encía(s); *vt* (*the intestine, etc.*) revestir, tapizar, recubrir; **to** — **up** alinear; *vi* **to** — **up** alinearse
lineage *n* estirpe *f*; **myeloid** —, **B** —, etc. estirpe mieloide, estirpe B, etc.
linezolid *n* linezolid *m*
liniment *n* linimento
lining *n* (*of the stomach, etc.*) recubrimiento, revestimiento
linked *adj* ligado, asociado; — **to cancer** asociado con (el) cáncer; **sex-linked** ligado al sexo; **X-linked** ligado al cromosoma X
linoleic acid *n* ácido linoleico
lip *n* labio; **lower** — labio inferior; **upper** — labio superior
lipase *n* lipasa
lipid *n* lípido
lipodystrophy *n* lipodistrofia
lipoma *n* lipoma *m*
lipoprotein *n* lipoproteína; **high density** — (**HDL**) lipoproteína de alta densidad; **low density** — (**LDL**) lipoproteína de baja densidad; **very low density** — (**VLDL**) lipoproteína de muy baja densidad
liposarcoma *n* liposarcoma *m*
liposuction *n* liposucción *f*
lipread *vi* (*pret & pp* **-read**) leer los labios
lipreading *n* (el) leer los labios
liquid *adj & n* líquido
lisinopril *n* lisinopril *m*
lisp *n* ceceo; *vi* cecear
listen *vi* escuchar; **I'm going to listen to your lungs**..Voy a escucharle los pulmones.
listeriosis *n* listeriosis *f*
listless *adj* apático (*debido a cansancio, enfermedad, etc.*)
liter *n* litro
lithium *n* litio
lithotripsy *n* litotricia, litotripsia (*esp. Mex*); **extracorporeal shock wave** — litotricia *or* litotripsia extracorpórea por ondas de choque
litter *n* (*stretcher*) camilla
little *adj* (*comp* **less**; *super* **least**) (*size*) pequeño, chico; (*quantity, degree*) poco; (*fam, sibling*) menor; **a little tumor**..un tumor pequeño...**a little milk**..un poco de leche...**little time**..poco tiempo... **my little brother**..mi hermano menor; *n* poco; — **by** — poco a poco
live *adj* (*virus, vaccine*) vivo; *vi* vivir; **to** — **with** vivir con, convivir con; **to live with smokers**..convivir con fumadores...**to live with diabetes**..vivir con (la) diabetes.. convivir con (la) diabetes...**Who do you live with?**..¿Con quién vive Ud.?
liver *n* hígado
liver spot *n* mancha parduzca en la piel que suele aparecerse en la vejez
lives *pl de* **life**
living will *n* testamento vital
load *n* carga; **viral** — carga viral
loaded *adj* (*fam*) borracho, intoxicado
lobar *adj* lobar, lobular
lobe *n* lóbulo
lobectomy *n* (*pl* **-mies**) lobectomía
lobelia *n* (*bot*) lobelia
lobotomy *n* (*pl* **-mies**) lobotomía
local *adj* local
localization *n* localización *f*
localized *adj* localizado
lochia *n* loquios, líquido que sale del útero después del parto
lockjaw *n* (*fam, ant*) tétanos
lodge *vi* alojarse; **The bullet lodged near the aorta**..La bala se alojó cerca de la aorta.
log *n* libreta, cuaderno, diario; **glucose** — libreta de autocontrol (*del diabético*), cuaderno *or* diario en que se anotan los niveles del azúcar
loner *n* solitario -ria *mf*
long *adj* largo; *adv* **How long have you had diabetes?**..¿Hace cuánto que tiene diabetes?...**How long were you unconscious?**..¿Por cuánto tiempo estuvo inconsciente?
long-acting *adj* de acción prolongada

longevity *n* longevidad *f*

long-term *adj* a largo plazo

look *vi* mirar; **Look upward**..Mire hacia arriba; **to — like** verse, parecerse; **What did this sore look like when you first noticed it?**..¿Cómo se veía esta herida cuando la vió por primera vez?...**She looks like her mother**..Se parece a su madre.

loop *n* (*IUD*) lazo; (*of bowel*) asa (*intestinal*)

loose *adj* suelto, flojo

loosen *vt* aflojar, soltar; **Loosen your belt please**..Afloje el cinturón por favor.

loperamide *n* loperamida

lopinavir *n* lopinavir *m*

loratadine *n* loratadina

lorazepam *n* lorazepam *m*

lordosis *n* lordosis *f*

losartan *n* losartán *m*

lose *vt* (*pret & pp* lost) perder; **to — consciousness** perder el conocimiento, perder la conciencia; **to — one's voice** perder la voz; **to — weight** perder peso, bajar de peso

loss *n* pérdida; **hair —** caída del cabello; **hearing —** ensordecimiento, pérdida de audición; **weight —** pérdida de peso

lost *pret & pp de* lose

lot *n* (*pharm*) lote *m*; **a — (fam)** mucho; **Do you sleep a lot?**..¿Duerme mucho? **a — of (fam)** mucho(s); **a lot of milk**..mucha leche...**a lot of pimples**..muchos granos

lotion *n* crema, loción *f*; **hand —** crema para manos; **suntan —** protector *m* solar, crema bronceadora

louse *n* (*pl* lice) piojo; **body —** piojo del cuerpo; **crab —** ladilla; **head —** piojo de la cabeza; **pubic —** ladilla, piojo del pubis, piojo púbico

lovastatin *n* lovastatina

love *n* amor *m*; **in — with** enamorado de; **to fall in — with** enamorarse de; *vt, vi* querer, amar

loved one *n* ser amado

loving *adj* cariñoso, afectuoso

low *adj* bajo; **low in calories**..bajo en calorías...**Your potassium is low**.. Su potasio está bajo; **low-fat, low-sodium, etc.** bajo en grasa, bajo en

sodio, etc.

low-dose *adj* a bajas dosis

lower (*comp de* low) *adj* más bajo; (*anat*) inferior (*form*), bajo, de abajo; **— than** más bajo que; (*a number*) inferior a, por debajo de; **lower than before**..más bajo que antes ...**lower than 140**..inferior a 140 ..por debajo de 140; **the — part** la parte baja *or* de abajo; *vt* bajar; **You need to lower your cholesterol**..Necesita bajar el colesterol... **Lower your arm**..Baje el brazo.

low-pitched *adj* grave, de tono bajo

lozenge *n* pastilla para chupar

LSD *V.* lysergic acid diethylamide.

lubricant *adj & n* lubricante *m*

lubricate *vt* lubricar

lubrication *n* lubricación *f*

Ludwig's angina *n* angina de Ludwig

lukewarm *adj* tibio

lumbar *adj* lumbar

lump *n* nódulo (*form*), bola, bolita, bulto (*esp. Esp*), (*due to trauma, esp. about the head*) chichón *m*

lumpectomy *n* (*pl* -mies) lumpectomía

lumpy *adj* (*comp* -ier; *super* -iest) nodular (*form*), que tiene bolas (*fam*)

lunch *n* almuerzo, comida (*esp. Mex*), comida del mediodía; **to have —** almorzar, comer (*esp. Mex*), tomar la comida del mediodía

lung *n* pulmón *m*

lupus *n* lupus *m*; **discoid —** lupus (eritematoso) discoide; **systemic — erythematosus (SLE)** lupus eritematoso sistémico

luteal *adj* lúteo, luteínico

lye *n* lejía

lying (*ger de* lie) **— down** acostado

lymph *n* linfa

lymphadenitis *n* linfadenitis *f*

lymphangitis *n* linfangitis *f*

lymphatic *adj* linfático

lymphedema *n* linfedema *m*

lymphocyte *n* linfocito; **B —, CD4 —, etc.** linfocito B, linfocito CD4, etc.

lymphogranuloma venereum (LGV) *n* linfogranuloma venéreo

lymphoid *adj* linfoide
lymphoma *n* linfoma *m*; **B cell** — linfoma de células B; **mucosa-associated lymphoid tissue (MALT)** — linfoma MALT, linfoma del tejido linfoide asociado a mucosas; **non-Hodgkin's** — linfoma no Hodgkin, linfoma no hodgkiniano;

T cell — linfoma de células T
lyophilized *adj* liofilizado
lysergic acid diethylamide (LSD) *n* dietilamida del ácido lisérgico (LSD)
lysine *n* lisina
lysis *n* lisis *f*; — **of adhesions** lisis de adherencias

M

MAC *V.* **Mycobacterium avium complex**.
macerate *vt* macerar
macrobiotic *adj* macrobiótico
macular degeneration *n* degeneración *f* macular
mad *adj* (*comp* **madder**; *super* **maddest**) enojado, enfadado (*esp. Esp*); (*crazy*) loco; **to get** — enojarse, enfadarse (*esp. Esp*)
made *pret & pp de* **make**
maggot *n* cresa, larva de mosca
magnesium *n* magnesio; — **sulfate** sulfato magnésico (*form*), sulfato de magnesio
magnifying glass *n* lupa, lente *m&f* de aumento
maintain *vt* mantener
maintenance *n* mantenimiento; **methadone** — mantenimiento con metadona
major *adj* (*anat, surgery*) mayor
make *vt* (*pret & pp* **made**) **to** — **love** hacer el amor
makeup *n* maquillaje *m*, cosmético(s)
malabsorption *n* malabsorción *f*
malaise *n* malestar *m*
malaria *n* paludismo, malaria
malathion *n* malatión *m*

male *adj* masculino, macho (*inv*); *n* varón *m*, hombre *m*
malformation *n* malformación *f*, anomalía, deformidad *f*; **arteriovenous** — malformación arteriovenosa
malignancy *n* malignidad *f* (*form*), cáncer *m*
malignant *adj* maligno
malinger *vi* hacerse el enfermo (*para evitar el trabajo, obtener compensación, etc.*)
malleolus *n* maléolo
malnourished *adj* desnutrido
malnutrition *n* desnutrición *f*
malocclusion *n* maloclusión *f*
malpractice *n* negligencia médica
mammaplasty *n* (*pl* -ties) mamoplastia
mammary *adj* mamario
mammogram *n* mamografía (*estudio imagenológico*)
mammography *n* mamografía (*técnica imagenológica*); **digital** — mamografía digital
mammoplasty *V.* **mammaplasty**.
man *n* (*pl* **men**) hombre *m*
manage *vt* manejar
managed care *n* cuidado médico ges-

tionado con fines de contener costos

management n manejo; **pain** — manejo del dolor

mandible n mandíbula

maneuver n maniobra; **Heimlich** — maniobra de Heimlich; vt, vi maniobrar

manganese n manganeso

manhood n edad f viril; masculinidad f, virilidad f

mania n manía

manic adj maníaco

manic-depressive adj maníaco-depresivo

manicure n manicura

manifestation n manifestación f

manipulate vt manipular

manipulation n manipulación f

manipulative adj manipulador

manometry n manometría

manual adj manual

manubrium n manubrio

many adj (comp **more**; super **most**) muchos; **many times**..muchas veces

margarine n margarina

margin n margen m

marijuana n marihuana, mariguana (Mex), hierba (fam), mota (Mex, CA; fam)

marital adj marital, matrimonial

mark n marca

marker n marcador m

married adj casado

marrow n médula; **bone** — médula ósea

marshmallow n (bot) malvavisco

mascara n rímel m

masculine adj masculino

masculinity n masculinidad f

mash n (crushing injury) machucón m; vt machucar, apachurrar

mask n máscara, (for oxygen) mascarilla, (protective) careta; **surgical** — mascarilla quirúrgica, cubrebocas(s) m (Mex), barbijo (SA); vt (signs, symptoms) enmascarar

masochism n masoquismo

masochist n masoquista mf

mass n masa, tumor m; **bone** — masa ósea; **muscle** — masa muscular

massage n masaje m; **cardiac** — masaje cardíaco; **to give a** — dar un masaje, dar masaje (esp. Mex); vt masajear, sobar (Amer)

massive adj masivo

MAST V. military anti-shock trousers.

mastectomy n (pl -mies) mastectomía; **modified radical** — mastectomía radical modificada

mastitis n mastitis f

mastocytosis n mastocitosis f

mastoid adj mastoideo

mastoidectomy n (pl -mies) mastoidectomía

mastoiditis n mastoiditis f

masturbate vt, vi masturbar(se)

masturbation n masturbación f

match vt (blood, tissue) ser compatible con; **Your sister's tissue type matches your own**..El tipo de tejido de su hermana es compatible con el suyo.

material n material m

maternal adj materno; (motherly) maternal; — **grandfather** abuelo materno; — **instinct** instinto maternal

maternity n maternidad f

matrix n matriz f; **nail** — matriz ungueal

matter n materia, sustancia; **gray** — sustancia gris; **white** — sustancia blanca

mattress n colchón m

mature adj maduro; vi madurar

maturity n madurez f

maxilla n (pl -lae) maxilar m superior

maxillary adj maxilar

maxillofacial adj maxilofacial

maximal adj máximo

maximize vt maximizar

maximum adj & n (pl -mums) máximo

MDA V. methylene dioxyamphetamine.

MDMA V. methylene dioxymethamphetamine.

MD, M.D. V. Doctor of Medicine.

meal n comida; **Meals on Wheels** programa m para repartir comidas a domicilio a ancianos o descapacitados

mean *adj* (*stat*) medio; (*cruel*) cruel; *n* media, promedio
measles *n* sarampión *m*
measure *n* medida; **heroic measures** medidas heroicas; *vt* medir
measurement *n* medida
measuring tape *n* cinta métrica
meat *n* carne *f*; **organ meats** vísceras; **red** — carne roja
meatus *n* (*pl* **meatus**) meato
mebendazole *n* mebendazol *m*
mechanic *n* mecánico -ca *mf*
mechanical *adj* mecánico
mechanism *n* mecanismo; **defense** — mecanismo de defensa
meclizine *n* meclozina; [*Note: the* o *is not a misprint.*]
meconium *n* meconio
medial *adj* (*anat*) interno, medial
median *n* (*nerve*) mediano; *n* (*stat*) mediana; — **age** mediana de edad
mediastinal *adj* mediastínico
mediastinoscopy *n* mediastinoscopia, mediastinoscopía (*Amer, esp. spoken*)
mediastinum *n* mediastino
medic *n* miembro de un cuerpo militar de sanidad
medical *adj* médico; — **savings account** (*US*) cuenta de ahorro dedicada a los gastos médicos
medicate *vt* medicar
medicated *adj* (*shampoo, etc.*) medicado, medicinal
medication *n* medicamento
medicinal *adj* medicinal
medicine *n* (*field*) medicina; (*medication*) medicina, medicamento; **addiction** — medicina de la adicción *or* de las addiciones; **allergy** —, **ulcer** —, etc. antialérgico, antiulceroso, etc.; **alternative** — medicina alternativa; **evidence-based** — medicina basada en la evidencia; **family** — medicina de familia *or* familiar; **folk** — medicina popular *or* tradicional, curanderismo; **herbal** — fitoterapia; **internal** — medicina interna; — **dropper** gotero (*Amer*), cuentagotas *m*; **nuclear** — medicina nuclear; **numbing** — (*fam*) anestésico (local); **occupational** — medicina laboral *or* del

trabajo; **physical** — medicina física; **preventive** — medicina preventiva; **socialized** — medicina socializada; **sports** — medicina deportiva; **veterinary** — medicina veterinaria, veterinaria
medicine chest, medicine cabinet *n* botiquín *m*
medicine dropper *n* gotero
medicolegal *adj* medicolegal
meditate *vi* meditar
meditation *n* meditación *f*
medium *adj* mediano; *n* medio; **contrast** — medio de contraste, contraste *m* (*fam*)
medroxyprogesterone *n* medroxiprogesterona
medulla *n* (*pl* **-lae**) bulbo raquídeo; (*of the adrenal gland*) médula
medullary *adj* medular
mefloquine *n* mefloquina
megacolon *n* megacolon *m*
megadose *n* megadosis *f*
megestrol *n* megestrol *m*
meglumine *n* meglumina
melancholy *n* melancolía
melanin *n* melanina
melanoma *n* melanoma *m*
melarsoprol *n* melarsoprol *m*
melasma *n* melasma *m*, cloasma *m*, paño (*fam*), manchas en la cara que aparecen durante el embarazo
melatonin *n* melatonina
melphalan *n* melfalán *m*
member *n* (*limb*) extremidad *f* (*form*), miembro; (*fam, penis*) pene *m*, miembro *m* (*fam*)
membrane *n* membrana; **mucous** — membrana mucosa; **tympanic** — membrana timpánica
memory *n* (*pl* **-ries**) memoria; **long-term** — memoria a largo plazo; **short-term** — memoria a corto plazo
men *pl de* **man**
menarche *n* menarquia, menarca (*Amer*), primera menstruación
meninges *pl de* **meninx**
meningioma *n* meningioma *m*
meningitis *n* meningitis *f*
meningocele *n* meningocele *m*
meningococcal *adj* meningocócico
meningococcus *n* (*pl* **-ci**) meningo-

coco
meninx *n* (*pl* **meninges**) (*frec. pl*) meninge *f*
meniscal *adj* meniscal
meniscectomy *n* (*pl* **-mies**) meniscectomía
meniscus *n* (*pl* **-ci**) menisco; **torn —** rotura de menisco
menopausal *adj* menopáusico
menopause *n* menopausia
men's room *n* baño de hombres
menstrual *adj* menstrual
menstruate *vi* menstruar
menstruation *n* menstruación *f*
mental *adj* mental; (*pertaining to chin*) mentoniano
menthol *n* mentol *m*
meperidine *n* meperidina, petidina (*OMS*)
mercaptopurine *n* mercaptopurina
mercury *n* mercurio
mercy killing *n* eutanasia, muerte piadosa
mesalamine *n* mesalazina; [*Note: the z is not a misprint.*]
mescal *n* mezcal *m*
mescaline *n* mescalina
mesenteric *adj* mesentérico
mesentery *n* mesenterio
mesh *n* malla
mesothelioma *n* mesotelioma *m*
mesotherapy *n* mesoterapia
metabolic *adj* metabólico
metabolism *n* metabolismo; **basal —** metabolismo basal
metacarpal *adj* & *n* metacarpiano
metal *n* metal *m*; **heavy —** metal pesado
metallic *adj* metálico
metaproterenol *n* orciprenalina, metaproterenol *m*
metastasis *n* (*pl* **-ses**) metástasis *f*
metastasize *vi* metastatizar, diseminarse
metastatic *adj* metastásico
metatarsal *adj* & *n* metatarsiano
metaxalone *n* metaxalona
meter *n* metro; (*measuring device*) aparato medidor, medidor *m*; (**blood**) **glucose —** glucómetro, medidor *m* de glucosa, aparato para medir el azúcar en la sangre (*fam*); **square —** metro cuadrado

metformin *n* metformina
meth (*fam*) *V.* **methamphetamine.**
methacholine *n* metacolina
methadone *n* metadona
methamphetamine *n* metanfetamina
methane *n* metano
methanol *n* metanol *m*, alcohol metílico
methaqualone *n* metacualona
methicillin *n* meticilina
methimazole *n* metamizol *m*, metimazol *m*
methionine *n* metionina
methocarbamol *n* metocarbamol *m*
method *n* método
methotrexate *n* metotrexato
methyl alcohol *n* alcohol metílico, metanol *m*
methylcellulose *n* metilcelulosa
methyldopa *n* metildopa
methylene blue *n* azul *m* de metileno
methylene dioxyamphetamine (MDA) *n* metilendioxianfetamina (MDA), droga *or* píldora del amor (*fam*)
methylene dioxymethamphetamine (MDMA) *n* metilendioximetanfetamina (MDMA), éxtasis *m* (*fam*)
methylphenidate *n* metilfenidato
methysergide *n* metisergida
metoclopramide *n* metoclopramida
metolazone *n* metolazona
metoprolol *n* metoprolol *m*
metric system *n* sistema métrico
metronidazole *n* metronidazol *m*
mice *pl de* **mouse**
miconazole *n* miconazol *m*
microalbuminuria *n* microalbuminuria
microbe *n* microbio
microbial *adj* microbiano
microbiology *n* microbiología, estudio de los microbios
microgram *n* microgramo
micrometastasis *n* (*pl* **-ses**) micrometástasis
micronutrient *n* micronutriente *m*
microorganism *n* microorganismo, microbio
microscope *n* microscopio; **electron —** microscopio electrónico; **light —** microscopio de luz
microscopic *adj* microscópico

microscopy *n* microscopia *or* microscopía

microsurgery *n* microcirugía

microvascular *adj* microvascular

microwave *n* microondas [*Note: in Spanish the plural form is more common.*]

mid *adj* medio; **mid-cycle** medio ciclo

midbrain *n* mesencéfalo (*form*), cerebro medio

middle *adj* (*finger*) medio; *n* mitad *f*, medio; **the middle of your arm**..la mitad del brazo...**in the middle of your hand**..en medio de la mano

midget *n* (*ant*) enano -na *mf*

midlife *adj* de (la) mediana edad

midline *n* línea media (del cuerpo)

midodrine *n* midodrina

midwife *n* (*pl* **-wives**) partera, comadrona; **male —** comadrón *m*

migraine (*fam*) **migraine headache**. *V.* **headache**.

mild *adj* (*soap, etc.*) suave; (*illness*) leve

mildew *n* moho

milia *n* milia, puntitos blanquecinos que tienden a ocurrir en la cara

miliaria *n* miliaria, sarpullido (*fam*), salpullido (*esp. Mex, fam*)

miliary *adj* miliar

milk *n* leche *f*; **breast —** leche materna; **condensed —** leche condensada; **cow's —** leche de vaca; **evaporated —** leche evaporada; **goat's —** leche de cabra; **lactose-free —** leche sin lactosa; **low-fat —** leche baja en grasas; **— product** producto lácteo *or* de la leche; **non-fat —** leche descremada *or* desnatada; **pasteurized —** leche pasteurizada; **powdered —** leche en polvo; **raw —** leche cruda; **skim —** leche descremada *or* desnatada; **soy —** leche de soja; **whole —** leche entera

milk of magnesia *n* leche *f* de magnesia

milk thistle *n* (*bot*) cardo mariano

milky *adj* lechoso

millisecond *n* milisegundo

milligram *n* miligramo

milliliter *n* mililitro

millimeter *n* milímetro

mimic *vt* (*pret & pp* **-icked**; *ger* **-icking**) imitar

mind *n* mente *f*; **to lose one's —** perder la razón, volverse loco; *vt* (*obey*) obedecer, hacer(le) caso; **He doesn't mind me**..No me obedece..No me hace caso.

miner *n* minero -ra *mf*

mineral *adj & n* mineral *m*

minimal *adj* mínimo

minimize *vt* minimizar

minimum *adj & n* (*pl* **-mums**) mínimo

minocycline *n* minociclina

minor *adj* (*anat, surgery*) menor; *n* menor *mf* (de edad); **emancipated — menor emancipado**

minoxidil *n* minoxidil *m*

mint *n* (*bot*) menta

minute *n* minuto

miracle *n* milagro

mirror *n* espejo

mirtazapine *n* mirtazapina

miscarriage *n* aborto (espontáneo)

miscarry *vi* (*pret & pp* **-ried**) abortar (*sin intención*), sufrir un aborto

mischievous *adj* travieso

misery *n* miseria

miss *vt* (*work, an appointment, etc.*) faltar a; (*dose of medication*) no tomar, dejar de tomar; (*a loved one, etc.*) extrañar; **Did you miss work?**..¿Faltó al trabajo?...**Try not to miss this appointment**..Trate de no faltar a esta cita...**Don't miss a single dose of this medicine**..No deje de tomar una sola dosis de esta medicina...**Have you missed a period?**..¿Le ha faltado la regla?..¿No le ha venido la regla?...**Do you miss your husband?**..¿Extraña a su esposo?

missing (*ger of* **miss**) *adj* **Ten pills are missing**..Faltan diez pastillas.

mistreat *vt* maltratar

mistreatment *n* maltrato

mite *n* ácaro; **dust —** ácaro del polvo

mitral *adj* mitral

mittelschmerz *n* dolores pélvicos que aparecen con la ovulación

mix *vt* mezclar

mixed *adj* (*in medical nomenclature*) mixto

mixture n mezcla
moan n gemido; vi gemir
mobile adj móvil; mobile MRI unit ..unidad f móvil de RMN
mobility n movilidad f
mobilization n movilización f; passive — movilización pasiva
mobilize vt movilizar
moderate adj moderado
moderation n moderación f
modification n modificación f; behavior — modificación de (la) conducta
modified adj modificado
modifier n modificador m; biological response — modificador de la respuesta biológica
modify vt (pret & pp -fied) modificar
modulator n modulador m; selective estrogen receptor — modulador selectivo de los receptores estrogénicos or de estrógenos
moist adj húmedo
moisten vt humedecer, mojar un poco
moisture n humedad f
moisturize vt humedecer, (skin) hidratar
moisturizing adj hidratante, humectante (esp. Amer)
molar adj (dent, obst) molar; n molar m (form), muela
mold n (dent) molde m; (fungus) moho; vt moldear
mole n lunar m; (obst) mola; hidatidiform — mola hidatiforme
molecular adj molecular
molecule n molécula
molest vt molestar (sexualmente)
molluscum contagiosum n molusco contagioso
mom n mamá
mommy n (pl -mies) mami f, mamita
mometasone n mometasona
monitor n monitor m; blood pressure — tensiómetro (form), esfigmomanómetro (form), aparato para medir la presión (de la sangre) (fam); cardiac — monitor cardíaco; fetal heart — cardiotocógrafo (form), monitor fetal; (blood) glucose — glucómetro, medidor m de glucosa, aparato para medir el azúcar en la sangre (fam); Holter —

Holter m; vt monitorear (Amer), monitorizar (Esp), seguir
monitoring n monitoreo (Amer), monitorización f (Esp)
mono (fam) V. mononucleosis.
monoclonal adj monoclonal
monogamous adj monógamo
monogamy n monogamia
mononucleosis n mononucleosis f
monosodium glutamate (MSG) n glutamato monosódico
monounsaturated adj monoinsaturado
mons pubis n monte m de Venus
monster n monstruo
montelukast n montelukast m
month n mes m
mood n estado de ánimo, humor m; — swing oscilación f del ánimo or humor, cambio repentino del estado de ánimo; to be in a bad — estar de mal humor; to be in a good — estar de buen humor
moral support n apoyo moral
morbid adj (path) mórbido, patológico; — obesity obesidad mórbida
morbidity n morbilidad f
more (comp de much y many) adj más; a few more days..unos días más; adv (comp de much) más; more difficult..más difícil; n más; — than más que, (a number) más de; more than usual..más que de costumbre...more than 200..más de 200
morgue n depósito de cadáveres, morgue f
morning n mañana
morphea n morfea, esclerodermia localizada
morphine n morfina
morphology n morfología
mortal adj mortal, fatal
mortality n mortalidad f; infant — mortalidad infantil
mortuary n (pl -ries) funeraria
mosquito n (pl -toes o -tos) mosquito
most adj (super de much o many) más, mayoría de; in most cases..en la mayoría de casos; adv (super de much) más; the most effective drug..el medicamento más eficaz
mother n madre f

motherhood *n* maternidad *f*
mother-in-law *n* (*pl* **mothers-in-law**) suegra
motility *n* motilidad *f*, movilidad *f*; **sperm** — motilidad espermática (*form*), movilidad *f* de los espermatozoides
motion *n* movimiento; — **sickness** mareo (producido por el movimiento); **range of** — rango de movimiento
motivate *vt* motivar
motivation *n* motivación *f*
motor *adj* (*nerve, etc.*) motor
motorcycle *n* motocicleta, moto *f* (*fam*)
mountain *n* montaña
mountaineering *n* montañismo, alpinismo
mouse *n* (*pl* **mice**) ratón *m*
moustache *n* bigote *m*
mouth *n* boca; **by** — por vía oral (*form*), por la boca; **mouth-to-mouth** boca a boca
mouthful *n* (*pl* **-fuls**) bocado
mouthpiece *n* boquilla
mouthwash *n* colutorio (*form*), enjuague *m* bucal
move *vt* mover, (*a patient*) trasladar; **We have to move you to another room**..Tenemos que trasladarlo a otro cuarto; **to** — **one's bowels** defecar (*form*), ir al baño (*euph*), hacer del baño (*Mex*), dar del cuerpo (*Carib*), hacer popó (*fam*), hacer caca (*fam or vulg*); *vi* moverse; **Don't move**..No se mueva.
movement *n* movimiento; **periodic limb movements during sleep** movimientos periódicos de las piernas durante el sueño; **rapid eye** — **(REM)** movimientos oculares rápidos
moxibustion *n* moxibustión *f*
MRI *abbr* **magnetic resonance imaging**. *V.* **imaging**.
MRSA *abbr* **methicillin-resistant Staphylococcus aureus**. *V.* **Staphylococcus aureus**.
MSG *V.* **monosodium glutamate**.
much *adj & adv* mucho
mucinous *adj* mucinoso
mucocele *n* mucocele *m*

mucocutaneous *adj* mucocutáneo
mucolytic *adj & n* mucolítico
mucormycosis *n* mucormicosis *f*
mucosa *n* mucosa
mucous *adj* mucoso
mucus *n* mucosidad *f*, moco
mullein *n* (*bot*) gordolobo
multidisciplinary *adj* multidisciplinario (*Amer*), multidisciplinar (*Esp*)
multifactorial *adj* multifactorial
multifocal *adj* multifocal
multinodular *adj* multinodular
multiple *adj* múltiple
multiply *vt, vi* (*pret & pp* **-plied**) multiplicar(se)
multivitamin *adj* multivitamínico; *n* multivitamínico, polivitamínico (*Esp*)
mumps *n* parotiditis *f* (*form*), paperas
mupirocin *n* mupirocina
murmur *n* (*card*) soplo; **heart** — soplo cardíaco
muscle *n* músculo; **biceps** — músculo bíceps, bíceps *m*; **deltoid** — músculo deltoides, deltoides *m*; **gastrocnemius** — músculo gastrocnemio, gastrocnemio; **gluteus** — músculo glúteo, glúteo; **pectoral** — músculo pectoral, pectoral *m*; **psoas** — músculo psoas, psoas *m*; **quadriceps** — músculo cuádriceps, cuádriceps *m*; **smooth** — músculo liso; **soleus** — músculo sóleo, sóleo; **trapezius** — músculo trapecio, trapecio; **triceps** — músculo tríceps, tríceps *m*
muscular *adj* muscular; (*person*) musculoso; — **dystrophy** distrofia muscular
musculoskeletal *adj* musculoesquelético
mushroom *n* hongo
musician *n* músico -ca *mf*
mutant *adj & n* mutante *m*
mutation *n* mutación *f*
mute *adj & n* mudo -da *mf*
mutilate *vt* mutilar
mutilation *n* mutilación *f*
mutism *n* mutismo, mudez *f*; **elective** — mutismo selectivo *or* electivo
myalgia *n* mialgia
myasthenia gravis *n* miastenia gravis

Mycobacterium avium complex (MAC) *n* complejo Mycobacterium avium

mycosis fungoides *n* micosis *f* fungoides

mycotic *adj* micótico

myelin *n* mielina

myelogram *n* mielografía (*estudio imagenológico*)

myelography *n* mielografía (*técnica imagenológica*)

myeloma *n* mieloma *m*; **multiple —** mieloma múltiple

myelomeningocele *n* mielomeningocele *m*

myeloproliferative *adj* mieloproliferativo

myocardial *adj* miocárdico

myocarditis *n* miocarditis *f*

myocardium *n* miocardio

myoglobin *n* mioglobina

myoma *n* mioma *m*; **uterine —** mioma uterino

myopathy *n* miopatía

myopia *n* miopía, dificultad *f* para ver los objetos lejanos

myopic *adj* miope, que tiene dificultad para ver los objetos lejanos

myositis *n* miositis *f*

myringitis *n* miringitis *f*

myringoplasty *n* (*pl* **-ties**) miringoplastia

myxedema *n* mixedema *m*

myxoma *n* mixoma *m*

N

nabumetone *n* nabumetona

nadolol *n* nadolol *m*

nagging *adj* (*pain*) persistente

nail *n* (*anat*) uña; (*carpentry*) clavo; **ingrown —** uña encarnada, uña enterrada (*Mex, CA, Carib*); **— clippers** cortauñas; **— file** lima de uñas; **— polish** esmalte *m* para uñas, esmalte de uñas (*Esp*); **— scissors** tijeras de uñas; **to bite** *o* **chew one's nails** comerse las uñas

naked *adj* desnudo

nalidixic acid *n* ácido nalidíxico

naloxone *n* naloxona

name *n* nombre *m*; **first —** nombre; **last —** apellido

nap *n* siesta; *vi* (*pret & pp* **napped**; *ger* **napping**) (*también* **to take a —**) dormir una siesta, tomar una siesta (*esp. Mex*)

napalm *n* napalm *m*

naproxen *n* naproxeno

naratriptan *n* naratriptán

narcissism *n* narcisismo

narcissist *n* narcisista *mf*

narcissistic *adj* narcisista

narcolepsy *n* narcolepsia

narcotic *adj & n* narcótico

narrow *adj* estrecho

narrowing *n* estenosis *f* (*form*), estrechamiento, estrechez *f*

nasal *adj* nasal; **— passages** conductos nasales; **— voice** voz nasal, voz gangosa

nasogastric *adj* nasogástrico

nasopharynx *n* nasofaringe *f*

natural *adj* natural

nature *n* naturaleza

naturopath *n* naturista *mf*, naturópata *mf*

naturopathic *adj* naturista, naturopático

naturopathy *n* naturismo, naturopatía

nausea *n* náusea (*frec. pl*); — **and vomiting** náuseas y vómitos

nauseate *vt* producir náuseas

nauseated *adj* **to be** — tener náuseas; **Do you feel nauseated?**.. ¿Tiene náuseas?

nauseating *adj* nauseabundo, que produce náuseas

nauseous *adj* que tiene náuseas; que produce náuseas

navel *n* ombligo

near *adv* cerca de

nearsighted *adj* miope (*form*), que tiene dificultad para ver los objetos lejanos

nearsightedness *n* miopía, dificultad *f* para ver los objetos lejanos

nebulization *n* nebulización *f*

nebulizer *n* nebulizador *m*

neck *n* cuello; **back of the** — nuca

necrobiosis lipoidica diabeticorum *n* necrobiosis lipoídica (diabeticorum)

necrolysis *n* necrólisis *f*; **toxic epidermal** — necrólisis epidérmica tóxica

necrophilia *n* necrofilia

necrophobia *n* necrofobia

necrosis *n* necrosis *f*

necrotic *adj* necrótico

necrotizing *adj* necrotizante, necrosante

nedocromil *n* nedocromilo

need *n* necesidad *f*; **special needs** necesidades especiales; *vt* necesitar, hacer(le) falta (a uno); **You need iron**..Necesita hierro..Le hace falta hierro

needle *n* aguja; **butterfly** — aguja con aletas, aguja mariposa; — **exchange** intercambio de agujas

needlestick *n* pinchazo con aguja, piquete *m* con aguja (*Mex*)

negative *adj* & *n* negativo; **false** — falso negativo; **true** — verdadero negativo

neglect *n* negligencia, descuido; *vt* descuidar, desatender

negligence *n* negligencia

negligent *adj* negligente

neighbor *n* vecino -na *mf*

neighborhood *n* vecindad *f*

nelfinavir *n* nelfinavir *m*

neoadjuvant *adj* neoadyuvante

neomycin *n* neomicina

neonatal *adj* neonatal

neonate *n* neonato, recién nacido -da *mf*

neonatologist *n* neonatólogo -ga *mf*, médico -ca *mf* especialista en los recién nacidos, especialista *mf* de los bebés (*fam*)

neonatology *n* neonatología, rama de la pediatría que se ocupa de los recién nacidos

neoplasia *n* neoplasia (*proceso*)

neoplasm *n* neoplasia (*tumor*)

neoplastic *adj* neoplásico

neostigmine *n* neostigmina

nephew *n* sobrino

nephrectomy *n* (*pl* -**mies**) nefrectomía

nephritis *n* nefritis *f*

nephrolithiasis *n* nefrolitiasis *f*

nephrogenic *adj* nefrogénico

nephrologist *n* nefrólogo -ga *mf*, médico -ca *mf* especialista en el riñón y sus enfermedades, especialista *mf* del riñón (*fam*)

nephrology *n* nefrología, estudio del riñón y sus enfermedades

nephroma *n* hipernefroma *m*

nephropathy *n* nefropatía; **diabetic** — nefropatía diabética

nephrosis *n* nefrosis *f*

nephrostomy *n* (*pl* -**mies**) nefrostomía

nephrotic *adj* nefrótico

nerve *n* nervio; **acoustic** — nervio auditivo *or* acústico; **cranial** — par *m* craneal, par; **entrapped** — atrapamiento del nervio; **facial** — nervio facial; **femoral** — nervio crural *or* femoral; **median** — nervio mediano; **optic** — nervio óptico; **phrenic** — nervio frénico; **pinched** — (*fam*) atrapamiento del nervio; **radial** — nervio radial; **sciatic** — nervio ciático; **spinal** — nervio espinal *or* raquídeo; **trigeminal** — nervio trigémino; **ulnar** — nervio cubital; **vagus** — nervio vago

nerve gas *n* gas nervioso
nervous *adj* nervioso; **to be —** estar nervioso
nervousness *n* nerviosismo
nettle *n* (*bot*) ortiga
network *n* red *f*; **network of hospitals**..red de hospitales
neural *adj* neural
neuralgia *n* neuralgia; **postherpetic —** neuralgia postherpética; **trigeminal —** neuralgia del trigémino
neuritis *n* neuritis *f*
neuroblastoma *n* neuroblastoma *m*
neurofibroma *n* neurofibroma *m*
neurofibromatosis *n* neurofibromatosis *f*
neurogenic *adj* neurogénico *or* neurógeno
neuroleptic *adj & n* neuroléptico
neurological, neurologic *adj* neurológico
neurologist *n* neurólogo -ga *mf*, médico -ca *mf* especialista en el sistema nervioso y sus enfermedades
neurology *n* neurología, estudio del sistema nervioso y sus enfermedades
neuroma *n* neurinoma *m*, neuroma *m*; **acoustic —** neurinoma del acústico, neuroma acústico (*esp. Mex*); **Morton's —** neuroma de Morton
neuromuscular *adj* neuromuscular
neuron *n* neurona
neuro-ophthalmology *n* neuro-oftalmología
neuropathy *n* neuropatía *f*; **diabetic —** neuropatía diabética; **peripheral —** neuropatía periférica; **sensory —** neuropatía sensitiva, neuropatía sensorial (*esp. Mex*)
neurophysiology *n* neurofisiología
neurosis *n* (*pl* -**ses**) (*ant*) neurosis *f*
neurosurgeon *n* neurocirujano -na *mf*
neurosurgery *n* (*pl* -**ries**) neurocirugía
neurosyphilis *n* neurosífilis *f*
neurotic *adj & n* (*ant*) neurótico -ca *mf*
neutral *adj* (*chem, etc.*) neutro
neutralize *vt* neutralizar
neutropenia *n* neutropenia
neutrophil *n* neutrófilo
never *adv* nunca

nevi *pl de* **nevus**
nevirapine *n* nevirapina
nevus *n* (*pl* **nevi**) nevo; **dysplastic —** nevo displásico
newborn *n* recién nacido -da *mf*; **premature —** recién nacido prematuro, prematuro -ra *mf* (*fam*)
next *adj* próximo, siguiente; **the — injection** la próxima inyección
niacin *n* niacina, ácido nicotínico
nicardipine *n* nicardipino, nicardipina (*esp. SA*)
nick *n* cortada pequeña, (*during surgery*) perforación *f*
nickel *n* níquel *m*
niclosamide *n* niclosamida
nicotine *n* nicotina
nicotinic acid *n* ácido nicotínico
niece *n* sobrina
nifedipine *n* nifedipino, nifedipina (*esp. SA*)
nifurtimox *n* nifurtimox *m*
night *adj* nocturno; **— terrors** terrores nocturnos; *n* noche *f*; **in the —** por la noche, durante la noche, en la noche; **last —** anoche
nightlight *n* lámpara *or* lamparita de noche
nightmare *n* pesadilla
nighttime *n* noche *f*; **at —** por la noche
nimodipine *n* nimodipino, nimodipina (*esp. SA*)
nipple *n* (*female*) pezón *m*; (*male*) tetilla; (*of a baby bottle*) tetina, mamila, tetilla (*Esp*); **— shield** pezonera
nit *n* liendre *f*
nitrate *n* nitrato
nitric acid *n* ácido nítrico
nitrite *n* nitrito
nitro (*fam*) *V.* **nitroglycerin**.
nitrofurantoin *n* nitrofurantoína
nitrogen *n* nitrógeno; **liquid —** nitrógeno líquido
nitroglycerin *n* nitroglicerina
nitrous oxide *n* óxido nitroso
nizatidine *n* nizatidina
nocardiosis *n* nocardiosis *f*
nocturnal *adj* nocturno; **— emission** polución nocturna
nod *vt* (*pret & pp* **nodded**; *ger* **nodding**) (*también* **to — one's head**)

mover la cabeza arriba y abajo; **Nod your head up and down to say yes**..Mueva la cabeza arriba y abajo para decir sí; **to — out** (*fam, as on heroin*) cabecear

node *n* (*card*) nódulo *or* nodo; (*lymph*) ganglio; **atrioventricular — nódulo *or* nodo auriculoventricular; **lymph — ganglio linfático; **sentinel — gánglio centinela; **sinoatrial** *or* **sinus — nódulo *or* nodo sinusal

nodular *adj* nodular

nodule *n* nódulo

noise *n* ruido

nonabsorbable *adj* no absorbible

nonflammable *adj* incombustible, que no se quema

noninvasive *adj* (*procedure, surgery*) no invasivo; (*disease*) no invasor

nonketotic *adj* no cetósico; [*Note: the s is correct even though* ketotic *translates as* cetónico *with an* n.]

nonprofit *adj* (*también* **not-for-profit**) sin fines de lucro

nonspecific *adj* inespecífico

nonsteroidal *adj* no esteroideo

nontender *adj* no dolorido

nontoxic *adj* no tóxico

noon *n* mediodía *m*

norepinephrine *n* noradrenalina, norepinefrina (*OMS*)

norfloxacin *n* norfloxacino, norfloxacina (*esp. Amer*)

norgestimate *n* norgestimato

norm *n* norma

normal *adj* normal

normalize *vt* normalizar

normally *adv* normalmente

nortriptyline *n* nortriptilina

nose *n* nariz *f*; **to blow one's —** sonarse la nariz, soplarse la nariz (*Carib*); **to pick one's —** sacarse los mocos, meterse el dedo en la nariz (para sacarse los mocos), hurgarse la nariz (*Esp*)

nosebleed *n* hemorragia nasal (*form*), sangrado nasal, sangrado por la nariz (*fam*)

no-see-um *n* jején *m*

nostril *n* fosa nasal

notice *vt* darse cuenta, notar, fijarse en; **When did you notice there was blood in your stool?**.. ¿Cuándo se dio cuenta (notó) que había sangre en las heces?

nourish *vt* alimentar, nutrir

nourishing *adj* nutritivo

nourishment *n* nutrición *f*, alimentación *f*

NSAID *abbr* **nonsteroidal antiinflammatory drug**. *V.* **drug**.

nuclear *adj* nuclear

numb *adj* adormecido (*form*), dormido; **to become —** adormecerse (*form*), dormirse; *vt* (*también* **to — up**) anestesiar, adormecer, dormir; **I'm going to numb up your finger**..Le voy a anestesiar (adormecer, dormir) el dedo.

number *n* número, cifra; **— one** (*fam, urination*) (el) orinar; **— two** (*fam, defecation*) (el) defecar; **to do — one** orinar, hacer del uno (*fam*); **to do — two** defecar, hacer del dos (*fam*)

numbness *n* adormecimiento, falta de sensación

nurse *n* enfermera (enfermero *if male*); **charge — enfermera de turno, enfermera a cargo; **head — jefa (jefe *m if male*) de enfermeras; **home health — enfermera que hace visitas a la casa; *vt* (*to breastfeed*) amamantar (*form*), dar el pecho, dar de mamar; (*to care for patients*) cuidar; *vi* (*to suckle*) mamar

nurse practitioner *n* (*US*) enfermera (enfermero *if male*) que tiene entrenamiento adicional para diagnosticar y tratar enfermedades sencillas

nursery *n* (*pl* -ries) guardería infantil; **newborn — sala de neonatología (*form*), sala de recién nacidos; **— school** jardín *m* de infancia, jardín preescolar, jardín de niños (*Mex*)

nursing *n* enfermería

nursing home *n* (*fam*) asilo *or* residencia de ancianos; residencia para ancianos, enfermos, u otros descapacitados donde se ofrecen servicios de enfermería

nurture *vt* nutrir, alimentar

nut *n* nuez *f*

nutrient *n* nutriente *m*
nutrition *n* nutrición *f*; **enteral —** nutrición enteral; **parenteral —** nutrición parenteral; **total parenteral — (TPN)** nutrición parenteral total (NPT)
nutritional *adj* nutricional, nutritivo, alimenticio; **— state** estado nutricional; **— value** valor nutritivo *or* nutricional
nutritionist *n* nutricionista *mf*
nutritious *adj* nutritivo
nylon *n* nailon *m*
nystagmus *n* nistagmus (*form*), nistagmo
nystatin *n* nistatina

O

oatmeal *n* avena
OB *adj* & *n* (*fam*) *V*. **obstetrics, obstetrician, obstetrical**.
obese *adj* obeso
obesity *n* obesidad *f*; **central —** obesidad central
obey *vt* obedecer
observation *n* observación *f*
obsession *n* obsesión *f*
obsessive-compulsive *adj* obsesivo-compulsivo
obstetric, obstetrical *adj* obstétrico
obstetrician *n* obstetra *mf*, tocólogo -ga *mf*
obstetrics *n* obstetricia, tocología
obstruct *vt* obstruir, bloquear (*fam*)
obstruction *n* obstrucción *f*; **partial small bowel —** obstrucción intestinal parcial, obstrucción parcial del intestino delgado; **upper airway —** obstrucción de la vía aérea superior
obstructive *adj* obstructivo
occasionally *adv* de vez en cuando, a veces
occipital *adj* occipital
occlusion *n* oclusión *f*
occlusive *adj* oclusivo
occupation *n* ocupación *f*, trabajo

occupational *adj* laboral, ocupacional
ochronosis *n* ocronosis *f*
octogenarian *n* octogenario -ria *mf*
ocular *adj* ocular
odor *n* olor *m*; **body —** olor corporal; **foot —** olor de pies
odorless *adj* sin olor, inodoro
off *prep* (*drugs, a medication, etc.*) ya no usando, ya no tomando; **How long have you been off heroin?** ...¿Hace cuánto que no usa heroína? **...Are you off prednisone?** ...¿Ya no toma prednisona?
office *n* oficina, (*of a doctor*) consultorio
ofloxacin *n* ofloxacino, ofloxacina (*esp. Amer*)
often *adv* a menudo, frecuentemente, seguido (*esp. Mex*); **How often do you have chest pain?** ...¿Con qué frecuencia le da dolor de pecho?.. ¿Cada cuánto (tiempo) le da dolor de pecho?...¿Qué tan seguido le da dolor de pecho?
oil *n* aceite *m*; **castor —** aceite de ricino; **coconut —** aceite de coco; **cod-liver —** aceite de hígado de bacalao; **corn —** aceite de maíz;

fish — aceite de pescado; **mineral** — aceite mineral; **olive** — aceite de oliva; **palm** — aceite de palma; **peanut** — aceite de maní *m*, aceite de cacahuate *m* (*esp. Mex*), aceite de cacahuete *m* (*esp. Esp*); **rapeseed** — aceite de colza; **safflower** — aceite de cártamo; **tea tree** — aceite del árbol del té; **vegetable** — aceite vegetal

oily *adj* graso; — **complexion** cutis graso; — **hair** cabello graso; — **skin** piel grasa

ointment *n* ungüento, pomada

OK, okay *adj & adv* bien

olanzapine *n* olanzapina

old *adj* viejo, de edad avanzada; **How old are you?**..¿Cuántos años tiene Ud.? — **man** viejo, anciano, señor *m* de edad avanzada; — **woman** vieja, anciana, señora de edad avanzada; **to grow** — envejecer

older (*comp de* **old**) *adj* más viejo, mayor; — **sister** hermana mayor

olecranon *n* olécranon *m*

olfactory *adj* olfativo, olfatorio

olsalazine *n* olsalazina

ombudsman *n* ombudsman *mf*, defensor -ra *mf* del pueblo, persona que maneja disputas entre pacientes y personal de salud

omentum *n* epiplón *m*

omeprazole *n* omeprazol *m*

on *prep* (*drugs, a medication, etc.*) usando, tomando, bajo el efecto de (*drogas, un medicamento, etc.*); **Are you on lithium?**..¿Está tomando litio? **Were you on PCP when you kicked the policeman?**..¿Estaba bajo el efecto de la fenciclidina cuando le dio una patada al policía?

onchocerciasis *n* oncocercosis *f*

oncologist *n* oncólogo -ga *mf*, médico -ca *mf* especialista en los tumores; **radiation** — oncólogo radioterapeuta

oncology *n* oncología, estudio de los tumores; **radiation** — oncología radioterápica

one-armed *adj* manco

one-eyed *adj* tuerto

one-legged *adj* con una sola pierna

onion *n* cebolla

onset *n* inicio, comienzo; **age at** — edad *f* de inicio; **early-onset** de comienzo *or* inicio precoz; **juvenile-onset** de inicio juvenil; **late-onset** de inicio tardío

onychomycosis *n* onicomicosis *f*

oophorectomy *n* (*pl* **-mies**) ooforectomía, ovariectomía

opacity *n* (*pl* **-ties**) opacidad *f*

opaque *adj* opaco

open *vt, vi* abrir(se); **Open your mouth**..Abra la boca.

opening *n* abertura

operable *adj* operable, que se puede corregir con cirugía

operate *vt, vi* operar; **to operate machinery**..operar maquinaria...**We need to operate on your leg**..Tenemos que operarle (de) la pierna.

operation *n* operación *f*

operative *adj* operatorio

ophthalmic *adj* oftálmico

ophthalmologist *n* oftalmólogo -ga *mf*, médico -ca *mf* especialista en los ojos y sus enfermedades, médico de los ojos (*fam*)

ophthalmology *n* oftalmología, estudio de los ojos y sus enfermedades

ophthalmoscope *n* oftalmoscopio

opiate *adj & n* opiáceo

opinion *n* opinión *f*; **second** — segunda opinión

opioid *adj & n* opioide *m*

opium *n* opio

opportunistic *adj* oportunista

optical, optic *adj* óptico

optician *n* óptico -ca *mf*

optics *n* óptica

optimal *V.* **optimum.**

optimism *n* optimismo

optimistic *adj* optimista

optimize *vt* mejorar lo más posible

optimum *adj* óptimo

option *n* opción *f*; **treatment options** opciones de tratamiento

optometrist *n* optometrista *mf*

OR *abbr* **operating room.** *V.* **room.**

oral *adj* oral, bucal

orange *adj* naranja, de color naranja; *n* (*fruit*) naranja

orbit *n* (*anat*) órbita

orbital *adj* orbitario

orchidectomy *V.* **orchiectomy.**

orchiectomy *n* (*pl* **-mies**) orquiectomía
orchitis *n* orquitis *f*
order *n* (*medical*) indicación *f* (*form*), orden *f*; *vt* indicar (*form*), ordenar
orderly *n* (*pl* **-lies**) (*ant*) camillero
orf *n* ectima contagioso
organ *n* órgano, víscera; **hollow —** víscera hueca; **solid —** órgano sólido; **vital —** órgano vital
organic *adj* orgánico; **— food** alimento(s) orgánico(s)
organism *n* organismo, microorganismo; **genetically modified — (GMO)** organismo modificado genéticamente (OMG)
organization *n* organización *f*; **health maintenance — (HMO)** (*US*) plan integral de salud que procura disminuir costos al contratar médicos de acuerdo al número de pacientes que atienden; **World Health Organization (WHO)** Organización Mundial de la Salud (OMS)
organochlorate *n* organoclorado
organophosphate *n* organofosforado
orgasm *n* orgasmo
orientation *n* orientación *f*; **sexual —** orientación sexual
orifice *n* orificio
orlistat *n* orlistat *m*
oropharynx *n* (*pl* **-rynges** *o* **-rynxes**) orofaringe *f*
orphan *n* huérfano -na *mf*
orphanage *n* orfanato, orfanatorio
orthodontia *n* ortodoncia, tratamiento para corregir la alineación de la dentadura
orthodontic *adj* ortodóncico; *npl* ortodoncia, rama de la odontología que estudia la alineación de la dentadura y su tratamiento
orthodontist *n* ortodoncista *mf*
orthopedic, orthopaedic *adj* ortopédico
orthopedics, orthopaedics *n* ortopedia; (*surgical*) cirugía ortopédica, traumatología (*esp. Esp*)
orthopedist, orthopaedist *n* ortopedista *mf*, médico de los huesos (*fam*); (*surgeon*) cirujano -na *mf*

ortopédico -ca, traumatólogo -ga *mf* (*esp. Esp*), cirujano de los huesos (*fam*)
orthopod (*fam*) *V.* **orthopedist, orthopaedist**.
orthosis *n* (*pl* **-ses**) ortesis *f*
orthotic *adj* relativo a una ortesis; **— device** ortesis *f*
oseltamivir *n* oseltamivir *m*
osmosis *n* ósmosis *f*
osseous *adj* óseo
ossicle *n* (*of the ear*) huesecillo (*del oído*)
osteitis *n* osteítis *f*; **— fibrosa cystica** osteítis fibrosa quística
osteoarthritis *n* artrosis *f*
osteogenesis imperfecta *n* osteogénesis imperfecta
osteoma *n* osteoma *m*
osteomalacia *n* osteomalacia
osteomyelitis *n* osteomielitis *f*
osteonecrosis *n* osteonecrosis *f*
osteopath *n* osteópata *mf*
osteopathy *n* osteopatía, disciplina terapéutica manual
osteophyte *n* osteofito
osteoporosis *n* osteoporosis *f*
osteosarcoma *n* osteosarcoma *m*
ostomy *n* (*pl* **-mies**) ostomía
otic *adj* ótico
otitis *n* otitis *f*; **— externa** otitis externa; **— media** otitis media
otolaryngologist *n* otorrinolaringólogo -ga *mf*; médico -ca *mf* especialista del oído, nariz y garganta
otolaryngology *n* otorrinolaringología; estudio del oído, nariz y garganta y sus enfermedades
otosclerosis *n* otosclerosis *or* otoesclerosis *f*
otoscope *n* otoscopio
ouch *interj* ¡Ay!
ounce (oz.) *n* onza (onz.)
outbreak *n* brote *m*; (*derm*) erupción *f*
outcome *n* desenlace *m*, resultado
outdated, out of date *adj* (*pharm, etc.*) vencido, caducado
outdoors *n* aire *m* libre
outer *adj* externo, exterior
outgrow *vt* (*pret* **-grew**; *pp* **-grown**) (*a habit*) quitarse(le) (a uno) con el tiempo, perder con la edad; **She**

will **outgrow** it..Se le quitará con el tiempo..Lo perderá con la edad.

outlet *n* (*psych*) desahogo; (*electrical*) tomacorriente *m* (*Amer*), toma *m* (*Amer, fam*), toma eléctrica (*esp. Esp*); [*Note:* toma *is considered masculine in Latin America but feminine in Spain.*]

out of it, (*fam*) fuera de sí

outpatient *adj* de consulta externa, ambulatorio; — **clinic** clínica de consulta externa, clínica ambulatoria; — **procedure** procedimiento ambulatorio; *n* paciente *mf* ambulatorio

output *n* gasto; **cardiac** — gasto cardíaco; **urine** — gasto urinario

outreach *adj* dedicado a extender servicios y beneficios comunitarios a gente necesitada

outside *adj* exterior, externo; *n* exterior *m*; *prep* (*también* — **of**) fuera de

ova *pl de* **ovum**

ovarian *adj* ovárico

ovary *n* (*pl* -**ries**) ovario; **polycystic** — ovario poliquístico

over *adv* (*greater than*) superior a (*form*), por encima de, sobre; **Your sugar is over 500**..Su azúcar está por encima de (superior a, sobre) 500...**Your blood pressure is 150 over 80**..Su presión arterial es de 150 sobre 80.

overactive *adj* demasiado activo

overate *pret de* **overeat**

overbite *n* sobremordida

overcome *vt* (*pret* -**came**; *pp* -**come**) superar, vencer; **to overcome fears** ..superar *or* vencer miedos

overcompensate *vi* sobrecompensar

overdo *vt* (*pret* -**did**; *pp* -**done**) **to** — **it** (*fam*) excederse; **Don't overdo it**..No se exceda.

overdose *n* sobredosis *f*, dosis excesiva

overeat *vi* (*pret* -**ate**; *pp* -**eaten**) comer demasiado

overexcite *vt* sobreexcitar; **to become overexcited** sobreexcitarse

overexert *vt* **to** — **oneself** esforzarse demasiado

overexertion *n* esfuerzo excesivo

overgrowth *n* sobrecrecimiento

overload *n* sobrecarga; **iron** — sobrecarga de hierro; *vt* sobrecargar

overnight *adv* durante la noche, toda la noche, por la noche

overproduction *n* sobreproducción *f*

overreact *vi* sobrerreaccionar

over-the-counter *adj* (*pharm*) de venta sin receta (médica), que se vende sin receta (médica)

overuse *n* sobreuso; — **injury** lesión *f* por sobreuso

overutilization *n* sobreutilización *f*

overweight *adj* que tiene sobrepeso

ovulate *vi* ovular

ovulation *n* ovulación *f*

ovum *n* (*pl* **ova**) óvulo, (*esp. after fertilization*) huevo (*fam*)

owie *n* (*ped, fam*) herida

oxalate *n* oxalato

oxidant *n* oxidante *m*

oxide *n* óxido

oximetry *n* oximetría

oxybutynin *n* oxibutinina

oxycodone *n* oxicodona

oxygen *n* oxígeno; (*as therapy*) oxigenoterapia (*form*), oxígeno (*fam*); **home** — oxigenoterapia domiciliaria (*form*), oxígeno domiciliario, oxígeno en la casa (*fam*); **hyperbaric** — oxigenoterapia hiperbárica

oxytocin *n* oxitocina

oz. *V.* **ounce**.

ozone *n* ozono

P

PABA *V.* **paraaminobenzoic acid.**
PAC *abbr* **premature atrial contraction.** *V.* **contraction.**
pacemaker *n* marcapasos *m*
pacifier *n* chupete *m*, chupón *m*
pack *n* (*compress*) compresa; (*of cigarettes*) paquete *m*, cajetilla; **ice —** bolsa de hielo; **packs per day** paquetes diarios, cajetillas diarias
package insert *n* prospecto de envase (*form*), prospecto, instructivo impreso (*Mex, CA*), instrucciones *fpl* del medicamento
packing *n* (*act*) taponamiento; (*material*) material como gasa usado para llenar una cavidad, (*once packed*) taponamiento; **nasal —** taponamiento nasal
paclitaxel *n* paclitaxel *m*
pad *n* (*cushion*) cojín *m*, almohadilla; (*of the finger*) yema (*del dedo*); **alcohol —** pequeña gasa impregnada de alcohol; **heating —** almohadilla eléctrica, cojín eléctrico (*esp. Mex*); *vt* (*pret & pp* **padded**; *ger* **padding**) acolchar, acojinar
padded *adj* acolchado
padding *n* (*ortho, etc.*) acolchonado, acolchado, material *m* que sirve para acolchar alguna parte del cuerpo
page *n* (*overhead*) llamada por altavoz; (*by beeper*) llamada por biper *or* buscapersonas; *vt* llamar por altavoz, perifonear (*form*); llamar por biper *or* buscapersonas
pager *n* biper *m* (*Amer*), buscapersonas *m* (*Esp, SA*)
pain *n* dolor *m*; **a pain in the back..** un dolor de *or* en la espalda; **back —** dolor de espalda; **to be in —** tener dolor
painful *adj* doloroso; **— procedure** procedimiento doloroso
painkiller *n* (*fam*) analgésico (*form*), medicamento para aliviar el dolor
painless *adj* indoloro (*form*), sin dolor

paint *n* pintura; **lead-based —** pintura a base de plomo
palatable *adj* de sabor aceptable, que no sabe mal
palate *n* paladar *m*; **cleft —** fisura palatina; **hard —** paladar duro, bóveda palatina (*form*); **soft —** paladar blando, velo del paladar (*form*)
pale *adj* pálido
palliation *n* paliación *f*
palliative *adj* paliativo
pallidotomy *n* (*pl* -**mies**) palidotomía
pallor *n* palidez *f*
palmar *adj* palmar, de la palma
palpate *vt* palpar
palpitate *vi* palpitar
palpitation *n* palpitación *f*, latido rápido o fuerte del corazón
palsy *n* (*pl* -**sies**) parálisis *f*; **Bell's —** parálisis facial periférica (idiopática), parálisis de Bell; **cerebral —** parálisis cerebral; **facial —** parálisis facial
pamper *vt* mimar, consentir
pamphlet *n* folleto
pancreas *n* (*pl* -**creases**) páncreas *m*
pancreatectomy *n* (*pl* -**mies**) pancreatectomía
pancreatic *adj* pancreático
pancreatitis *n* pancreatitis *f*
pandemic *n* pandemia
pang *n* punzada, dolor breve y agudo; **hunger —** dolor *or* punzada de hambre
panhypopituitarism *n* panhipopituitarismo
panic *n* pánico
pant *vi* jadear
panties *npl* calzón *m* (*frec. pl*), pantaletas (*esp. Mex*), bloomer *m* (*esp. CA, frec. pl*), panties *mpl* (*esp. Carib*), bragas (*esp. Esp*)
pantoprazole *n* pantoprazol *m*
pants *npl* pantalones *mpl*
pantyhose *npl* pantimedias
paper *n* papel *m*
papilla *n* papila

papillary *adj* papilar
papillomavirus *n* papilomavirus *m*;
  human — (HPV) virus *m* del papiloma humano (VPH)
Pap smear *V.* **smear.**
paraaminobenzoic acid (PABA) *n*
  ácido paraaminobenzoico (PABA)
paracentesis *n* (*pl* **-ses**) paracentesis
  f
paracoccidioidomycosis *n* paracoccidioidomicosis *f*
paradoxical *adj* paradójico
paragonimiasis *n* paragonimiasis *f*
parainfluenza *n* parainfluenza
paralysis *n* parálisis *f*; **facial —** parálisis facial; **sleep —** parálisis del
  sueño
paralyze *vt* paralizar
paralyzing *adj* paralizante
paramedic *adj* paramédico; *n* paramédico -ca *mf*, persona con entrenamiento médico básico encargada
  de llevar heridos y enfermos al hospital
paranasal *adj* paranasal
paranoia *n* paranoia
paranoid *adj* paranoide, paranoico
paraparesis *n* paraparesia; **tropical**
  spastic — paraparesia espástica
  tropical
paraphimosis *n* parafimosis *f*
paraplegia *n* paraplejia *or* paraplejía
paraplegic *adj* & *n* parapléjico -ca *mf*
paraquat *n* paraquat *m*
parasite *n* parásito
parasitic *adj* parasitario
parasitology *n* parasitología, estudio
  de los parásitos y sus efectos en el
  organismo
paraspinal *adj* paraespinal
parasympathetic *adj* parasimpático
parathion *n* paratión *m*
parathyroid *adj* paratiroideo; *n* (*fam*)
  glándula paratiroidea, paratiroides
  f (*fam*)
parathyroidectomy *n* (*pl* **-mies**) paratiroidectomía
paratyphoid *n* paratifoidea
paregoric *n* paregórico, tintura de
  opio alcanforada
parent *n* padre *m*, madre *f*; *npl* padres
  mpl; **adoptive —** padres adoptivos;
  biological — padres biológicos

parental *adj* parental
parenteral *adj* parenteral
parenthood *n* paternidad *f*, maternidad *f*, (el) tener hijos
parenting *n* crianza de los niños; **—**
  education educación *f* parental,
  educación para padres (y madres);
  — skills habilidades *fpl* parentales;
  — workshop taller *m* para padres
  (y madres)
paresis *n* paresia
parietal *adj* parietal
Parkinsonism *n* parkinsonismo
paronychia *n* paroniquia
parotid *adj* parotídeo; *n* (*fam*) glándula parótida, parótida (*fam*)
parotitis *n* parotiditis *f*
paroxetine *n* paroxetina
paroxysm *n* paroxismo
paroxysmal *adj* paroxístico
part *n* parte *f*
partial *adj* parcial
participation *n* participación *f*
particle *n* partícula
partner *n* (*sexual, gay*) pareja; (*professional*) socio -cia *mf*
parvovirus *n* parvovirus *m*
pass *n* paso; *vt* (*parasites, a stone,
  etc.*) eliminar, expulsar, botar (*esp.
  Carib, fam*); **Have you ever passed a stone?**..¿Ha eliminado (expul-
  sado, botado) alguna vez una piedra
  (al orinar)? **to — (away)** (*euph*)
  morir, fallecer; **to — gas** expulsar
  gas, ventosear; *vi* **to — out** desmayarse, perder el conocimiento *or*
  la conciencia
passage *n* conducto; **nasal passages**
  conductos nasales
passion flower *n* (*bot*) pasionaria,
  pasiflora
passive *adj* pasivo
passive-aggressive *adj* pasivo-agresivo
paste *n* pasta
pasteurized *adj* pasteurizado
pastime *n* pasatiempo
pat *n* palmada *or* palmadita, golpeci-
  to; *vt* (*pret & pp* **patted**; *ger* **pat-
  ting**) dar palmadas *or* palmaditas,
  dar golpecitos
patch *n* parche *m*; **nicotine —** parche de nicotina

patella n (pl **-lae**) rótula
paternal adj paterno
paternity n paternidad f
path (fam) V. **pathology.**
pathological, pathologic adj patológico; **pathological liar** mentiroso -sa mf compulsivo
pathologist n patólogo -ga mf, anatomopatólogo -ga mf, médico -ca mf que estudia tejidos y líquidos con fines diagnósticos; **speech** — logopeda mf (form), fonoaudiólogo -ga mf, terapeuta mf del lenguaje, especialista mf en trastornos del lenguaje
pathology n patología, anatomía patológica, estudio de los tejidos y líquidos con fines diagnósticos
patient adj paciente; n paciente mf, enfermo -ma mf
pattern n patrón m
paunch n barriga, panza, panzón m
pavillion n pabellón m
PCB V. **polychlorinated biphenyl.**
PCP V. **phencyclidine.**
PCR abbr **polymerase chain reaction.** V. **reaction.**
peak n pico, valor máximo; — (**expiratory**) **flow** flujo espiratorio máximo; vi alcanzar el pico or valor máximo
peanut n maní m, cacahuate m (esp. Mex), cacahuete m (esp. Esp); — **butter** mantequilla de maní, crema or mantequilla de cacahuate
pectoral adj & n pectoral m
pediatric adj pediátrico, infantil
pediatrician n pediatra mf
pediatrics n pediatría
pediculosis n pediculosis f
pedicure n pedicura, pedicure m
pedophilia n paidofilia or pedofilia
pee (fam) n pis m (fam or vulg), pipí m (esp. ped, fam); vi hacer pis (fam or vulg), hacer pipí (esp. ped, fam)
pee pee n (ped, fam, penis) pene m, pipí m
peel vi (skin) descamarse (form), pelarse, despellejarse (fam); **I'm peeling** o **My skin is peeling**..Me estoy pelando (despellejando).
peeling n exfoliación f (form), descamación f (form), (el) pelarse; (procedure) dermoabrasión f
peer n igual mf, par mf; (V. también **group** y **pressure.**)
PEG abbr **percutaneous endoscopic gastrostomy.** V. **gastrostomy.**
PEG abbr **polyethylene glycol** V. **polyethylene.**
peginterferon n peginterferón m
pegylated adj pegilado
pellagra n pelagra
pelvic adj pélvico, pelviano
pelvis n pelvis f
pemphigoid n penfigoide m
pemphigus n pénfigo
pen n insulin — pluma or bolígrafo de insulina, dispositivo tipo pluma para la inyección de insulina
penciclovir n penciclovir m
pending adj pendiente
penetrate vt penetrar
penetrating adj penetrante
penetration n penetración f
penicillamine n penicilamina
penicillin n penicilina
penile adj peneano
penis n pene m, miembro (fam)
pentachlorophenol n pentaclorofenol m
pentamidine n pentamidina
pentoxifylline n pentoxifilina
people n personas, gente f; **little** — (euph, dwarfs) enanos -nas mfpl
pep n (fam) energía, vigor m
pepper n pimienta
peppermint n (bot) hierbabuena or yerbabuena
pepsin n pepsina
peptic adj péptico
per prep por; **beats** — **minute** latidos por minuto
percent n por ciento
percentage n porcentaje m
perception n percepción f; **depth** — percepción de la profundidad
perchlorate n perclorato
percutaneous adj percutáneo
perfectionism n perfeccionismo
perfectionist adj & n perfeccionista mf
perforate vt perforar
perforated adj perforado
perforation n perforación f
performance n rendimiento, des-

empeño; **peformance-enhancing drugs** drogas para mejorar el rendimiento

perfume *n* perfume *m*

perfusion *n* perfusión *f*

perianal *adj* perianal

pericardial *adj* pericárdico

pericarditis *n* pericarditis *f*; **constrictive** — pericarditis constrictiva

pericardium *n* pericardio

perinatal *adj* perinatal

perineal *adj* perineal

perinephric *adj* perirrenal

period *n* período *or* periodo; (*menstrual*) período (*menstrual*), regla; **Do you still have periods?**..¿Todavía tiene períodos (la regla)?... **Are you on your period?**..¿Está en su período (regla)?...**When was your last period?**..¿Cuándo fue su último período (última regla)? **incubation** — período de incubación

periodic *adj* periódico

periodontal *adj* periodontal

periodontics *n* periodoncia

periodontist *n* periodoncista *mf*

perioral *adj* perioral

periorbital *adj* periorbitario

peripheral *adj* periférico

periphery *n* periferia

peristalsis *n* peristaltismo, peristalsis *f*

peritoneal *adj* peritoneal

peritoneum *n* peritoneo

peritonitis *n* peritonitis *f*

periungual *adj* periungueal

perleche *n* queilitis *f*, boqueras (*fam*)

permanent *adj* permanente

permethrin *n* permetrina

permission *n* permiso

peroneal *adj* peroneo

peroxide *n* peróxido

persist *vi* persistir

persistent *adj* persistente

person *n* persona, individuo; **blind** — ciego -ga *mf*; **deaf** — sordo -da *mf*; **disabled** — descapacitado -da *mf*; **little** — (*euph, dwarf*) enano -na *mf*; **old** — viejo -ja *mf*, anciano -na *mf*, persona de edad avanzada; — **with HIV** persona con VIH; **sick** — enfermo -ma *mf*; **wounded** — herido -da *mf*; **young** — joven *mf*

personal *adj* personal

personality *n* (*pl* **-ties**) personalidad *f*; **antisocial** — personalidad antisocial; **borderline** — personalidad límite *or* borderline; **cyclothymic** — personalidad ciclotímica; **histrionic** — personalidad histriónica; **narcissistic** — personalidad narcisista; **obsessive-compulsive** — personalidad obsesivo-compulsiva; **paranoid** — personalidad paranoide; **passive-aggressive** — personalidad pasivo-agresiva; **schizoid** — personalidad esquizoide; **type A** — personalidad tipo A

personnel *n* personal *m*; **health** — personal de salud

perspiration *n* (*form*) transpiración *f* (*form*), sudor *m*

perspire *vi* (*form*) transpirar (*form*), sudar

pertussis *n* tos ferina, coqueluche *m&f* (*fam*)

pessary *n* (*pl* **-ries**) pesario, aparato que se coloca en la vagina para corregir el descenso de la matriz

pessimism *n* pesimismo

pessimistic *adj* pesimista

pesticide *n* plaguicida *m*, pesticida *m*

PET *abbr* **positive emission tomography.** *V.* **tomography.** (*V. también* **scan.**)

pet *n* mascota

petroleum *n* petróleo; — **jelly** vaselina, petrolato

pewterwort *n* (*bot*) cola de caballo

peyote *n* peyote *m*

pH *n* pH *m*

phallic *adj* fálico

phalloplasty *n* faloplastia

phallus *n* falo

phantom pain *n* dolor *m* fantasma

pharmaceutical *adj* farmacéutico; *n* fármaco

pharmacist *n* farmacéutico -ca *mf*, boticario -ria *mf*

pharmacological, pharmacologic *adj* farmacológico

pharmacologist *n* farmacólogo -ga *mf*, especialista *mf* en los medicamentos

pharmacology *n* farmacología, estudio de los medicamentos

pharmacopoeia *n* farmacopea

pharmacy *n* (*pl* **-cies**) farmacia, botica

pharyngeal *adj* faríngeo

pharynges *pl de* **pharynx**

pharyngitis *n* faringitis *f*

pharynx *n* (*pl* **-rynges** *o* **-rynxes**) faringe *f*

phase *n* fase *f*

phenazopyridine *n* fenazopiridina

phencyclidine (PCP) *n* fenciclidina (PCP)

phenobarbital *n* fenobarbital *m*

phenol *n* fenol *m*

phenolphthalein *n* fenolftaleína

phenomenon *n* fenómeno; **Raynaud's** — fenómeno de Raynaud

phenothiazine *n* fenotiazina

phenotype *n* fenotipo

phentermine *n* fentermina

phenylalanine *n* fenilalanina

phenylephrine *n* fenilefrina

phenylketonuria (PKU) *n* fenilcetonuria

phenylpropanolamine *n* fenilpropanolamina

phenytoin *n* fenitoína, difenilhidantoína

pheochromocytoma *n* feocromocitoma *m*

phimosis *n* (*pl* **-ses**) fimosis *f*

phlebitis *n* flebitis *f*

phlebotomist *n* flebotomista *mf*, flebotomiano -na *mf* (*esp. Esp*), sangrador *m*, persona que saca sangre

phlebotomy *n* flebotomía, extracción *f* de sangre de una vena; (*therapeutic*) flebotomía (terapéutica), sangría

phlegm *n* flema (*frec. pl*)

phlegmon *n* flemón *m*

phobia *n* fobia, temor morboso y obsesivo; **social** — fobia social

phosphate *n* fosfato

phosphorus *n* fósforo

photoallergy *n* (*pl* **-gies**) fotoalergia

photocoagulation *n* fotocoagulación *f*

photosensitive *adj* fotosensible

photosensitivity *n* fotosensibilidad *f*

phototherapy *n* fototerapia

phototoxic *adj* fototóxico

phrenic *adj* frénico

physiatrist *n* fisiatra *mf*, médico -ca *mf* especialista en medicina física y rehabilitación

physiatry *n* fisiatría, medicina física y rehabilitación

physical *adj* físico; *n* (*fam*) examen físico

physician *n* médico -ca *mf*, doctor -ra *mf*; **attending** — médico tratante; **family** — médico de cabecera, médico de la familia; **family practice** — médico de familia, médico familiar (*esp. Mex*); **on-call** — (*también* — **on call**) médico de guardia; **personal** — médico de cabecera, médico personal; **primary care** — médico de atención primaria, médico de cabecera; **private** — médico privado; **treating** — médico tratante

physiological, physiologic *adj* fisiológico

physiologist *n* fisiólogo -ga *mf*

physiology *n* fisiología

physiotherapist *n* fisioterapeuta *mf*

physiotherapy *n* fisioterapia

physique *n* físico

physostigmine *n* fisostigmina

picaridin *n* picaridina

PICC *abbr* **peripherally-inserted central catheter**. *V.* **catheter.**

pick *vt* (*a scab, etc.*) rascarse, quitarse; **to** — **one's nose** sacarse los mocos, meterse el dedo en la nariz (para sacarse los mocos), hurgarse la nariz (*Esp*)

PID *abbr* **pelvic inflammatory disease**. *V.* **disease.**

piece *n* pedazo

pierce *vt* perforar

piercing *adj* (*pain*) punzante (*dolor*); *n* piercing *m*, perforación *f* de partes del cuerpo con fines estéticos

pigeon-toed *adj* con los pies torcidos hacia dentro

pigment *n* pigmento

pigmentation *n* pigmentación *f*

pigmented *adj* pigmentado

pilar *adj* pilar

piles *npl* (*ant*) hemorroides *fpl*, almorranas

pill *n* pastilla, píldora; **birth control** — píldora anticonceptiva; **morning after** — píldora postcoital (*form*), píldora del día siguiente *or* del día después; **pain** — analgésico (*form*), pastilla para aliviar el dolor; — **cutter** cortapastillas *m*, maquinita para cortar pastillas; — **organizer** caja dividida en secciones para organizar pastillas de acuerdo con el día y la hora de tomarlas; **sleeping** — somnífero (*form*), pastilla para dormir; **the** — (*fam, oral contraceptive*) la píldora anticonceptiva, la píldora (*fam*); **water** — (*fam*) diurético (*form*), pastilla para eliminar agua

pillow *n* almohada

pillowcase *n* funda de almohada

pilonidal *adj* pilonidal

pimple *n* grano, barro, espinilla

pin *n* alfiler *m*; (*ortho*) clavo

pinch *vt, vi* (*to bind*) apretar

pindolol *n* pindolol *m*

pineal *adj* pineal

pineapple *n* piña

pinguecula *n* pinguécula

pink *adj* rosado

pinkeye *n* (*fam*) conjuntivitis *f*, ojo rojo (*fam*)

pins and needles *npl* (*sensation*) hormigueo

pint *n* unidad *f* de medida equivalente a aproximadamente medio litro

pinta *n* mal *m* del pinto, infección *f* tropical que causa manchas en la piel

pinworm *n* oxiuro, pequeña lombriz blanca que afecta en particular a los niños

pioglitazone *n* pioglitazona

pipe *n* (*for smoking*) pipa

piroxicam *n* piroxicam *m*

piss (*vulg*) *n* orina, pis *m* (*fam or vulg*); *vi* orinar, hacer pis (*fam or vulg*), mear (*vulg*)

pitch *n* (*sound*) tono

pitcher *n* jarra

pituitary *adj* hipofisario, pituitario

pityriasis *n* pitiriasis *f*; — **alba** pitiriasis alba; — **rosea** pitiriasis rosada

PKU *V.* **phenylketonuria**.

place *vt* colocar, poner; **Place your hands on your hips..**Coloque (Ponga) las manos en la cintura.

placebo *n* (*pl* **-bos** *o* **-boes**) placebo

placement *n* colocación *f*

placenta *n* (*pl* **-tas** *o* **-tae**) placenta; — **previa** placenta previa

placental *adj* placentario; — **abruption** desprendimiento prematuro de placenta

plague *n* peste *f*; **bubonic** — peste bubónica

plan *n* plan *m*; **written action** — plan escrito para el paciente con el manejo de diferentes situaciones relacionadas a su enfermedad

plane *n* plano

planned parenthood *n* planificación *f* familiar

plant *n* (*bot*) planta

plantar *adj* plantar

plaque *n* (*dent*) placa (bacteriana); (*card*) placa (de ateroma)

plasma *adj* plasmático; — **potassium** potasio plasmático; *n* plasma *m*; **fresh frozen** — plasma fresco congelado

plasmapheresis *n* plasmaféresis *f*

plaster *n* (*for a cast*) yeso; (*ant, medicinal*) cataplasma, emplasto

plastic *adj & n* plástico

plate *n* (*dent*) prótesis *f* dental (*form*), dentadura postiza; (*surg*) placa

platelet *n* plaqueta

platinum *n* platino

pleasure *n* placer *m*

plethysmography *n* pletismografía

pleura *n* (*pl* **-rae**) pleura

pleural *adj* pleural

pleurisy *n* pleuresía

pleuritic *adj* pleurítico

pleuritis *n* pleuritis *f*

plexus *n* (*pl* **-xi** *o* **-xuses**) plexo; **brachial** — plexo braquial

plug *n* tapón *m*

plunger *n* (*of a syringe*) émbolo

PMS *abbr* **premenstrual syndrome**. *V.* **syndrome**.

pneumococcus *n* (*pl* **-ci**) neumococo

pneumoconiosis *n* (*pl* **-ses**) neumoconiosis *f*

pneumonectomy *n* (*pl* **-mies**) neumonectomía

pneumonia *n* neumonía, pulmonía (*fam*); **aspiration** — neumonía por aspiración; **community-acquired** — neumonía adquirida en la comunidad

pneumonitis *n* neumonitis *f*; **hypersensitivity** — neumonitis por hipersensibilidad

pneumothorax *n* neumotórax *m*

pockmark *n* cacaraña, hoyo en el rostro producido por la viruela

podiatrist *n* podólogo -ga *mf*

podiatry *n* podología

podophyllin *n* podofilina

point *n* (*anat*) punto

poison *n* veneno; **ant** — hormiguicida *m*, veneno para hormigas; **Poison Control Center** Centro de Toxicología; **rat** — raticida *m*, veneno para ratas; *vt* envenenar

poisoning *n* envenenamiento, intoxicación *f*

poison ivy *n* hiedra venenosa

poison oak *n* roble venenoso

poisonous *adj* venenoso

policy *n* (*pl* **-cies**) (*insurance*) póliza (*de seguro*)

polio (*fam*) *V.* poliomyelitis.

poliomyelitis *n* poliomielitis *f*, polio *f* (*fam*)

polish *vt* (*dent, etc.*) pulir

pollen *n* polen *m*

polluted *adj* contaminado

pollution *n* contaminación *f*; **air** — contaminación atmosférica, contaminación del aire; **water** — contaminación del agua

polyarteritis nodosa *n* poliarteritis nodosa *or* nudosa

polychlorinated biphenyl (PCB) *n* bifenilo policlorado (BPC)

polyclonal *adj* policlonal

polycystic *adj* poliquístico

polycythemia *n* policitemia; **vera** — policitemia vera

polyethylene *n* polietileno; **glycol (PEG)** polietilenglicol *m*

polymyalgia rheumatica *n* polimialgia reumática

polymyositis *n* polimiositis *f*

polymyxin B *n* polimixina B

polyp *n* pólipo; **adenomatous** — pólipo adenomatoso; **juvenile** — pólipo juvenil; **nasal** — pólipo nasal

polypectomy *n* (*pl* **-mies**) polipectomía

polyposis *n* poliposis *f*; **familial adenomatous** — poliposis adenomatosa familiar

polypropylene *n* polipropileno

polysomnography *n* polisomnografía

polyunsaturated *adj* poliinsaturado

polyurethane *n* poliuretano

polyvinyl chloride *n* cloruro de polivinilo

pons *n* puente *m*, protuberancia

pool *n* (*genetics*) acervo; **gene** — acervo genético; *vi* (*blood*) acumularse, estancarse (*la sangre*)

poo poo *n* (*ped, fam*) popó (*fam*), caca (*fam or vulg*); **to go** — — hacer popó *or* caca

poorly *adv* mal

popliteal *adj* poplíteo

population *n* población *f*

porcelain *n* porcelana

porcine *adj* porcino

pore *n* poro

pork *n* carne *f* de cerdo *or* puerco

porphyria *n* porfiria; **cutanea tarda** porfiria cutánea tarda

portable *adj* portátil

portal *adj* portal; (*vein*) porta

portion *n* porción *f*

Portuguese man-of-war *n* fragata portuguesa, carabela portuguesa (*Esp*), tipo de medusa

port-wine stain *n* mancha en vino de Oporto

position *n* posición *f*; **fetal** — posición fetal; **missionary** — posición misionera; *vt* poner en posición, colocar

positive *adj & n* positivo; **false** — falso positivo; **true** — verdadero positivo

possibility *n* posibilidad *f*

possible *adj* posible

post- *pref* post- *or* pos-; [*Note: when applying the Spanish prefix* post-, *the Real Academia Española recommends dropping the* t *when it is to be followed by a consonant, although in practice the* t *is included more often than not.*]

posterior *adj* posterior

postexposure *adj* postexposición
postictal *adj* postictal
postmenopausal *adj* postmenopáusico *or* posmenopáusico
postmortem *adj & adv* post mortem
postnasal *adj* postnasal *or* posnasal; — **drip** goteo postnasal *or* posnasal
postnatal *adj* postnatal *or* posnatal
postoperative *adj* postoperatorio
postpartum *adj & adv* postparto *or* posparto (*inv*); **the second week postpartum**..la segunda semana postparto *or* posparto
postpone *vt* posponer
postprandial *adj* posprandial
posttraumatic *adj* postraumático
postural *adj* postural
posture *n* postura
pot (*fam*) marihuana, mariguana (*Mex*), hierba (*fam*), mota (*Mex, CA; fam*)
potable *adj* potable, que se puede beber
potassium *n* potasio; — **chloride** cloruro potásico (*form*), cloruro de potasio; — **hydroxide** hidróxido potásico (*form*), hidróxido de potasio
potato *n* (*pl* **-toes**) papa, patata (*Esp*)
potbelly *n* barriga, panza, panzón *m*
potency *n* (*pl* **-cies**) potencia
potent *adj* potente
potential *adj & n* potencial *m*; **evoked —** potencial evocado
potty *n* (*pl* **-ties**) (*ped*) inodoro (para niños)
pouch *n* (*surg*) reservorio; **ileal —** reservorio ileal
poultice *n* (*ant*) cataplasma, emplasto
poultry *n* aves *fpl* de corral
pound (lb) *n* libra (lb)
poverty *n* pobreza
povodine-iodine *n* povidona yodada
powder *n* polvo
powdered *adj* en polvo
power *n* poder *m*; **durable — of attorney for health care** (*US*) poder notarial duradero para la atención médica; — **of attorney** poder *m* notarial
powerful *adj* (*medication, etc.*) potente, fuerte

PPD *abbr* **purified protein derivative.** *V.* **derivative.**
practice *n* práctica; **Dr. Ho has a large practice**..El doctor Ho tiene muchos pacientes; **clinical —** práctica clínica; *vt* (*medicine*) ejercer, practicar; *vi* practicar
practitioner *n* practicante *mf*; (*physician*) clínico -ca *mf*; **general —** médico -ca *mf* general *or* generalista
pramipexole *n* pramipexol *m*
pramlintide *n* pramlintida
pravastatin *n* pravastatina
praziquantel *n* praziquantel *m*, prazicuantel *m* (*OMS*)
prazosin *n* prazosina
prebiotic *n* prebiótico
precancerous *adj* precanceroso
precaution *n* precaución *f*; **as a precaution**..por precaución; **air-borne precautions** precauciones de transmisión aérea; **contact precautions** precauciones de contacto; **droplet precautions** precauciones de transmisión por gotas; **standard precautions** precauciones estándar; **universal precautions** (*ant*) precauciones universales (*ant*)
precise *adj* preciso
precision *n* precisión *f*
precocious *adj* precoz
precordial *adj* precordial
precursor *n* precursor *m*
predict *vt* predecir, pronosticar; **I can't predict how much longer she will live**..No puedo predecir cuánto más va a vivir.
predispose *vt* predisponer
predisposed *adj* predispuesto, propenso
predisposing *adj* predisponente
predisposition *n* predisposición *f*, propensión *f*
prednisolone *n* prednisolona
prednisone *n* prednisona
preeclampsia *n* preeclampsia
preemie *n* (*fam*) recién nacido -da *mf* prematuro -ra, prematuro -ra *mf* (*fam*)
pre-existing *adj* preexistente
prefilled *adj* prellenado; — **syringe** jeringa *or* jeringuilla prellenada

pregnancy *n* (*pl* **-cies**) embarazo; **ectopic** — embarazo ectópico; **tubal** — embarazo tubárico; **unwanted** — embarazo no deseado

pregnant *adj* embarazada, encinta (*fam*); **You are three months pregnant**..Ud. Tiene tres meses de embarazo; **to get** *o* **become** — embarazarse, quedarse embarazada (*esp. Esp*)

preliminary *adj* preliminar

premalignant *adj* premaligno

premature *adj* prematuro, precoz

premedication *n* premedicación *f*

premenopausal *adj* premenopáusico

premenstrual *adj* premenstrual

premolar *adj* & *n* premolar *m*

prenatal *adj* prenatal

preoperative *adj* preoperatorio

prep *n* (*fam*) preparación quirúrgica, preparación del paciente para un procedimiento o una cirugía

preparation *n* preparación *f*; (*pharm*) preparado

prepare *vt* preparar

prepubertal *adj* prepuberal

presbycusis *n* presbiacusia

presbyopia *n* presbicia, vista cansada (*fam*)

preschool *n* jardín *m* preescolar, jardín infantil, jardín de niños (*Mex*)

prescribe *vt* recetar, prescribir

prescription *n* receta (médica), prescripción *f*

presence *n* presencia

presentation *n* presentación *f*; **breech** — presentación pelviana (*form*), presentación pélvica (*esp. Mex, form*), presentación de nalgas (*fam*)

preservative *n* conservante *m*, conservador *m* (*esp. Mex*)

preserve *vt* conservar; **to preserve cognitive function**..conservar la función cognitiva

press *vt* presionar; **Does it hurt when I press here?**...¿Le duele cuando presiono aquí?

pressure *n* presión *f*, opresión *f*; **like a pressure over your chest**..como una opresión en el pecho; **bi-level positive airway** — **(BiPAP)** presión positiva (de la vía aérea) a dos

niveles; **blood** — presión arterial (*form*), presión sanguínea (*form*), presión (de la sangre) (*fam*); **continuous positive airway** — **(CPAP)** presión positiva continua (en la vía aérea); **diastolic** — presión diastólica; **high blood** — hipertensión *f* (*form*), presión alta (*fam*); **You have high blood pressure**..Ud. tiene hipertensión (presión alta); **peer** — presión de grupo; **systolic** — presión sistólica

pressure point *n* punto de presión

preterm *adj* pretérmino (*inv*); **preterm newborns**..recién nacidos pretérmino

prevalence *n* prevalencia

prevent *vt* (*disease, etc.*) prevenir; **to prevent cavities**..prevenir la caries

preventable *adj* prevenible; — **disease** enfermedad *f* prevenible

prevention *n* prevención *f*

preventive *adj* preventivo

previous *adj* anterior, previo; **your previous doctor**..su médico -ca *mf* anterior..su médico previo

priapism *n* priapismo

prick *n* pinchazo, piquete *m* (*Mex*); (*vulg, penis*) pene *m*; *vt* pinchar, picar (*Mex*); **to** — **oneself** pincharse, picarse (*Mex*)

prickle *vi* hormiguear, picar

prickly heat *n* sudamina, sarpullido, salpullido (*esp. Mex*), erupción *f* por calor, erupción por sudar en exceso durante tiempos de calor

priest *n* sacerdote *m*, padre *m*, cura *m*

primaquine *n* primaquina

primary *adj* primario; — **care** atención primaria

primitive *adj* primitivo

principle *n* principio; **pleasure** — principio del placer

prion *n* prión *m*

prison *n* cárcel *f*, prisión *f*

privacy *n* privacidad *f*, intimidad *f*

private *adj* privado, íntimo; — **doctor** médico -ca *mf* privado; — **parts** (*fam*) genitales *mpl*, partes íntimas (*fam*)

PRK *abbr* **photorefractive keratectomy**. *V.* **keratectomy**.

probability *n* (*pl* **-ties**) probabilidad

f
probably *adv* probablemente
probenecid *n* probenecid *m*
probiotic *n* probiótico
problem *n* problema *m*
probucol *n* probucol *m*
procainamide *n* procainamida
procaine *n* procaína
procedure *n* procedimiento; **loop electrosurgical excision — (LEEP)** conización *f* con asa diatérmica
process *n* proceso; (*anat*) apófisis *f*; **mastoid —** apófisis mastoides; **xiphoid —** apófisis xifoides
processed *adj* (*food*) procesado, industrializado
pro-choice *adj* pro-elección, a favor de la legalización del aborto voluntario
proctitis *n* proctitis *f*
prodrome *n* pródromo, malestar *m* que precede a una enfermedad
produce *vt* producir
product *n* producto
professional *adj* profesional; **— courtesy** cortesía profesional; *n* profesional *mf*; **health —** profesional de la salud, profesional sanitario (*Esp*)
profile *n* perfil *m*
progeria *n* progeria
progesterone *n* progesterona
prognosis *n* (*pl* -ses) pronóstico
prognostic *adj* pronóstico
program *n* programa *m*
progress *n* progreso; *vi* progresar
progression *n* progresión *f*
progressive *adj* progresivo
proguanil *n* proguanil *m*
projectile *n* proyectil *m*; **— vomiting** vómito(s) en proyectil, vómitos en escopetazo (*Esp*), vómitos fuertes
projection *n* (*psych, etc.*) proyección *f*
prolactin *n* prolactina
prolactinoma *n* prolactinoma *m*
prolapse *n* prolapso; **mitral-valve —** prolapso de la válvula mitral; **rectal —** prolapso rectal *or* de recto; **uterine —** prolapso uterino *or* de útero
pro-life *adj* pro-vida, en contra de la legalización del aborto voluntario

proliferate *vi* proliferar
proliferation *n* proliferación *f*
proliferar *vi* to proliferate
proliferative *adj* proliferativo
proline *n* prolina
prolong *vt* prolongar; **to prolong death**..prolongar la muerte...**to prolong life**..prolongar la vida
prolongation *n* prolongación *f*
promethazine *n* prometazina
prominence *n* prominencia; **bony —** prominencia ósea
prone *adj* (*facedown*) decúbito prono (*form, inv*), boca abajo; (*predisposed*) propenso, predispuesto; **accident-prone** propenso a sufrir accidentes
prongs *n* **nasal —** cánula nasal
proper *adj* adecuado, apropiado
prophylactic *adj* profiláctico; *n* (*ant*) preservativo, condón *m*
prophylaxis *n* profilaxis *f*; **postexposure —** profilaxis postexposición
proportion *n* proporción *f*
propoxyphene *n* propoxifeno
propranolol *n* propranolol *m*
proprioception *n* propiocepción *f*
proprioceptive *adj* propioceptivo
proptosis *n* proptosis *f*
propylene glycol *n* propilenglicol *m*
propylthiouracil *n* propiltiouracilo
prostaglandin *n* prostaglandina
prostate *n* (*fam*) glándula prostática, próstata (*fam*)
prostatectomy *n* (*pl* -mies) prostatectomía
prostatic *adj* prostático
prostatitis *n* prostatitis *f*
prosthesis *n* (*pl* -ses) prótesis *f*
prosthetic *adj* protésico, postizo
prostitute *n* prostituto -ta *mf*
protease *n* proteasa
protect *vt* proteger; **Protect your skin**..Proteja su piel; **to — against** proteger de; **to — oneself** protegerse
protection *n* protección *f*
protective *adj* protector
protector *n* protector *m*; **hearing —** protector auditivo
protein *adj* proteico; *n* proteína (*frec. pl*); **— supplement** suplemento

proteico *or* de proteínas
protocol *n* protocolo
protozoan *n* protozoo
protrude *vi* protruir, sobresalir, proyectar hacia adelante
protuberance *n* protuberancia
provide *vt* proveer, proporcionar
provider *n* proveedor -ra *mf*; **health
care** — proveedor de salud
provisional *adj* provisional
provoke *vt* provocar
proximal *adj* próximo
prune *n* ciruela pasa
pruritis *n* prurito
PSA *abbr* **prostate-specific antigen.**
V. **antigen.**
pseudo- *pref* pseudo- *or* seudo-;
[*Note: when translating the English prefix* pseudo- *the Real Academia Española recommends* seudo-
over pseudo-, *although the latter is
more common.*]
pseudoaneurysm *n* pseudoaneurisma
or seudoaneurisma *m*
pseudocyst *n* pseudoquiste *or* seudoquiste *m*; **pancreatic** — pseudoquiste *or* seudoquiste pancreático
pseudoephedrine *n* pseudoefedrina
or seudoefedrina
pseudogout *n* pseudogota *or* seudogota
pseudohypoparathyroidism *n* pseudohipoparatiroidismo *or* seudohipoparatiroidismo
pseudotumor *n* pseudotumor *or* seudotumor *m*; — **cerebri** pseudotumor *or* seudotumor cerebral
psilocybin *n* psilocibina
psittacosis *n* psitacosis *f*
psoas *n* psoas *m*
psoralen *n* psoraleno; — **plus ultraviolet A (PUVA)** psoraleno más
radiación ultravioleta A (PUVA)
psoriasis *n* psoriasis *f*
psoriatic *adj* psoriásico
psyche *n* psique *f*, psiquis *f*
psychiatric *adj* psiquiátrico
psychiatrist *n* psiquiatra *mf*
psychiatry *n* psiquiatría; **child** —
paidopsiquiatría (*form*), psiquiatría
de niños
psychoactive *adj* psicoactivo
psychoanalysis *n* psicoanálisis *m*,

análisis *m* (*fam*)
psychoanalyst *n* psicoanalista *mf*,
analista *mf* (*fam*)
psychoanalyze *vt* psicoanalizar
psychogenic *adj* psicógeno
psychological *adj* psicológico
psychologist *n* psicólogo -ga *mf*
psychology *n* psicología
psychomotor *adj* psicomotor
psychopath *n* psicópata *mf*
psychosis *n* (*pl* **-ses**) psicosis *f*
psychosocial *adj* psicosocial
psychosomatic *adj* psicosomático
psychotherapist *n* psicoterapeuta *mf*
psychotherapy *n* psicoterapia
psychotic *adj* & *n* psicótico -ca *mf*
psychotropic *adj* & *n* psicotrópico
psyllium *n* psilio
PTCA *abbr* **percutaneous transluminal coronary angioplasty.** *V.*
angioplasty.
PTH *abbr* **parathyroid hormone.** *V.*
hormone.
pterygium *n* pterigión *m*, carnosidad
f (*en el ojo*)
ptomaine *n* tomaína
ptosis *n* ptosis *f*
PT *abbr* **prothrombin time.** *V.* **time.**
PTT *abbr* **partial thromboplastin
time.** *V.* **time.**
pubertal *adj* puberal
puberty *n* pubertad *f*; **precocious** —
pubertad precoz
pubic *adj* púbico, pubiano; — **area**
pubis *m*
public *adj* público
pudendal *adj* pudendo
puerperal *adj* puerperal
puerperium *n* puerperio
puff *n* (*fam, on an inhaler*) inhalación *f*, puff *m* (*Ang*)
puffy *adj* (*comp* **-fier**; *super* **-fiest**)
hinchado
puke (*vulg*) *V.* **vomit.**
pull *n* tirón *m*; **muscle** — (*también*
pulled muscle) distensión *f* (muscular), tirón (muscular) (*fam*); *vt* **to**
— **a muscle** sufrir una distensión
(muscular), sufrir un tirón (muscular)
pulmonary *adj* pulmonar
pulmonic *adj* pulmonar
pulmonologist *n* neumólogo -ga *mf*,

neumonólogo -ga *mf* (*SA*), médico -ca *mf* especialista en los pulmones y sus enfermedades, especialista *mf* de los pulmones (*fam*)

pulmonology *n* neumología, neumonología (*SA*), estudio de los pulmones y sus enfermedades

pulsation *n* pulsación *f*

pulse *n* pulso; **I'm going to take your pulse**..Voy a tomarle el pulso; **carotid —, radial —**, etc. pulso carotídeo, pulso radial, etc.

pulse oximetry *n* oximetría de pulso (*Amer*), pulsioximetría (*Esp*)

pumice stone *n* piedra pómez

pump *n* bomba; **breast —** sacaleches *m*, tiraleche *m* (*esp. Mex*); **insulin —** bomba de insulina; *vt* (*blood*) bombear, impulsar (*la sangre*)

puncture *n* punción *f* (*form*), pinchazo, piquete *m* (*Mex*); **lumbar —** punción lumbar; *vt* puncionar (*form*), punzar, pinchar, picar (*Mex*)

pupil *n* (*of the eye*) pupila (*del ojo*)

pure *adj* puro

purée *n* puré *m*

purgative (*ant*) *adj* purgante; *n* purgante *m*, purga

purge *n* (*ant*) purga

purification *n* purificación *f*, depuración *f*

purified *adj* purificado, depurado

purifier *n* purificador *m*, depurador *m*

purify *vt* (*pret & pp* **-fied**) purificar, depurar

purine *n* purina

purple *adj* morado

purpura *n* púrpura; **Henoch-Schönlein —** púrpura de Schönlein-Henoch; **idiopathic thrombocytopenic — (ITP)** púrpura trombocitopénica idiopática (PTI); **throm-**botic thrombocytopenic — (TTP) púrpura trombocitopénica trombótica (PTT)

purse *vt* (*one's lips*) fruncir (*los labios*)

pus *n* pus *m*

push *vi* (*obst*) pujar, empujar; **Take a deep breath and push!**..¡Respire profundo y puje!

push-up *n* flexión *f* (de brazo *or* pecho), lagartija

pustule *n* pústula

put *vt* (*pret & pp* **put**; *ger* **putting**) **to — on** (*clothing*) ponerse (*ropa*); **Put on this gown so that it opens over your back**..Póngase esta bata con la abertura hacia atrás; **to — on lipstick** pintarse los labios; **to — on makeup** maquillarse; **to — on nail polish** pintarse las uñas

PUVA *abbr* **psoralen plus ultraviolet A**. *V*. **psoralen**.

PVC *abbr* **premature ventricular contraction**. *V*. **contraction**.

pyelogram *n* urografía (*estudio imagenológico*); **intravenous — (IVP)** urografía intravenosa

pyelography *n* urografía (*técnica imagenológica*)

pyelonephritis *n* pielonefritis *f*

pyloric *adj* pilórico

pyloroplasty *n* (*pl* **-ties**) piloroplastia

pylorus *n* píloro

pyoderma gangrenosum *n* pioderma gangrenoso

pyogenic *adj* piógeno

pyorrhea *n* piorrea

pyrantel *n* pirantel *m*

pyrazinamide *n* pirazinamida

pyrethrin *n* piretrina

pyridoxine *n* piridoxina, vitamina B_6

pyrimethamine *n* pirimetamina

Q

quack n (*fam*) matasanos *mf*, charlatán -tana *mf*
quadrant n cuadrante *m*
quadriceps n cuádriceps *m*
quadriplegia n tetraplejía, cuadriplejía (*esp. SA*)
quadriplegic adj & n tetrapléjico -ca *mf*, cuadripléjico -ca *mf* (*esp. SA*)
quadruplet n cuatrillizo -za *mf*
quality n (*pl* -ties) calidad *f*; — of life calidad de vida
quantity n cantidad *f*
quarantine n cuarentena; *vt* poner en cuarentena
quart n cuarto (de galón)
quarter n cuarta parte, cuarto; **a quarter of a tablet**..la cuarta parte de una tableta
queasy adj (*comp* -ier; *super* -iest) con un poco de náusea, que tiene

náuseas; **I feel queasy** o **My stomach is queasy**..Siento un poco de náusea.
quetiapine n quetiapina
quickening n primeros movimientos fetales percibidos por la embarazada
quiet vi **to — down** tranquilizarse, calmarse
quinacrine n quinacrina, mepacrina (*OMS*)
quinapril n quinapril *m*
quinidine n quinidina
quinine n quinina
quintuplet n quintillizo -za *mf*
quit vt (*pret & pp* quit; *ger* quitting) dejar de, (*to discontinue*) suspender; **You need to quit drinking**.. Tiene que dejar de beber (tomar).

R

rabeprazole n rabeprazol *m*
rabid adj rabioso, con el mal de rabia
rabies n rabia
raccoon n mapache *m*
race n (*of people*) raza; *vi* (*one's heart*) latir rápido (el corazón)
radial adj (*anat*) radial
radiate vi (*pain*) irradiarse, (*heat*) irradiar
radiation n radiación *f*; **ionizing —** radiación ionizante

radical adj radical
radiculopathy n radiculopatía; **cervical —** radiculopatía cervical
radii *pl de* radius
radioactive adj radiactivo
radioactivity n radiactividad *f*
radiography n radiografía
radioiodine n radioyodo
radioisotope n radioisótopo
radiologist n radiólogo -ga *mf*, médico -ca *mf* especialista en las imáge-

nes diagnósticas

radiology *n* radiología, estudio de las imágenes diagnósticas

radionuclide *n* radionúclido

radiotherapy *n* radioterapia

radium *n* radio

radius *n* (*pl* **radii**) radio

radon *n* radón *m*

rage *n* ira, furia; furia en la carretera (*se aplica a conductores furiosos que pierden el control de sus emociones y atacan a otros automovilistas*)

ragweed *n* (*bot*) ambrosía

raise *vt* levantar, elevar; (*a child*) criar; **Raise your leg**..Levante su pierna...**This medicine may raise your sugar**..Esta medicina le puede elevar el azúcar.

raloxifene *n* raloxifeno

ramipril *n* ramipril *m*

ran *pret de* **run**

random *adj* aleatorio; **in random fashion**..en forma aleatoria; **at —** al azar

range *n* rango; **in normal —** en rango normal; **— of motion** rango de movimiento; **— of values** rango de valores

ranitidine *n* ranitidina

rape *n* violación *f* (*sexual*); **date —** violación por acompañante (*de cita*); *vt* violar

rapid *adj* rápido

rare *adj* raro, poco común; (*meat*) poco cocido *or* cocinado, poco hecho (*Esp*)

rarely *adv* raras veces

rash *n* erupción cutánea (*form*), erupción de la piel, (*esp. due to heat or chafing*) sarpullido (*fam*), salpullido (*esp. Mex, fam*); **diaper —** dermatitis *f* del pañal

rat *n* rata

rate *n* tasa, frecuencia; **basal metabolic —** tasa de metabolismo basal; **birth —** tasa de natalidad, natalidad *f*; **death —** tasa de mortalidad, mortalidad *f*; **heart —** frecuencia cardíaca; **infant mortality —** tasa de mortalidad infantil; **respiratory —** frecuencia respiratoria

ratio *n* (*math*) razón *f*; **international**

normalized — (INR) razón internacional normalizada (INR)

ration *n* ración *f*

rationalization *n* (*psych*) racionalización *f*

rationalize *vi* (*psych*) racionalizar

rattlesnake *n* serpiente *f* de cascabel

raw *adj* (*food*) crudo; (*skin, mucous membrane*) excoriado (*form*), pelado

ray *n* rayo; **the sun's rays** los rayos del sol

Raynaud's phenomenon *n* fenómeno de Raynaud

razor *n* navaja (de afeitar), rasuradora, rastrillo (*Mex*), cuchilla (de afeitar) (*esp. Esp*); **— blade** hoja de afeitar

RDA *V.* **recommended dietary allowance**.

reach *n* alcance *m*; **out of — of children** fuera del alcance de los niños; *vt, vi* alcanzar

react *vi* reaccionar

reaction *n* reacción *f*; **adverse —** reacción adversa; **allergic —** reacción alérgica; **conversion —** histeria de conversión; **cross —** reacción cruzada; **delayed —** reacción tardía; **polymerase chain — (PCR)** reacción en cadena de la polimerasa; **transfusion —** reacción transfusional

reactivate *vt* reactivar

reactivation *n* reactivación *f*

reactive *adj* reactivo

reactivity *n* reactividad *f*

read *vt, vi* (*pret & pp* **read**) leer; **to — lips** leer los labios

reading *n* (*of an instrument*) lectura

reagent *n* reactivo

reality *n* (*pl* **-ties**) realidad *f*

reason *n* razón *f*

reattach *vt* reconectar, recolocar, volver a unir

rebound *n* rebote *m*; **— hypertension** hipertensión *f* de rebote

recall *n* recuerdo, memoria a corto plazo, capacidad *f* para recordar; (*of a defective product*) retirada (*de un producto defectuoso*); *vt* recordar; (*a defective product*) retirar

receding hairline *n* entradas

recently *adv* recientemente, últimamente

receptionist *n* recepcionista *mf*

receptor *n* receptor *m*; **estrogen receptor-positive** positivo para receptores de estrógeno

recessive *adj* recesivo

recipient *n* (*of a transfusion, transplant, etc.*) receptor -ra *mf* (*de una transfusión, un trasplante, etc.*)

recognition *n* reconocimiento

recognize *vt* reconocer

recombinant *adj* recombinante

recommend *vt* recomendar

recommendation *n* recomendación *f*

recommended dietary allowance (RDA) *n* dosis diaria recomendada

reconnect *vt* reconectar

reconsitution *n* reconstitución *f*; **immune** — reconstutición inmunológica *or* inmune

reconstruct *vt* reconstruir

reconstruction *n* reconstrucción *f*

reconstructive *adj* reconstructivo

record *n* (*medical*) historia clínica, historial médico, expediente (clínico) (*Mex, CA*); (*of temperatures, etc.*) registro; **electronic medical** — historia clínica electrónica

recourse *n* recurso

recover *vt, vi* recuperar(se)

recovery *n* recuperación *f*

recreation *n* recreación *f*, (*esp. during school*) recreo

recreational *adj* recreacional; — **use of drugs** uso recreacional de drogas

recta *pl de* **rectum**

rectal *adj* rectal; *n* (*fam*) tacto rectal

rectocele *n* rectocele *m*

rectum *n* (*pl* **-ta** *o* **-tums**) recto

recumbent *adj* decúbito (*form, inv*), recostado

recuperate *vi* recuperarse

recuperation *n* recuperación *f*

recur *vi* (*pret & pp* **recurred**; *ger* **recurring**) recurrir (*form*), volver a ocurrir

recurrence *n* recidiva (*form*), recurrencia

recurrent *adj* recurrente, recidivante (*Esp, form*)

recycle *vt* reciclar

recycling *n* reciclaje *m*

red *adj* (*comp* **redder**; *super* **reddest**) rojo; **Red Crescent** Media Luna Roja; **Red Cross** Cruz Roja

reddish *adj* rojizo

redness *n* rubor *m* (*form*), enrojecimiento

reduce *vt* reducir, disminuir, bajar; (*ortho*) reducir; *vi* (*fam, to lose weight*) perder peso, bajar de peso

reducible *adj* reductible, reducible (*esp. Esp*)

reduction *n* reducción *f*

reevaluate *vt* reevaluar

refeeding *n* realimentación *f*

refer *vt* (*pret & pp* **referred**; *ger* **referring**) (*a patient*) referir, remitir (*esp. Esp*), mandar a ver a un especialista

reference *n* referencia

referral *n* remisión *f*

referred *adj* (*pain*) referido

refill (*pharm*) *n* renovación *f*, relleno (*Ang*), refill *m* (*Ang*), nuevo surtido, nuevo surtido de medicamento autorizado anteriormente en la receta médica, autorización *f* para surtidos adicionales en el futuro; **Why didn't you get a refill?**..¿Por qué no obtuvo un nuevo surtido de medicamento (autorizado anteriormente en la receta médica)?...**I'm giving you three refills so you won't have to see me for four months**.. Le estoy dando tres autorizaciones para surtidos nuevos para que no necesite consultarme durante cuatro meses; *vt* renovar, rellenar (*Ang*), refill (*Ang*); (*pharmacist as subject*) surtir(le) (*un medicamento*) de nuevo (de acuerdo con una receta hecha previamente); (*physician as subject*) autorizar un nuevo surtido (*de medicamento*); **The pharmacist can refill your digoxin without your having to see me**.. El farmacéutico puede surtirle de nuevo su digoxina sin que Ud. necesite consultarme...**Dr. Jones can refill your atenolol**..La doctora Jones le puede autorizar un nuevo surtido de su atenolol; [*Note:The U.S. system of authorizing future refills of me-*

dication is rare in Latin America and often requires considerable explanation. Eventually the English word refill *will probably become universal among Spanish-speaking persons living in the U.S.*]

reflex *n* reflejo; **conditioned** — reflejo condicionado; **gag** — reflejo nauseoso; **patellar** — reflejo rotuliano; — **hammer** martillo de reflejos; **startle** — reflejo de sobresalto

reflexology *n* reflexología

reflux *n* reflujo; **acid** — reflujo de ácido; **esophageal** — reflujo gastroesofágico

refraction *n* refracción *f*

refractive error *n* defecto de refracción

refractory *adj* resistente al tratamiento

refrigerate *vt* refrigerar

refrigeration *n* refrigeración *f*

refrigerator *n* refrigerador *m*

regain *vt* recuperar; **to** — **consciousness** volver en sí, recobrar el conocimiento; **to** — **weight** recuperar peso

regenerate *vi* regenerarse

regeneration *n* regeneración *f*

regimen *n* régimen *m*

region *n* región *f*

regional *adj* regional

registry *n* registro; **tumor** — registro de tumores

regression *n* (*psych, oncology, etc.*) regresión *f*

regular *adj* regular

regurgitate *vt* regurgitar, vomitar sin esfuerzo

regurgitation *n* regurgitación *f*; (*insufficiency*) insuficiencia; **aortic** —, **mitral** —, **etc.** insuficiencia aórtica, insuficiencia mitral, etc.

rehabilitate *vt* rehabilitar; **to become rehabilitated** rehabilitarse

rehabilitation *n* rehabilitación *f*

rehydrate *vt* rehidratar

rehydration *n* rehidratación *f*

reinfected *adj* reinfectado, infectado de nuevo

reinfection *n* reinfección *f*

reinforce *vt* reforzar

reinforcement *n* refuerzo

reject *vt* rechazar

rejection *n* rechazo

rejuvenate *vt* rejuvenecer; **to become rejuvenated** rejuvenecerse

relapse *n* recidiva (*form*), recaída; *vi* recaer

related *adj* emparentado; **She is related to me**..Es pariente mía; — **donor** donante emparentado, donante que es familiar de uno

relation *n* relación *f*; (*relative*) familiar *m*, pariente *mf*

relationship *n* relación *f*

relative *n* familiar *m*, pariente *mf*; **blood** — pariente consanguíneo (*form*), pariente de sangre

relax *vt* relajar, aflojar; **Relax your leg**..Relaje (Afloje) la pierna; *vi* relajar(se); **Relax**..Relájese.

relaxant *n* relajante *m*; **muscle** — relajante muscular

relaxation *n* relajación *f*, (*rest*) descanso; — **techniques** técnicas de relajación

relaxing *adj* relajante

release *n* liberación *f*; **carpal tunnel** — liberación del túnel carpiano; **controlled-release** de liberación controlada; **extended-release** de liberación prolongada; **slow-release** de liberación prolongada or lenta; **sustained-release** de liberación sostenida; **timed-release** de liberación controlada; *vt* liberar; **copper-releasing, hormone-releasing, etc.** liberador de cobre, liberador de hormona, etc.

reliability *n* fiabilidad *f*

reliable *adj* confiable, fiable

relief *n* alivio; (*aid*) ayuda, socorro, auxilio

relieve *vt* aliviar

REM *abbr* **rapid eye movement**. *V.* **movement**.

remedy *n* (*pl* -**dies**) remedio; **cough** — remedio para la tos; **home** — remedio casero

remember *vt* recordar

remission *n* remisión *f*; **complete** — remisión completa; **partial** — remisión parcial; **to go into** — entrar en remisión

remodeling *n* remodelamiento, remodelación *f*; **bone** — remodelamiento óseo, remodelación ósea; **cardiac** — remodelamiento cardíaco, remodelación cardíaca

remorse *n* remordimiento

removable *adj* removible, que se puede quitar

removal *n* extracción *f*, eliminación *f*, retirada; **tattoo** — eliminación de tatuajes

remove *vt* extraer (*form*), remover, quitar, sacar, (*a catheter, monitor, etc.*) retirar

renal *adj* renal

renew *vt* renovar

renovascular *adj* renovascular

repair *n* reparación *f*; *vt* reparar, arreglar (*fam*)

repeat *vt* repetir

repellent *n* repelente *m*; **insect** — repelente de insectos

repetition *n* repetición *f*

repetitive *adj* repetitivo

replace *vt* reemplazar, sustituir (*V. también* **substitute**.)

replacement *n* sustitución *f*, (*joint*) artroplastia; **aortic valve** —, **mitral valve** —, **etc.** sustitución valvular aórtica, sustitución valvular mitral, etc; **total hip** — prótesis *f* total de cadera; **total knee** — prótesis *f* total de rodilla

report *vt* reportar, declarar; **The law requires me to report your condition to the Public Health Department**..La ley me exige reportar su enfermedad al Departamento de Salud Pública.

reportable *adj* (*disease*) de declaración obligatoria

repress *vt* (*psych*) reprimir

repression *n* (*psych*) represión *f*

reproduce *vt, vi* reproducir(se)

reproduction *n* reproducción *f*; **assisted** — reproducción asistida

reproductive *adj* reproductivo, reproductor

reschedule *vt* (*an appointment*) reprogramar, cambiar (*una cita*) para otra fecha

rescue *n* rescate *m*, salvamento; **air** — rescate aéreo; *vt* rescatar, salvar

rescuer *n* socorrista *mf*, rescatador -ra *mf*

research *n* investigación *f*; **stem cell** — investigación de células madres

resect *vt* extirpar, resecar, quitar con cirugía

resection *n* resección *f*; **lymph node** — vaciamiento ganglionar; **transurethral** — **of the prostate (TURP)** resección transuretral de (la) próstata

reserpine *n* reserpina

reserve *n* reserva

reservoir *n* reservorio

resident *n* residente *mf*; (*physician*) médico -ca *mf* residente, residente *mf*; **family practice** —, **surgical** —, **etc.** residente de medicina familiar, residente de cirugía, etc.

residual *adj* residual

residue *n* residuo

resin *n* resina

resist *vt* resistir

resistance *n* resistencia; **cross-resistance** resistencia cruzada; **insulin** — resistencia a la insulina

resistant *adj* resistente; **methicillin-resistant** resistente a la meticilina

resolution *n* resolución *f*; **high** — alta resolución

resolve *vi* resolverse

resorb *vt* reabsorber; **to get resorbed** reabsorberse

resorption *n* reabsorción *f*

resort *n* recurso; **last** — último recurso

resource *n* recurso

respect *n* respeto; *vt* respetar

respiration *n* respiración *f*

respirator *n* mascarilla *or* máscara (para filtrar el aire); (*ventilator*) respirador *m*, ventilador *m*, aparato para suministrar respiración artificial

respiratory *adj* respiratorio

respire *vt, vi* respirar

respond *vi* responder

response *n* respuesta; **complete** — respuesta completa; **immune** — respuesta inmune; **partial** — respuesta parcial; **sustained** — respuesta sostenida

rest *n* descanso, reposo; (*remaining portion*) demás, resto; **the rest of**

the pills..las demás pastillas..el resto de las pastillas; **at** — en reposo; **bed** — reposo en cama; *vt, vi* descansar, reposar

restenosis *n* reestenosis *f*

resting *adj* en reposo; — **heart rate** frecuencia cardíaca en reposo

restless *adj* inquieto, intranquilo

restoration *n* (*dent, surg*) restauración *f*

restorative *adj* (*dent, surg*) restaurativo

restore *vt* restablecer, (*dent, surg*) restaurar

restrain *vt* (*a patient*) sujetar (*a un paciente*)

restraints *npl* (*también* **physical** —) ataduras, cintas para limitar los movimientos de un paciente agitado

restrict *vt* restringir, limitar

restriction *n* restricción *f*, limitación *f*; (**medical**) **work** — limitación de trabajo (por indicaciones médicas)

restroom *n* baño

result *n* resultado

resume *vt* reanudar, volver a tomar *or* hacer

resurfacing *n* exfoliación (profunda); **laser skin** — exfoliación por láser

resuscitate *vt* reanimar, resucitar; **Do Not Resuscitate (DNR)** no reanimar (NR); **DNR order** orden *f* de no reanimar (ONR)

resuscitation *n* reanimación *f*; **cardiopulmonary** — **(CPR)** reanimación cardiopulmonar (RCP)

resynchronization *n* resincronización *f*; **cardiac** — resincronización cardíaca

retain *vt* retener; **to** — **water** retener agua

retainer *n* (*orthodontia*) retenedor *m*

retardation *n* retraso, retardo; **intrauterine growth** — retraso *or* retardo del crecimiento intrauterino, crecimiento intrauterino retardado (*Esp*); **mental** — (*ant*) retraso mental

retarded *adj* retrasado; **mentally** — (*ant*) retrasado mental

retch *vi* vomitar sin nada que expulsar

retching *n* arcadas (*form*), vómito sin nada que expulsar

retention *n* retención *f*; **urinary** — retención urinaria

reticulocyte *n* reticulocito

retina *n* (*pl* **-nas** *o* **-nae**) retina; **detached** — desprendimiento de retina

retinal *adj* retiniano

retinitis *n* retinitis *f*; — **pigmentosa** retinitis pigmentaria *or* pigmentosa

retinoblastoma *n* retinoblastoma *m*

retinoic acid *n* ácido retinoico

retinoid *n* retinoide *m*

retinol *n* retinol *m*

retinopathy *n* retinopatía; **diabetic** — retinopatía diabética

retraining *n* reentrenamiento

retrograde *adj* retrógrado

retroperitoneal *adj* retroperitoneal

retroviral *adj* retroviral

retrovirus *n* retrovirus *m*

reusable *adj* reusable

revaccination *n* revacunación *f*

revascularization *n* revascularización *f*

reversal *n* reversión *f*; **vasectomy** — reversión de vasectomía

reversible *adj* reversible

review of systems *n* revisión *f* por sistemas

revision *n* revisión *f*

revitalize *vt* revitalizar

revitalizing *adj* revitalizante, revitalizador

revive *vt* reanimar; *vi* reanimar(se), revivir

rhabdomyolysis *n* rabdomiólisis *or* rabdomiolisis *f*

rhabdomyoma *n* rabdomioma *m*

rhabdomyosarcoma *n* rabdomiosarcoma *m*

rheumatic *adj* reumático

rheumatism *n* reumatismo, reuma *m*; **palindromic** — reumatismo palindrómico

rheumatoid *adj* reumatoide

rheumatologist *n* reumatólogo -ga *mf*, médico -ca *mf* especialista en las enfermedades que afectan las articulaciones, especialista *mf* de las coyunturas (*fam*)

rheumatology *n* reumatología, estudio de las enfermedades que afec-

tan las articulaciones
rhinitis *n* rinitis *f*; **allergic —** rinitis alérgica
rhinophyma *n* rinofima *m*
rhinoplasty *n* (*pl* **-ties**) rinoplastia
rhinovirus *n* rinovirus *m*
rhythm *n* ritmo; **— method** abstinencia periódica, método del ritmo
rib *n* costilla; **— cage** caja torácica
ribavirin *n* ribavirina
riboflavin *n* riboflavina, vitamina B_2
ribonucleic acid (RNA) *n* ácido ribonucleico (ARN)
rice *n* arroz *m*
rich *adj* rico; (*food*) rico, rico en grasa; **— in protein** rico en proteínas
ricin *n* ricina
rickets *n* raquitismo
rifabutin *n* rifabutina
rifampin *n* rifampicina
rifamycin *n* rifamicina
rifaximin *n* rifaximina
right *adj* derecho; *n* (*right-hand side*) derecha; (*legal, moral*) derecho
right-handed *adj* diestro (*form*), que escribe con la mano derecha; **Are you right-handed or left-handed?** ..¿Escribe Ud. con la mano derecha o la izquierda?
rigid *adj* rígido
rigidity *n* rigidez *f*
rigor mortis *n* rigor mortis *m*
rimantadine *n* rimantadina
ring *n* anillo; **vaginal —** anillo vaginal
ringing *n* (*in ear, etc.*) zumbido
ringworm *n* tinea corporis (*form*), tiña del cuerpo
rinse *n* enjuage *m*; *vt* enjuagar
ripe *adj* (*fruit*) maduro
rise *n* aumento, elevación *f*; *vi* (*pret* **rose**; *pp* **risen**) subir(se), elevar(se); (*to get up*) levantarse; **Your sugar rose**..Su azúcar subió.
risedronate *n* risedronato
risk *n* riesgo; **calculated —** riesgo calculado; **high-risk** de alto riesgo; **low-risk** de bajo riesgo; **— factor** factor *m* de riesgo; **risks and benefits** riesgos y beneficios; **to run the — of** correr el riesgo de; **to take a — arriesgarse; *vt* arriesgar
risperidone *n* risperidona

ritonavir *n* ritonavir *m*
ritual *n* ritual *m*
rivalry *n* rivalidad *f*; **sibling —** rivalidad entre hermanos
rizatriptan *n* rizatriptán *m*
RNA *V.* **ribonucleic acid.**
roast *vt* asar
robotic *adj* robótico
rock climbing *n* escalada
rod *n* (*bacteria*) bacilo; (*of the eye*) bastón *m*; (*ortho*) barra; **Harrington —** barra de Harrington
rodent *n* roedor *m*
rodenticide *n* raticida *m*, veneno para ratas y animales parecidos
rofecoxib *n* rofecoxib *m*
role *n* papel *m*; **— model** modelo a seguir
roll *vi* **to — over** voltearse, darse vuelta; **Now roll over**..Ahora voltéese (dese vuelta); **to — up** (*one's sleeve, pants leg, etc.*) arremangarse, subirse la manga; **Roll up your sleeve**..Arremánguese..Súbase la manga.
roof of the mouth *n* paladar *m*
room *n* habitación *f*, cuarto, sala; **the patient's room**..la habitación (el cuarto) del paciente; **delivery —** sala de partos; **emergency — (ER)** sala de urgencias; **operating — (OR)** quirófano, sala de operaciones; **recovery —** sala de recuperación; **waiting —** sala de espera
root *n* raíz *f*; **hair —** raíz del pelo; **nerve —** raíz nerviosa; **— canal** (*fam*) root canal therapy, *V.* **therapy**; **tooth — o — of the tooth** raíz del diente
rosacea *n* acné rosácea (*form*), rosácea
rose *pret de* **rise**
rosemary *n* (*bot*) romero
roseola infantum *n* exantema súbito
rosiglitazone *n* rosiglitazona
rosuvastatin *n* rosuvastatina
rot *vt, vi* (*pret & pp* **rotted**; *ger* **rotting**) pudrir(se)
rotator cuff *n* manguito de los rotadores
rotten *adj* podrido
rough *adj* (*skin, etc.*) áspero
roughage *n* fibra

roughness *n* aspereza

round *adj* redondo; *npl* pase *m* de visita, rondas; **to make rounds** *o* **to round** pasar visita

roundworm *n* áscaris *m*, (tipo de) lombriz intestinal

rouse *vt* despertar, despertar agresivamente

route *n* vía; — **of administration** vía de administración

routine *adj* rutinario; *n* rutina; **daily** — rutina diaria

rub *vt* (*pret & pp* **rubbed**; *ger* **rubbing**) frotar; (*to massage*) masajear, sobar (*Amer*); (*to chafe*) rozar; *vi* rozar

rubber *n* goma, hule *m* (*esp. Mex, CA*); (*fam, condom*) preservativo, condón *m*

rubella *n* rubéola

rubeola *n* (*form*) sarampión *m*

rule *n* regla; *vt* **to** — **out** descartar; **Cancer was ruled out**..Se descartó el cáncer.

rum *n* ron *m*

run *vi* (*pret* **ran**; *pp* **run**; *ger* **running**) correr; **to** — **in one's family** venir de familia; **to** — **out** acabarse; **When did your medicine run out?**..¿Cuándo se le acabó la medicina? **to** — **over** atropellar, arrollar

runaway *n* niño -ña *mf* que ha abandonado el hogar

run down *adj* debilitado, agotado

runner *n* corredor -ra *mf*

runny *adj* (*comp* **-nier**; *super* **-niest**) líquido, de consistencia líquida; **to have a** — **nose** gotearle la nariz, tener flujo nasal, tener escurrimiento nasal (*esp. Mex*)

runs, the (*fam*) diarrea

rupture *n* ruptura, rotura; **premature** — **of membranes** ruptura *or* rotura prematura de membranas; *vt, vi* reventar(se); **ruptured appendix** ruptura del apéndice

rural *adj* rural

rusty *adj* oxidado; — **nail** clavo oxidado

Rx *n* receta

S

sac *n* (*anat*) saco

saccharin *n* sacarina

sacra *pl de* **sacrum**

sacral *adj* sacro

sacroiliac *adj* sacroilíaco, sacroiliaco (*esp. Mex*)

sacrum *n* (*pl* **-cra**) sacro

sad *adj* (*comp* **sadder**; *super* **saddest**) triste

sadism *n* sadismo

sadist *n* sádico -ca *mf*

sadistic *adj* sádico

sadness *n* tristeza

sadomasochism *n* sadomasoquismo

sadomasochist *n* sadomasoquista *mf*

safe *adj* seguro, sin riesgo

safety *n* seguridad *f*; — **pin** imperdible *m*, seguro (*Mex*)

sag *vi* (*pret & pp* **sagged**; *ger* **sagging**) caerse

sage *n* (*bot*) salvia

salad *n* ensalada

salbutamol *n* salbutamol *m*
salicylate *n* salicilato
salicylic acid *n* ácido salicílico
saline *adj* salino
saliva *n* saliva
salivary *adj* salival
salivation *n* salivación *f*
salmeterol *n* salmeterol *m*
salmonellosis *n* salmonelosis *f*
salpingitis *n* salpingitis *f*
salpingo-oophorectomy *n* (*pl* -**mies**) salpingooforectomía
salsalate *n* salsalato
salt *n* sal *f*; **Epsom** — sal de Epsom, sulfato de magnesio; **iodized** — sal yodada; **smelling salts** carbonato de amonio (*que se utiliza para reanimar a un desmayado*)
salted *adj* salado, que tiene sal
saltine *n* galleta salada
salty *adj* salado
salvage *adj* de rescate; — **therapy** tratamiento de rescate; *n* rescate *m*, salvamento; *vt* salvar, rescatar
salve *n* ungüento, pomada, bálsamo
sample *n* muestra
sanatorium *n* sanatorio
sandfly *n* (*pl* -**flies**) flebótomo, (tipo de) mosquito
sane *adj* cuerdo
sanitary *adj* higiénico; sanitario; — **napkin** toalla sanitaria *or* femenina
sanitation *n* saneamiento (ambiental), medidas sanitarias, sanidad *f*; **Department of Sanitation** Departamento de Sanidad
sanity *n* cordura, juicio
saphenous *adj* safeno
saquinavir *n* saquinavir *m*
sarcoidosis *n* sarcoidosis *f*
sarcoma *n* sarcoma *m*; **Ewing's** — sarcoma de Ewing; **Kaposi's** — sarcoma de Kaposi
sarin *n* sarín *m*
SARS *abbr* **severe acute respiratory syndrome** . *V.* **syndrome**.
sarsaparilla *n* (*bot*) zarzaparrilla
sassafras *n* (*bot*) sasafrás *m*
sat *pret & pp de* **sit**
satiety *n* saciedad *f*
saturate *vt* saturar
saturated *adj* saturado

sauna *n* sauna *m&f*
save *vt* salvar; **We want to save your leg**..Queremos salvar su pierna.
saw *pret de* **see**
saw palmetto *n* (*bot*) Serenoa repens, especie de palma nativa de los Estados Unidos
scab *n* costra
scabies *n* escabiosis *f* (*form*), sarna; **Norwegian** — sarna noruega
scald *n* escaldadura; *vt* escaldar; **to** — **oneself** escaldarse
scalding *n* escaldadura
scale *n* (*for weighing*) balanza, báscula; (*piece of skin*) escama; (*of measurement*) escala; **pain** — escala del dolor; **sliding** — escala móvil; *vt* (*dent*) eliminar el sarro
scaling *n* (*derm*) descamación *f*; (*dent*) eliminación *f* del sarro
scalp *n* cuero cabelludo
scalpel *n* bisturí *m*
scaly *adj* (*comp* -**ier**; *super* -**iest**) escamoso
scan *n* escán *m* (*Ang*); estudio por imagen utilizando tomografía, resonancia magnética *o* gammagrafía; **bone** — gammagrafía ósea, serie ósea; **CAT** *o* **CT** — (*fam*) tomografía axial computarizada, tomografía computarizada, TAC *m&f* (*fam*), TC *m&f* (*fam*); **gallium** — gammagrafía con galio; **nuclear** — gammagrafía; **PET** — (*fam*) tomografía por emisión de positrones, PET *m* (*fam*); **thallium** — gammagrafía con talio; *vt* (*pret & pp* **scanned**; *ger* **scanning**) escanear (*Ang*); realizar un estudio por imagen utilizando tomografía, resonancia magnética o gammagrafía
scanner *n* escáner *m* (*Ang*), aparato que produce imágenes del cuerpo
scapula *n* (*pl* -**lae**) escápula, omóplato *or* omoplato, paleta (*fam*)
scar *n* cicatriz *f*; **to leave a scar**.. dejar cicatriz
scare *n* susto
scarlatina *n* (*form*) escarlatina
scarring *adj* que deja cicatriz; *n* cicatrización *f*, cicatrices *fpl*
schedule *n* horario; **vaccination** — esquema de vacunación, calenda-

rio de vacunación (*Esp, SA*), calendario vacunal (*Esp*)

scheduled *adj* (*appointment etc.*) programado

schistosomiasis *n* esquistosomiasis *f*

schizoaffective *adj* esquizoafectivo

schizophrenia *n* esquizofrenia; **paranoid** — esquizofrenia paranoide

schizophrenic *adj & n* esquizofrénico -ca *mf*

school *n* escuela; **medical** — facultad *f* de medicina, escuela de medicina (*fam*)

sciatic *adj* ciático

sciatica *n* ciática

scientific *adj* científico

scientist *n* científico -ca *mf*

scissors *npl* tijeras; **a pair of scissors**..unas tijeras

sclera *n* (*pl* -rae) esclerótica

scleritis *n* escleritis *f*

scleroderma *n* esclerodermia

sclerosing *adj* esclerosante

sclerosis *n* esclerosis *f*; **amyotrophic lateral** — esclerosis lateral amiotrófica; **multiple** — esclerosis múltiple; **progressive systemic** — esclerosis sistémica progresiva; **tuberous** — esclerosis tuberosa

sclerotherapy *n* escleroterapia

scoliosis *n* escoliosis *f*

scooter *n* motoneta

scopolamine *n* escopolamina

score *n* índice *m*, valor *m*, puntaje *m*, valoración *f*; **Apgar** — índice *or* puntaje de Apgar, valoración de Apgar (*Mex*), Apgar *m* (*fam*); **T-score** valor T; **Z-score** valor Z

scored *adj* (*pharm*) ranurado

scorpion *n* alacrán *m* (*esp. Amer*), escorpión *m* (*esp. Esp*)

scrape *n* abrasión *f* (*form*), raspadura (*fam*); *vt* raspar

scratch *n* rasguño, (*by claws*) arañazo; *vt* rasguñar, arañar; (*an itch, etc.*) rascarse; **How did you scratch yourself?**..¿Cómo se rasguñó?...**You have to quit scratching**..Tiene que dejar de rascarse.

screen *n* (*también* **screening test**) examen *m* de detección; *vt, vi* realizar un examen de detección, realizar exámenes en personas que no

tienen síntomas para buscar afecciones ocultas

screening *n* cribado (*form*), despistaje *m*, detección *f*, realización de exámenes de detección; — **for cancer** (*también* **cancer** —) cribado (despistaje, detección) del cáncer

screw *n* tornillo

script (*fam*) *V*. **prescription**.

scrofula *n* escrófula

scrotal *adj* escrotal

scrotum *n* escroto

scurvy *n* escorbuto

seasickness *n* mareo (en barco)

season *n* (*winter, spring, etc.*) estación *f*; (*for a disease, etc.*) temporada; **flu** — temporada gripal (*form*), temporada de la gripe

seasonal *adj* estacional

seat *n* asiento; **Have a seat**..Siéntese.. Tome asiento; **infant car** — asiento para bebé (para el coche), asiento infantil (para vehículo) (*esp. Esp*); — **belt** cinturón *m* de seguridad

sea urchin *n* erizo de mar

sebaceous *adj* sebáceo

seborrhea *n* seborrea

seborrheic *adj* seborréico

sebum *n* sebo

second *adj* segundo; *n* segundo

secondary *adj* secundario

secretary *n* (*pl* -ries) secretario -ria *mf*

secrete *vt* segregar (*form*), secretar

secretion *n* secreción *f*

secretory *adj* secretorio

section *n* sección *f*; **frozen** — biopsia por congelación

sedate *vt* sedar, dar un sedante

sedation *n* sedación *f*; **conscious** — sedación consciente

sedative *adj & n* sedante *m*, calmante *m*

sedentary *adj* sedentario

sediment *n* sedimento

see *vt, vi* (*pret* **saw**; *pp* **seen**) ver, (*a doctor*) consultar; **When was the last time you saw an eye doctor?** ..¿Cuándo fue la última vez que consultó a un médico de los ojos?

seek *vt* **to** — **medical attention** acudir al médico

seen *pp de* **see**

segment *n* segmento

seize *vi* convulsionar (*form*), tener convulsiones, tener una convulsión, tener un ataque (epiléptico) (*fam*)

seizure *n* convulsión *f*, crisis epiléptica (*form*), ataque (epiléptico) (*fam*); **Did you have a seizure?**..¿Tuvo convulsiones?..¿Tuvo una convulsión?..¿Tuvo un ataque (epiléptico)? **absence** — crisis de ausencia; **complex partial** — crisis parcial compleja; **febrile** — convulsión febril; **focal** — crisis parcial; **generalized** — convulsión generalizada; **gran mal** — (*ant*) convulsión generalizada, crisis de gran mal (*ant*); **partial** — crisis parcial; **petit mal** — (*ant*) crisis de ausencia, (crisis de) pequeño mal (*ant*); **psychomotor** — (*ant*) crisis parcial compleja; **temporal lobe** — crisis del lóbulo temporal, crisis parcial compleja; **tonic-clonic** — convulsión *or* crisis tónico-clónica

selective *adj* selectivo

selegiline *n* selegilina

selenium *n* selenio

self-absorbed *adj* ensimismado

self-awareness *n* autoconciencia, autoconocimiento

self-catheterization *n* autosondaje *m*, colocación *f* de una sonda en la vejiga por uno mismo

self-centered *adj* egocéntrico

self-confidence *n* autoconfianza, seguridad *or* confianza en uno mismo

self-conscious *adj* cohibido

self-control *n* autocontrol *m*, control *m* de uno mismo

self-destructive *adj* autodestructivo

self-discipline *n* autodisciplina

self-esteem *n* autoestima

self-examination *n* autoexploración *f* (*form*), autoexamen *m*

self-help *n* autoayuda

self-image *n* autoimagen *f*

self-inflicted *adj* autoinfligido, provocado, hecho por uno mismo

self-limited *adj* autolimitado, que se cura solo

self-medicate *vi* automedicarse

self-prescribe *vt* autorrecetarse

self-realization *n* autorrealización *f*

self-respect *n* autorrespeto, respeto de uno mismo

self-treatment *n* autotratamiento

semen *n* semen *m*

semicircular canal *n* conducto *or* canal *m* semicircular

seminal *adj* seminal

seminoma *n* seminoma *m*

senile *adj* senil

senior citizen *n* (*US*) persona anciana, persona que recibe ciertos derechos debido a su edad mayor

senna *n* (*bot*) sen *m*

sensation *n* sensación *f*; **light touch** — tacto fino, sensibilidad *f*; — **of pain** sensación de dolor

sense *n* sentido; — **of balance** sentido del equilibrio; — **of hearing** sentido del oído; — **of sight** sentido de la vista; — **of smell** sentido del olfato; — **of taste** sentido del gusto; — **of touch** sentido del tacto

sensitive *adj* sensible; **a test sensitive for**..una prueba sensible para

sensitivity *n* (*pl* **-ties**) sensibilidad *f*

sensitize *vt* sensibilizar; **to become sensitized** sensibilizarse

sensory *adj* (*nerve*) sensitivo; (*perception*) sensorio

separate *adj* separado; *vt* separar; **Separate your legs**..Separe las piernas.

sepsis *n* sepsis *f*

septa *pl de* **septum**

septic *adj* séptico

septicemia *n* septicemia

septoplasty *n* (*pl* **-ties**) septoplastia

septum *n* (*pl* **-ta**) tabique *m*, septo; **deviated** — desviación *f* septal (*form*), tabique desviado; **interatrial** — septo *or* tabique interauricular; **interventricular** — septo *or* tabique interventricular; **nasal** — tabique nasal

sera *pl de* **serum**

serial *adj* seriado

series *n* (*pl* **series**) serie *f*

serine *n* serina

serious *adj* (*illness, condition*) grave, serio

seroconversion *n* seroconversión *f*

serological, serologic *adj* serológico

serology *n* (*pl* -gies) serología; (*test*) prueba serológica

seronegative *adj* seronegativo

seropositive *adj* seropositivo

serotonin *n* serotonina

serotype *n* serotipo

sertaconazole *n* sertaconazol *m*

sertraline *n* sertralina

serum *adj* sérico; — **sodium** sodio sérico; *n* (*pl* sera) suero

service *n* servicio; **medical services** servicios médicos; **social services** servicios sociales

serving *n* porción *f*, ración *f*; **amount per** — cantidad *f* por porción *or* ración; — **size** tamaño de porción *or* ración; **servings per container** porciones *or* raciones por envase

set *n* — **of teeth** dentadura; *vt* (*pret & pp* set; *ger* setting) (*fam, a fracture*) reducir

sever *vt* cortar, cortar completamente

severe *adj* severo, grave, (*pain*) severo, intenso

severity *n* gravedad *f*, (*pain, etc.*) intensidad *f*

sew *vt* (*pp* sewn) (*fam, to suture*) suturar, coser (*fam*)

sewage *n* aguas residuales, aguas negras

sex *n* sexo, relaciones sexuales; **oral** — sexo oral; **safe** — sexo seguro, sexo sin riesgo de infección; — **change** cambio de sexo; **to have** — tener relaciones (sexuales)

sexual *adj* sexual

sexuality *n* sexualidad *f*

shaft *n* (*hair, penis*) tallo

shake *vt* (*pret* shook; *pp* shaken) agitar, sacudir; **Shake well before using**..Agítese bien antes de usar(se) ...**You shouldn't shake your child** ..No debe sacudir a su hijo; **Shake your head from side to side to say no**..Mueva la cabeza de lado a lado para decir no; *vi* (*to tremble*) temblar

shakes, the (*fam*) temblores *mpl*

shaky *adj* (*fam*) tembloroso

shaman *n* chamán *m*, hechicero -ra *mf*, brujo -ja *mf*

shame *n* vergüenza

shampoo *n* (*pl* -poos) champú *m*; *vt, vi* (*pret & pp* -pooed) lavarse el pelo

shape *n* forma; (*condition*) condición *f*, estado; **in** — en forma, en buen estado físico; **to keep in** — mantenerse en forma

share *vt* compartir; **to** — **needles** compartir agujas, compartir jeringas, compartir jeringuillas (*Carib, Esp*)

shark *n* tiburón *m*

sharp *adj* (*pain*) agudo; (*object*) punzante, cortante, punzocortante (*esp. Mex*); (*pointed*) puntiagudo; **Sharp or dull?**..¿Puntiagudo o romo?.. ¿Pincha o no? — **object** objeto punzante, objeto cortante, objeto punzocortante

shave *vt, vi* afeitar(se)

shaver *n* (*también* electric —) máquina de afeitar, afeitadora (eléctrica), rasuradora (eléctrica) (*esp. Mex*), maquinilla de afeitar (*Esp*)

shaving *n* (*metal, etc.*) viruta

shaving cream *n* crema de afeitar

sheath *n* vaina; **nerve** — vaina nerviosa

shed *vt* (*pret & pp* shed; *ger* shedding) (*viruses, parasites, etc.*) eliminar, liberar

sheepskin *n* piel de cordero *or* oveja

sheet *n* (*bed*) sábana

shellfish *n* (*pl* -fish *o* -fishes) marisco

shell shock *n* neurosis *f* de guerra

shelter *n* refugio, centro de acogida (*Esp*); **battered women's** — refugio para mujeres maltratadas or golpeadas, centro de acogida para mujeres maltratadas (*Esp*); **homeless** — refugio *or* centro de acogida para personas sin hogar

shigellosis *n* shigelosis *f*

shin *n* espinilla; — **splints** dolor *m* de espinilla debido a ejercicio excesivo

shinbone *n* (*anat*) tibia (*form*), espinilla, canilla

shingles *n* herpes *m* zoster

shirt *n* camisa

shiver *n* escalofrío; *vi* temblar

shock *n* shock *m*, choque *m* (*esp. Mex, CA*); **anaphylactic** — shock *or* choque anafiláctico; **cardiogenic** — shock *or* choque cardiogénico; **electric** — descarga eléctrica; **hypovolemic** — shock *or* choque hipovolémico; **neurogenic** — shock *or* choque neurogénico; **septic** — shock *or* choque séptico; — **wave** onda de choque

shoe *n* zapato; **orthopedic shoes** zapatos ortopédicos

shook *pret de* **shake**

shoot *vt, vi* (*pret & pp* **shot**) **to** — **up** (*fam*) inyectarse (*drogas*)

shooter *n* (*vulg*) persona que se inyecta drogas

shooting *adj* (*pain*) punzante

short *adj* (*stature*) bajo; (*dimension*) corto; (*time*) corto, breve; **to be** — **of breath** *V.* **breath.**

short-acting *adj* de acción corta

shortness *V.* **breath.**

short-term *adj* a corto plazo

shot *n* (*fam*) inyección *f*

shot *pret & pp de* **shoot**

shoulder *n* hombro; **frozen** — hombro congelado; — **blade** (*fam*) escápula, omóplato *or* omoplato, paleta (*fam*)

show *vt* mostrar, enseñar; **Show me your feet**..Muéstreme (Enséñeme) los pies.

shower *n* ducha, baño de regadera (*esp. Mex*); **to take a** — ducharse, tomar una ducha, tomar un baño de regadera

shrank *pret de* **shrink**

shrapnel *n* metralla

shrimp *n* camarón *m*

shrink *n* (*fam*) psiquiatra *mf*; *vt, vi* (*pret* **shrank**; *pp* **shrunk**) (*tumor, etc.*) reducir(se)

shrug *vi* (*pret & pp* **shrugged**; *ger* **shrugging**) **to** — **one's shoulders** encogerse de hombros, levantar los hombros; **Shrug your shoulders**.. Encójase de hombros.

shrunk *pp de* **shrink**

shunt *n* (*physio*) cortocircuito; (*surg*) derivación *f*; **portacaval** — derivación portocava; **transjugular intrahepatic portosystemic** — **(TIPS)** derivación portosistémica percutánea intrahepática; **ventri-**culoperitoneal** — derivación ventriculoperitoneal

shut-in *n* persona incapaz de abandonar el hogar (*debido a debilidad*)

shy *adj* (*comp* **shyer**; *super* **shyest**) tímido

shyness *n* timidez *f*

sialoadenitis *n* sialoadenitis *f*

sibling *n* hermano -na *mf*; **siblings** hermanos

sibutramine *n* sibutramina

sick *adj* enfermo; **to get** — enfermarse

sickbed *n* cama de enfermo

sickly *adj* (*comp* **-lier**; *super* **-liest**) enfermizo

sickness *n* enfermedad *f*, mal *m*; **decompression** — enfermedad por descompresión; **morning** — vómitos del embarazo; **motion** — mareo (producido por el movimiento); **mountain** — mal de montaña, soroche *m* (*SA*); **radiation** — enfermedad por radiación; **serum** — enfermedad del suero; **sleeping** — enfermedad del sueño

side *n* lado, (*anat*) costado; **on your father's side**..por el lado de su padre; **to sleep on one's** — dormir de lado *or* costado

sideache *n* dolor *m* de costado

side rail *n* (*of a bed*) baranda

SIDS *abbr* **sudden infant death syndrome.** *V.* **syndrome.**

sieve *n* colador *m*

sigh *n* suspiro; *vi* suspirar

sight *n* visión *f*, vista

sighted *adj* que puede ver

sigmoid *adj* sigmoideo, sigmoide

sigmoidoscope *n* sigmoidoscopio

sigmoidoscopy *n* (*pl* **-pies**) sigmoidoscopia, sigmoidoscopía (*Amer, esp. spoken*); **flexible** — sigmoidoscopia flexible

sign *n* (*of an illness*) signo; — **language** lenguaje *m or* lengua de señas (*Amer*), lenguaje *or* lengua de signos (*Esp*); **vital signs** signos vitales, constantes *fpl* vitales (*Esp*); **warning** — signo *or* señal *f* de alarma; *vt, vi* (*one's name*) firmar; (*deaf language*) comunicarse mediante el lenguaje de señas *or* sig-

nos
signature n firma
significance n significado
significant other n compañero -ra mf sentimental
sildenafil n sildenafilo, sildenafil m (Amer)
silicone n silicona
silicosis n silicosis f
silk n seda
silver n plata; — **nitrate** nitrato de plata
simethicone n simeticona
simvastatin n simvastatina
since adv desde; **since you were injured**..desde que se hirió; prep desde; **since your last visit**..desde su última visita
single adj (unmarried) soltero
sinoatrial adj (conduction, etc.) sinoauricular; (node) sinusal
sinus n seno, sinus m; **ethmoid** — seno etmoidal; **frontal** — seno frontal; **maxillary** — seno maxilar; **pilonidal** — sinus or seno pilonidal; — **tract** fístula (generalmente entre un quiste o abceso y la piel)
sinusitis n sinusitis f
sip n sorbo; **sip of water**..sorbo de agua; vt (pret & pp **sipped**; ger **sipping**) sorber
sister n hermana
sister-in-law n (pl **sisters-in-law**) cuñada
sit vi (pret & pp **sat**; ger **sitting**) (to remain seated) quedarse sentado; **You shouldn't sit for long periods of time**..No debe quedarse sentado por períodos prolongados; **to** — **down** sentarse; **to** — **up** (from a supine position) sentarse
site n sitio; **surgical** — sitio quirúrgico
sit-up n abdominal m
size n tamaño
skeletal adj esquelético
skeleton n esqueleto
skiing n esquí m
skill n habilidad f, destreza; **communication skills** habilidades comunicativas; **social skills** habilidades sociales
skin adj dérmico; n piel f; (of the face) cutis m, tez f; (of fruit) piel; — **tag** pequeño tumor benigno de la piel que tiende a ocurrir en el cuello y en las axilas; vt (pret & pp **skinned**; ger **skinning**) (to scrape) raspar; **How did you skin your knee?**..¿Cómo se raspó la rodilla?
skin popping n (fam) inyección f bajo la piel (de la heroína)
skip vt (pret & pp **skipped**; ger **skipping**) saltarse; **to** — **a meal** saltarse una comida
skirt n falda
skull n cráneo
skullcap n (bot) escutelaria
skunk n zorrillo (esp. Amer), mofeta (esp. Esp)
slam vt (pret & pp **slammed**; ger **slamming**) (fam) inyectarse (drogas)
slash vt cortar; **to slash one's wrists**.. cortarse las venas
SLE abbr **systemic lupus erythematosus**. V. **lupus**.
sleep n sueño; (eye secretions) lagaña (Amer), legaña (Esp); — **apnea** apnea del sueño; **to go to** — dormirse, quedarse dormido; **Do you have trouble going to sleep?**..¿Tiene dificultad para dormirse (quedarse dormido)?...**Does your arm go to sleep?**..¿Se le duerme el brazo? **to go without** — ir sin dormir, trasnochar, desvelarse (Mex); **to put to** — (to anesthetize) anestesiar, dormir; **We will put you to sleep for the operation**..Lo vamos a anestesiar (dormir) para la operación; vi (pret & pp **slept**) dormir
sleeper (fam) V. **sleeping pill**.
sleeping pill n somnífero (form), pastilla para dormir
sleepwalk vi caminar dormido
sleepwalking n sonambulismo (form), (el) caminar dormido
sleepy adj (comp -**ier**; super -**iest**) somnoliento; **to be** — tener sueño; **to make** — dar sueño
sleeve n manga; **long** — o **long-sleeved shirt** camisa de manga larga
slept pret & pp de **sleep**
sliding scale n escala móvil

slight *adj* leve, ligero

sling *n* cabestrillo

slip *vi* (*pret & pp* **slipped**; *ger* **slipping**) resbalar(se)

slippery elm *n* (*bot*) olmo americano

slitlamp *n* lámpara de hendidura

sliver *n* astilla

slouch *vi* sentarse o pararse con mala postura, encorvarse

slough *vi* (*también* **to — off**) desprenderse, caerse

slow *adj* lento

slur *vi* (*pret & pp* **slurred**; *ger* **slurring**) **to — one's words** *o* **speech** arrastrar las palabras

small *adj* pequeño, chico; **to get smaller** reducir(se), disminuir(se); *n* **— of the back** parte baja de la espalda

smallpox *n* viruela

smart *adj* inteligente, listo; *vi* doler, arder

smarting *n* dolor *m*, ardor *m*, quemazón *f*, escozor *m*

smear *n* (*micro*) frotis *m*; **Papanicolaou — (***form***) o Pap —** citología cervical (*form*), citología (*fam*), prueba de Papanicolaou, prueba que se hace durante el examen pélvico con el fin de detectar cáncer del cérvix

smegma *n* esmegma *m*

smell *n* olor *m*; *vt* oler; **Can you smell this?**..¿Puede oler esto? *vi* oler; **to — bad** oler mal; **to — like** oler a

smile *n* sonrisa; *vi* sonreír(se)

smog *n* aire contaminado, smog *m* (*Ang*)

smoke *n* humo; **secondhand tobacco —** humo ambiental del tabaco; *vt, vi* fumar

smoke detector *n* detector *m* de humo

smoker *n* fumador -ra *mf*

smoking *n* (el) fumar (tabaco); **No smoking**..Prohibido fumar

smooth *adj* (*surface*) liso; (*skin, etc.*) suave, terso, liso; (*hair*) liso, suave

smother *vt, vi* asfixiar(se) (*form*), ahogar(se)

snack *n* bocadillo, refrigerio, botana (*Mex*), merienda, algo que se come

entre comidas; *vi* comer entre comidas

snail *n* caracol *m*

snake *n* serpiente *f*

sneeze *n* estornudo; *vi* estornudar

sniff *vt* (*cocaine, glue, etc.*) aspirar (por la nariz), inhalar (por la nariz), esnifar (*Esp*) (*cocaína, pegamento, etc.*); *vi* aspirar por la nariz

sniffle *vi* sorber(se) los mocos; **to have the sniffles** (*fam*) gotearle la nariz, tener flujo nasal

snore *vi* roncar

snoring *n* ronquidos

snort *vt* (*fam, cocaine*) aspirar (por la nariz), inhalar (por la nariz), esnifar (*Esp*) (*cocaína*)

snot *n* (*vulg*) moco

snuff *n* (*tobacco*) rapé *m*, tabaco para inhalar

soak *n* (*cloth, etc.*) remojar; (*body part*) remojar, sumergir en agua (*por un período prolongado*)

soap *n* jabón *m*

sober *adj* sobrio; *vi* **to — up** recuperarse de la embriaguez, recuperarse de la borrachera (*fam*)

sobriety *n* sobriedad *f*

soccer *n* fútbol *m*

social *adj* social

socioeconomic *adj* socioeconómico

sock *n* calcetín *m*

socket *n* (*dent*) alvéolo *or* alveolo; **eye —** órbita (del ojo) (*form*), cuenca (del ojo)

sodium *n* sodio; **— benzoate** benzoato sódico (*form*), benzoato de sodio; **— bicarbonate** bicarbonato sódico (*form*), bicarbonato de sodio; **— chloride** cloruro sódico (*form*), cloruro de sodio; **— fluoride** fluoruro sódico (*form*), fluoruro de sodio; **— hydroxide** hidróxido sódico (*form*), hidróxido de sodio

sodomize *vt* sodomizar

sodomy *n* sodomía

soft *adj* blando, suave

soft drink *n* refresco

soften *vt* (*skin*) suavizar, ablandar

softening *adj* (*lotion, etc.*) suavizante

soil *vt* ensuciar; **to — oneself** ensu-

ciarse
solar *adj* solar
soldier *n* soldado
sole *n* (*of the foot*) planta; (*of a shoe*) suela
soleus *n* sóleo
solid *adj & n* sólido
soluble *adj* soluble
solution *n* solución *f*; **buffer** — solución amortiguadora, tampón (*esp. Esp*); **normal saline** — solución salina normal; **oral rehydration** — suero de rehidratación oral, suero oral (*fam*)
solvent *n* solvente *m*, disolvente *m*
somatic *adj* somático
somatization *n* somatización *f*
somatropin *n* somatropina
son *n* hijo
son-in-law *n* (*pl* **sons-in-law**) yerno
sonogram *n* sonograma *m*, sonografía (*estudio imagenológico*)
sonography *V.* **ultrasonography**.
soon *adv* pronto
soothe *vt* aliviar, calmar
sorbitol *n* sorbitol *m*
sore *adj* dolorido; — **throat** dolor *m* de garganta; *n* llaga, herida, úlcera; **pressure** — úlcera de decúbito (*form*), úlcera por presión, llaga debida a permanecer mucho tiempo sentado o encamado sin cambiar de posición
sorry *adj* **to be** — sentir, lamentar; **I'm sorry you had to wait so long** ..Lamento (Siento) que haya tenido que esperar tanto tiempo...**I'm sorry**..Lo siento.
sotalol *n* sotalol *m*
sound *n* sonido; **heart** — ruido cardíaco
soup *n* sopa
sour *adj* agrio
source *n* fuente *f*, origen *m*; — **of infection** fuente de infección; — **of protein** fuente de proteínas
soy *n* soja
spa *n* balneario, spa *m*
space *n* espacio
spaced out *adj* (*fam*) ido, distraído
spacer *n* espaciador *m*; (*for metered dose inhaler*) cámara espaciadora
spacey *adj* (*fam*) distraído, olvidadizo

spare *vt* preservar, conservar; **limb-sparing** con preservación de extremidad; **nerve-sparing** con preservación nerviosa
sparfloxacin *n* esparfloxacino, esparfloxacina (*esp. Amer*)
spasm *n* espasmo
spasmodic *adj* espasmódico
spastic *adj* espástico
spasticity *n* espasticidad *f*
spat *pret & pp de* **spit**
speak *vt, vi* (*pret* **spoke**; *pp* **spoken**) hablar
spearmint *n* (*bot*) hierbabuena
specialist *n* especialista *mf*; **heart** —, **liver** —, etc. especialista del corazón, especialista del hígado, etc; **infectious disease** — especialista *mf* en enfermedades infecciosas, infectólogo -ga *mf* (*esp. Amer*); — **in allergies,** — **in immunology, etc.** especialista en alergias, especialista en inmunología, etc.
specialty *n* (*pl* -**ties**) especialidad *f*
species *n* (*pl* -**cies**) especie *f*
specific *adj* específico; **a test specific for**..una prueba específica para
specimen *n* espécimen *m*, muestra
spectinomycin *n* espectinomicina
spectrum *n* (*pl* -**tra**) espectro
speculum *n* (*pl* -**la** *o* -**lums**) espéculo
speech *n* lenguaje *m*, habla, voz *f*; **esophageal** — voz esofágica; — **development** desarrollo del lenguaje
speed *n* (*fam*) metanfetamina
spell *n* ataque *m*, acceso
spell *vt* deletrear; **Can you spell 'world' backwards?**..¿Puede deletrear 'mundo' al revés?
sperm *n* (*individual spermatozoon*) espermatozoide *m*; (*semen*) esperma *m*
spermatocele *n* espermatocele *m*
spermatozoon *n* espermatozoide *m*
spermicidal *adj* espermicida
spermicide *n* espermicida *m*
SPF *abbr* **sun protection factor**. *V.* **factor**.
spherocytosis *n* esferocitosis *f*; **hereditary** — esferocitosis hereditaria
sphincter *n* esfínter *m*
sphincterotomy *n* (*pl* -**mies**) esfinte-

rotomía

spice *n* especia, condimento

spicy *adj* (*comp* **-ier**; *super* **-iest**) condimentado, picante

spider *n* araña; **brown recluse —** araña marrón, araña parda, araña violinista (*esp. Mex*)

spider angioma *n* angioma *m* en araña, araña vascular

spin *vi* (*pret & pp* **spun**; *ger* **spinning**) dar vueltas, girar; **Do you feel as though everything is spinning?**..¿Siente que todo le da vueltas?

spina bifida *n* espina bífida

spinach *n* espinaca (*frec. pl*)

spinal *adj* espinal, raquídeo

spine *n* columna vertebral, columna (*fam*); (*thorn*) espina; **cervical —** columna cervical; **lumbar —** columna lumbar; **lumbosacral —** columna lumbosacra; **thoracic —** columna dorsal *or* torácica

spirochete *n* espiroqueta

spirometer *n* espirómetro

spirometry *n* espirometría; **incentive —** espirometría incentivada

spironolactone *n* espironolactona

spit *n* saliva; *vt, vi* (*pret & pp* **spat**; *ger* **spitting**) escupir; **to — up** (*ped, fam*) regurgitar (*form*), volverse(le) (a uno) la comida (*fam*), vomitar un poquito

spleen *n* bazo

splenectomy *n* (*pl* **-mies**) esplenectomía

splenic *adj* esplénico

splint *n* tablilla, férula (*form; manufactured, often refers to removable cast*); *vt* entablillar, colocar una tablilla (férula) en

splinter *n* astilla

split *adj* partido, agrietado; *n* grieta, hendidura; *vt, vi* (*pret & pp* **split**; *ger* **splitting**) partir(se), agrietar(se)

spoil *vt* (*pret & pp* **spoiled**) (*a child*) consentir, mimar; *vi* (*food, etc.*) echarse a perder

spoke *pret de* **speak**

spoken *pp de* **speak**

spokesperson *n* representante *mf*; **We would like one family member to serve as spokesperson.**..Quisiéra-

mos que un solo familiar haga de representante.

spondylolysthesis *n* espondilolistesis *f*

spondylosis *n* espondilosis *f*

sponge *n* esponja

spontaneous *adj* espontáneo

spoonful *n* (*tablespoonful*) cucharada, (*teaspoonful*) cucharadita

sporadic *adj* esporádico

spore *n* espora

sporotrichosis *n* esporotricosis *f*

sport *n* deporte *m*; **contact —** deporte de contacto; **to play sports**..hacer deporte

spot *n* mancha

spotting *n* manchado, sangrado uterino leve (*que deja manchas en la ropa interior*)

spouse *n* esposo -sa *mf*

sprain *n* esguince *m* (*form*), torcedura; *vt* torcerse; **I sprained my wrist**..Se me torció la muñeca..Me torcí la muñeca.

spray *n* aerosol *m*, spray *m* (*Ang*); **nasal —** aerosol nasal; **pepper —** spray *m or* aerosol *m* de pimienta

spread *n* (*person to person*) propagación *f*; (*within the body*) diseminación *f* (*form*); *vt, vi* (*pret & pp* **spread**) propagar(se), diseminar(se)

spring, springtime *n* primavera

sprue *n* esprue *m*; **celiac** *o* **nontropical —** esprue celiaco *or* no tropical; **tropical —** esprue tropical

spun *pret & pp de* **spin**

spur *n* (*ortho*) espolón *m*

spurt *V.* **growth.**

sputum *n* esputo, flema (*fam*)

squamous *adj* escamoso

square *adj* cuadrado; **— meter** metro cuadrado

squat *vi* (*pret & pp* **squatted**; *ger* **squatting**) ponerse en cuclillas

squeeze *vt* apretar; **Squeeze my fingers as hard as you can**..Apriete mis dedos lo más fuerte que pueda.

squint *vt* entrecerrar; *vi* entrecerrar los ojos

stabbing *adj* (*pain*) punzante

stability *n* estabilidad *f*

stabilization *n* estabilización *f*

stabilize *vt, vi* estabilizar(se)

stabilizer *n* estabilizador *m*; **mood —** estabilizador del ánimo *or* humor

stable *adj* estable

stage *n* (*disease, etc.*) estadio, etapa; (*cancer*) estadio; (*sleep*) etapa; (*puberty*) estadio, estadío

stagger *vi* tambalear(se)

staging *n* (*tumor*) estadificación *f*

stain *n* mancha; (*micro*) tinción *f*, coloración *f*; **Gram's —** tinción *or* coloración de Gram; **port-wine —** mancha en vino de Oporto

stamina *n* vigor *m*, resistencia

stammer *vi* tartamudear

stand (*pret & pp* stood) *vt* (*to endure*) aguantar, tolerar; *vi* (*to be standing*) estar de pie, estar parado; (*to stand up*) levantarse, pararse, ponerse de pie; **Avoid standing for long periods of time.**.Evite estar de pie por períodos largos...**Now stand (up).**. Ahora levántese.

standard *adj & n* estándar *m*

standing *adj* de pie, parado; **— order** orden *f* que no expira

stapedectomy *n* (*pl* **-mies**) estapedectomía

staph (*fam*) estafilococo

Staphylococcus aureus, Staphylococcus aureus; **methicillin-resistant — — (MRSA)** Staphylococcus aureus resistente a meticilina (SARM)

staple *n* (*surg*) grapa

starch *n* almidón *m*

stare *vi* fijar la vista; **Stare at that point on the wall.**.Fije la vista en ese punto en la pared.

starvation *n* inanición *f*

starve *vi* morir de hambre

stasis *n* estasis *m&f*; **venous —** estasis venosa, estasis venoso (*esp. Esp*)

state *n* estado, condición *f*; **hypercoagulable —** estado de hipercoagulabilidad; **— of the art** estado del arte

statin *n* estatina

station *n* estación *f*, central *f*; **nursing —** estación de enfermería, central *f* de enfermeras (*esp. Mex*)

statistic *n* estadística; *npl* (*branch of math*) estadística

status *n* estado; **mental —** estado mental; **— asthmaticus** estado asmático; **— epilepticus** estado epiléptico

stavudine *n* estavudina

stay *n* estancia, estadía (*esp. SA*); **hospital —** estancia *or* estadía hospitalaria; *vi* **to — in bed** guardar cama

STD *abbr* **sexually transmitted disease.** *V.* **disease.**

steak *n* bistec *m*

steam *n* vapor *m*; *vt* (*to cook by steaming*) cocer al vapor

steel *n* acero; **stainless —** acero inoxidable

stenosis *n* (*pl* **-ses**) estenosis *f*; **aortic —, mitral —, etc.** estenosis aórtica, estenosis mitral, etc.

stenotic *adj* estenótico

stent *n* stent *m*, malla cilíndrica para mantener abierto una arteria o un conducto

step *n* paso; **the next —** el próximo paso; *vi* (*pret & pp* **stepped**; *ger* **stepping**) (*también* **to take a —**) dar un paso

stepbrother *n* hermanastro

stepchild *n* (*pl* **-children**) hijastro -tra *mf*

stepdaughter *n* hijastra

stepfather *n* padrastro

stepmother *n* madrastra

stepsister *n* hermanastra

stepson *n* hijastro

sterile *adj* estéril

sterility *n* esterilidad *f*

sterilization *n* esterilización *f*

sterilize *vt* esterilizar

sterna *pl de* **sternum**

sternal *adj* esternal

sternum *n* (*pl* **-na**) esternón *m*

steroid *adj* esteroideo; *n* esteroide *m*

stethoscope *n* estetoscopio

stibogluconate, stibamine glucoside (*OMS*) *n* estibogluconato, estibamina glucósido (*OMS*)

stick *n* (*prick*) pinchazo, piquete *m* (*Mex*); **You are going to feel a stick.**.Va a sentir un pinchazo (piquete); *vt* (*pret & pp* **stuck**) pinchar, picar (*Mex*); **to — oneself** pincharse, picarse (*Mex*); **to — out one's tongue** sacar la lengua; **Stick out your tongue**..Saque la lengua; *vi* **to — out** sobresalir, proyectar hacia adelante

sticker *n* (*bot*) espina

sticky *adj* (*comp* -**ier**; *super* -**iest**) pegajoso

sties *pl de* **sty**

stiff *adj* rígido, tieso; **Do your hands feel stiff in the morning?**..¿Siente sus manos rígidas (tiesas) en la mañana?

stiffness *n* rigidez *f*

stillbirth *n* nacimiento de un niño muerto

stillborn *adj* mortinato (*form*), nacido muerto

stimulant *adj & n* estimulante *m*

stimulate *vt* estimular

stimulating *adj* estimulante

stimulation *n* estimulación *f*; **digital — estimulación digital; transcutaneous electrical nerve — (TENS)** estimulación nerviosa eléctrica transcutánea (ENET)

stimulus *n* (*pl* -**li**) estímulo

sting *n* punzada, (*of an insect*) picadura, piquete *m* (*esp. Mex*); **Did you feel a sting?**..¿Sintió una picadura (un piquete)? **bee — picadura** *or* piquete de abeja; *vt* (*pret & pp* **stung**) picar; *vi* arder, doler; **The numbing medication will sting a little bit**..El anestésico le va a arder (doler) un poco.

stinger *n* aguijón *m*

stinging *n* punzadas

stingray *n* raya

stirrup *n* (*anat, gyn, etc.*) estribo

stitch *n* punto (de sutura); (*pain in side*) dolor *m* de costado; *vt* (*también* **to — up**) suturar (*form*), coser

St. John's wort *n* (*bot*) hipérico, hierba de San Juan

stocking *n* media; **compression stockings** medias de compresión *or* compresivas

stocky *adj* robusto, fornido

stoic *adj* (*patient*) con alta tolerancia al dolor, que no se queja mucho

stoma *n* estoma *m*, abertura artificial entre un órgano y el exterior del cuerpo

stomach *adj* estomacal; *n* estómago; (*fam*) abdomen *m*; **acid — (*fam*)** acidez estomacal; **pit of the — boca del estómago; to be sick to one's — (*fam*)** tener náusea(s)

stomachache *n* dolor *m* de estómago

stomatitis *n* estomatitis *f*

stone *n* cálculo (*form*), piedra; **kidney — cálculo renal (*form*)**, piedra del *or* en el riñón

stood *pret & pp de* **stand**

stool *n* heces *fpl* (fecales) (*form*), popó (*fam*), caca (*fam or vulg*), deposición *f* (*Esp, SA*), evacuación *f*, excremento; **loose stools** heces pastosas o líquidas; **— softener** laxante *m* emoliente, emoliente *m*, ablandador *m* de heces

stoop *vi* (*también* **to — over**) agacharse, doblarse

stooped *adj* encorvado; **to become — encorvarse**

stop *vt* (*pret & pp* **stopped**; *ger* **stopping**) (*a habit, etc.*) dejar de; (*a medication, etc.*) suspender; *vi* **to — up** obstruir (*form*), tapar; **My nose is stopped up**..Tengo la nariz tapada.

store *n* reserva; **the body's store of iron**..la reserva de hierro del organismo; *vt* almacenar

strabismus *n* estrabismo

straight *adj* recto, derecho

straighten *vt, vi* enderezar(se); **Straighten your leg**..Enderece la pierna.

strain *n* tensión *f*; (*of bacteria, etc.*) cepa; (*muscle, ligament, etc.*) lesión muscular debida a uso excesivo o incorrecto; *vt* (*a muscle or ligament*) lastimar por uso excesivo o incorrecto (*un músculo o un ligamento*); (*one's eyes, one's voice*) forzar (*la vista, la voz*); (*urine for stones*) filtrar, colar (*la orina para buscar piedras*); *vi* esforzarse, hacer un gran esfuerzo; (*at stool*) pujar

straitjacket *n* camisa de fuerza

strangle *vt, vi* estrangular(se)

strangulated *adj* estrangulado

strangulation *n* estrangulación *f*

strap *n* correa, tira
strawberry *n* (*pl* **-ries**) fresa
streak *n* raya, línea
stream *n* (*urine*) chorro miccional (*form*), chorro (de la orina)
strength *n* fuerza; **the strength in your hand**..la fuerza de su mano.. **your strength**..su(s) fuerza(s); **double-strength** de doble fuerza, de doble dosis; **extra-strength** de fuerza extra; **physical —** fuerza física; [*Note: the plural* fuerzas *is often used when referring to one's strength in general.*]
strengthen *vt* (*muscles, bones, etc.*) fortalecer
strenuous *adj* intenso, vigoroso; **strenuous activities** actividades intensas
strep *n* (*fam*) estreptococo; **— throat** faringitis producida por el estreptococo
streptokinase *n* estreptoquinasa *or* estreptocinasa
streptomycin *n* estreptomicina
stress *n* estrés *m*; **Are you under a lot of stress?**..¿Está bajo mucho estrés? **job —** estrés laboral *or* del trabajo; *vt* **to — (one) out** *o* **put — on (one)** estresar; *vi* **to — out** estresarse
stressed *adj* estresado
stressful *adj* estresante
stressor *n* estresor *m*
stretch *vt, vi* estirar(se)
stretcher *n* (*litter*) camilla
stretching *n* estiramiento
stretch mark *n* estría
strict *adj* estricto
stricture *n* estenosis *f*, estrechez *f*
strike *vt* (*pret & pp* **struck**) pegar, golpear
strip *V.* **test strip**.
stroke *n* (*blow*) golpe *m*; (*cerebrovascular event*) ictus *m* (*form*), accidente *m* cerebrovascular (*form*), ataque *m* cerebral, derrame *m* (*fam*), embolia (*fam*); (*ischemic*) infarto cerebral; (*embolic*) embolia cerebral; (*hemorrhagic*) derrame cerebral
strong *adj* fuerte
strongyloidiasis *n* estrongiloidiasis *f*

struck *pret & pp de* **strike**
structural *adj* estructural
strung out *adj* (*fam, on drugs*) adicto
strychnine *n* estricnina
stub *vt* (*pret & pp* **stubbed**; *ger* **stubbing**) **to — one's foot (against)** tropezar (con)
stuck *pret & pp de* **stick**
student *n* estudiante *mf*; **medical —** estudiante *mf* de medicina
study *n* (*pl* **-dies**) estudio; **double-blind —** estudio doble ciego; **sleep —** estudio del sueño
stuffy, stuffed up *adj* (*fam*) con congestión nasal (*form*), con la nariz tapada (*fam*)
stumble *vi* tropezar, dar un traspié
stump *n* (*anat*) muñón *m*
stun *vt* (*pret & pp* **stunned**; *ger* **stunning**) aturdir, dejar brevemente incapacitado; **to become stunned** aturdirse, quedarse brevemente incapacitado
stung *pret & pp de* **sting**
stun gun *n* paralizador *m* (*Amer*), pistola paralizante (*Esp*)
stunt *vt* (*growth*) impedir (*el crecimiento*)
stupor *n* estupor *m*
stutter *vi* tartamudear
sty, stye *n* (*pl* **styes**) orzuelo, perrilla (*Mex, fam*)
subacromial *adj* subacromial
subacute *adj* subagudo
subarachnoid *adj* subaracnoideo
subclavian *adj* subclavio
subclinical *adj* subclínico
subconjunctival *adj* subconjunctival
subconscious *adj* subconsciente; *n* subconsciencia *or* subconciencia
subcutaneous *adj* subcutáneo
subdural *adj* subdural
sublethal *adj* subletal
sublimation *n* (*psych*) sublimación *f*
sublingual *adj* sublingual
subluxation *n* subluxación *f*
submandibular *adj* submandibular
submental *adj* submentoniano
subnormal *adj* subnormal
subspecialist *n* subespecialista *mf*
subspecialty *n* (*pl* **-ties**) subespecialidad *f*
substance *n* sustancia

substitute *n* sustituto; **salt —** sustituto de la sal; *vt* sustituir; **You can substitute tortillas for bread**..Puede sustituir el pan por las tortillas; [*Note: the order of the two objects* tortillas *and* bread *is reversed when translating to Spanish. It may be helpful to think of* sustituir *as a synonym for the English verb to* replace. *The sentence above would then read*: You can replace bread with tortillas..Puede sustituir el pan por las tortillas.]

substitution *n* sustitución *f*

subtotal *adj* subtotal

subtract *vt, vi* (*arith*) restar; **Subtract 7 from 100**..Réste 7 a 100.

subungual *adj* subungueal

suck *vt, vi,* (*at mother's breast*) mamar; **to — one's thumb** chuparse el dedo

suckle *vt* amamantar; *vi* mamar

sucralfate *n* sucralfato

suction *n* succión *f*; **— curettage** legrado por succión

sudden *adj* súbito

suddenly *adv* de repente, súbitamente

sue *vt, vi* presentar una demanda (contra), demandar

sufentanil *n* sufentanilo

suffer *vi* sufrir; **to — from** padecer; **She suffers from arthritis**..Ella padece artritis.

sufferer *n* persona que padece; **asma — persona** que padece asma

suffering *n* sufrimiento; **to prevent suffering**..prevenir el sufrimiento

sufficient *adj* suficiente

suffocate *vt, vi* asfixiar(se) (*form*), ahogar(se)

suffocation *n* asfixia, sofocación *f*

sugar *n* azúcar *m&f*

sugar-coated *adj* cubierto de azúcar

sugarless *adj* sin azúcar

suicidal *adj* suicida, con tendencias suicidas, que piensa en suicidarse

suicide *n* suicidio; **assisted —** suicidio asistido; **— attempt** intento de suicidio; **— gesture** gesto suicida; **to commit —** suicidarse

suitable *adj* adecuado, apropiado, idóneo; **a suitable donor**..un donante adecuado

suite *n* sala; **endoscopy —** sala de endoscopia

sulfacetamide *n* sulfacetamida

sulfadiazine *n* sulfadiazina *or* sulfadiacina

sulfa drugs *n* sulfas [*Note: the Spanish term* sulfas *is rarely used in the singular.*]

sulfamethoxazole *n* sulfametoxazol *m*

sulfasalazine *n* sulfasalazina

sulfate *n* sulfato

sulfite *n* sulfito

sulfonamide *n* sulfonamida

sulfur *n* azufre *m*; **— dioxide** dióxido de azufre

sulindac *n* sulindaco

sumatriptan *n* sumatriptán *m*

summer *n* verano

sun *n* sol *m*; **to get —** tomar el sol, asolearse

sunburn *n* quemadura solar *or* de sol; *vi* (*también* **to get sunburned**) quemarse (con el sol); **Do you sunburn easily?** *o* **Do you get sunburned easily?**..¿Se quema fácilmente (con el sol)?

sunglasses *npl* lentes *or* anteojos oscuros, gafas de sol (*esp. Esp*)

sunlamp *n* lámpara de rayos ultravioleta

sunlight *n* luz *f* del sol

sunscreen *n* filtro solar, protector *m* solar

sunstroke *n* insolación *f*

suntan *n* bronceado; **to get a —** broncearse

superego *n* (*pl* **-gos**) (*psych*) superyó

superficial *adj* superficial

superior *adj* (*anat*) superior

supernumerary *adj* supernumerario

supine *adj* supino, acostado boca arriba

supper *n* cena

supple *adj* ágil

supplement *n* suplemento

supplemental, supplementary *adj* suplementario

supply *n* (*pl* **-plies**) abastecimiento, surtido; **medical supplies** suministros médicos, insumos médicos (*Amer*)

support *n* (*physical*) soporte *m*; (*so-*

cial) apoyo; **advanced cardiac life —** soporte vital avanzado; **arch —** plantilla; **basic life —** soporte vital básico; **life —** soporte vital; **nutritional —** soporte nutricional; **— group** grupo de apoyo; *vt* sostener, soportar; (*social sense*) apoyar

suppository *n* (*pl* **-ries**) supositorio; **vaginal —** óvulo, supositorio vaginal

suppress *vt* suprimir

suppressant *n* supresor *m*; **appetite —** supresor del apetito

suppression *n* supresión *f*

suppressive *adj* supresor

suppurative *adj* supurativo

suramin *n* suramina

sure *adj* seguro; **to be** *o* **make —** asegurarse, estar seguro; **Be sure to keep the wound clean.**.Asegúrese de mantener limpia la herida.

surface *n* superficie *f*

surfactant *n* surfactante *m*

surgeon *n* cirujano -na *mf*; **general —** cirujano general; **oral —** cirujano oral; **orthopedic —** cirujano ortopédico, traumatólogo -ga *mf* (*esp. Esp*); **thoracic —** cirujano torácico; **vascular —** cirujano vascular

surgery *n* cirugía; **ambulatory —** cirugía ambulatoria; **bariatric —** cirugía bariátrica; **breast reduction —** mamoplastia de reducción, cirugía para reducir el tamaño de las mamas; **cosmetic —** cirugía estética; **elective —** cirugía electiva; **general —** cirugía general; **laparoscopic —** cirugía laparoscópica; **major —** cirugía mayor; **maxilofacial —** cirugía maxilofacial; **minor —** cirugía menor; **open heart —** cirugía a corazón abierto; **oral —** cirugía oral *or* bucal; **orthopedic —** cirugía ortopédica, traumatología (*esp. Esp*); **outpatient —** cirugía ambulatoria, cirugía sin ingreso; **plastic —** cirugía plástica; **radical —** cirugía radical; **reconstructive —** cirugía reconstructiva; **robotic —** cirugía robótica; **thoracic —** cirugía torácica

surgical *adj* quirúrgico

surrogate mother *n* madre subrogada, madre de alquiler (*fam*)

surrounding *adj* circundante

surveillance *n* vigilancia

survival *n* supervivencia

survive *vt, vi* sobrevivir

survivor *n* superviviente *mf*, sobreviviente *mf*; **cancer —** superviviente *or* sobreviviente del cáncer

susceptibility *n* susceptibilidad *f*

susceptible *adj* susceptible

suspend *vt* (*treatment, etc.*) suspender

suspension *n* suspensión *f*

sustain *vt* sostener

suture *n* sutura; **absorbable —** sutura reabsorbible; *vt* suturar, coser (*fam*)

swab *n* hisopo, bastoncillo de algodón (*Esp*), palillo con punta de algodón

swaddle *vt* envolver (*un bebé*) con ropa apretada

swallow *n* trago; *vt* tragar, pasar (*fam*); *vi* (*dry swallow*) tragar, tragar saliva, pasar saliva (*fam*); **Swallow please.**.Trague por favor ..Trague saliva por favor..Pase saliva por favor.

swam *pret de* **swim**

sweat *n* sudor *m*; **night sweats** sudoración nocturna; *vi* (*pret & pp* **sweat** *o* **sweated**) sudar

sweating *n* sudoración *f*

sweaty *adj* sudoroso

sweet *adj* dulce; **to have a — tooth** (*fam*) gustar(le) (a uno) los dulces, ser goloso (*esp. Esp*); *npl* dulces *mpl*, caramelos, golosinas

sweetener *n* edulcorante *m*; **artificial —** edulcorante artificial

swell *vi* (*pret* **swelled**; *pp* **swelled** *o* **swollen**) (*también* **to — up**) hincharse; **Do your feet swell (up)?**.. ¿Se le hinchan los pies?

swelling *n* hinchazón *f*

swim *vi* (*pret* **swam**; *pp* **swum**; *ger* **swimming**) nadar; **to go swimming** ir a bañarse, ir a nadar

swimmer's ear *n* (*fam*) otitis externa

swimmer's itch *n* (*fam*) dermatitis *f* por cercarias

swimming *n* natación *f*

swish *vt* enjuagar; — **and spit** enjuagar y escupir; — **and swallow** enjuagar y tragar

swollen (*pp de* **swell**) *adj* hinchado

swum *pp de* **swim**

symmetric, symmetrical *adj* simétrico

symmetry *n* simetría

sympathectomy *n* (*pl* -mies) simpatectomía

sympathetic *adj* compasivo, comprensivo; (*neuro*) simpático

sympathy *n* compasión *f*

symphysis *n* (*pl* -ses) sínfisis *f*

symptom *n* síntoma *m*

symptomatic *adj* sintomático

synapse *n* sinapsis *f*

synchronize *vt* sincronizar

syncope *n* síncope *m*

syndrome *n* síndrome *m*; **acquired immunodeficiency** — (**AIDS**) síndrome de inmunodeficiencia adquirida (SIDA *or* sida *m*); **adult respiratory distress** — (**ARDS**) síndrome de dificultad respiratoria del adulto (SDRA); **antiphospholipid** — síndrome antifosfolípido; **Asherman's** — síndrome de Asherman; **battered child** — síndrome del niño maltratado; **blind loop** — síndrome del asa ciega; **carcinoid** — síndrome carcinoide; **carpal tunnel** — síndrome del túnel carpiano; **chronic fatigue** — síndrome de fatiga crónica; **compartmental** — síndrome compartimental; **complex regional pain** — síndrome de dolor regional complejo; **Cushing's** — síndrome de Cushing; **Down's** — síndrome de Down; **Ehlers-Danlos** — síndrome de Ehlers-Danlos; **empty nest** — síndrome del nido vacío; **Felty's** — síndrome de Felty; **fetal alcohol** — síndrome alcohólico fetal; **Gilbert's** — síndrome de Gilbert; **Gilles de la Tourette** — síndrome de Gilles de la Tourette; **Guillain-Barré** — síndrome de Guillain-Barré; **hemolytic-uremic** — síndrome hemolítico-urémico; **hepatorenal** — síndrome hepatorrenal; **irritable bowel** — síndrome de intestino irritable; **Klinefelter's** — síndrome de Klinefelter; **Marfan's** — síndrome de Marfán; **Ménière's** — enfermedad *f* de Ménière; **metabolic** — síndrome metabólico; **Munchausen** — síndrome de Munchausen; **myelodysplastic** — síndrome mielodisplásico; **nephrotic** — síndrome nefrótico; **neuroleptic malignant** — síndrome neuroléptico maligno; **overuse** — síndrome de sobrecarga, lesión *f* por sobrecarga; **Peutz-Jeghers** — síndrome de Peutz-Jeghers; **Pickwickian** — síndrome de Pickwick; **polycystic ovary** — síndrome de ovario poliquístico; **postconcussional** — síndrome conmocional; **post-polio** — síndrome post-polio; **premenstrual** — (**PMS**) síndrome premenstrual; **Reiter's** — síndrome de Reiter; **Rendu-Osler-Weber** — enfermedad *f* de Rendu-Osler-Weber; **restless legs** — síndrome de piernas inquietas; **Reye's** — síndrome de Reye; **severe acute respiratory** — (**SARS**) síndrome respiratorio agudo severo (SRAS); **Sheehan's** — síndrome de Sheehan; **short bowel** — síndrome de intestino corto; **Sjögren's** — síndrome de Sjögren; **staphylococcal scalded skin** — síndrome de la piel escaldada estafilocócica; **Stevens-Johnson** — síndrome de Stevens-Johnson; **sudden infant death** — (**SIDS**) síndrome de la muerte súbita infantil (*Amer*), síndrome de la muerte súbita del lactante (*Esp*); **toxic shock** — síndrome de shock tóxico, síndrome de choque tóxico (*esp. Mex, CA*); **Turner's** — síndrome de Turner; **wasting** — síndrome de desgaste; **Wernicke-Korsakoff** — síndrome de Wernicke-Korsakoff; **Wolff-Parkinson-White** — síndrome de Wolff-Parkinson-White

synergy *n* sinergia

synovial *adj* sinovial

synovitis *n* sinovitis *f*

synthesis *n* síntesis *f*

synthesize *vt* sintetizar

synthetic *adj* sintético
syphilis *n* sífilis *f*
syphilitic *adj* sifilítico
syringe *n* jeringa, jeringuilla (*Carib, Esp*); **bulb** — pera de goma
syringomyelia *n* siringomielia
syrup *n* jarabe *m*; **cough** — jarabe para la tos
system *n* sistema *m*; **autonomic nervous** — sistema nervioso autónomo; **cardiovascular** — sistema cardiovascular; **central nervous** — (**CNS**) sistema nervioso central (SNC); **digestive** — aparato digestivo; **endocrine** — sistema endocrino; **immune** — sistema inmunológico *or* inmune; **metric** — sistema métrico; **musculoskeletal** — aparato locomotor; **parasympathetic nervous** — sistema nervioso parasimpático; **peripheral nervous** — sistema nervioso periférico; **reproductive** — aparato reproductor; **respiratory** — aparato respiratorio; **skeletal** — sistema esquelético; **sympathetic nervous** — sistema nervioso simpático
systemic *adj* sistémico
systolic *adj* sistólico

T

table *n* mesa; **exam** — mesa de exploración (*form*), mesa (*fam*), camilla (*SA*); **operating** — mesa de operaciones; **tilt** — mesa basculante
tablespoonful *n* cucharada (grande)
tablet *n* tableta
taboo *adj & n* (*pl* **taboos**) tabú *m*
tachycardia *n* taquicardia
tacrine *n* tacrina
tacrolimus *n* tacrolimus *m*, tacrolimús *m* (*OMS*)
tadalafil *n* tadalafilo
taenia *n* tenia
tailbone *n* (*fam*) coxis *m* (*form*) cóccix *m* (*form*), colita (*Amer, fam*), rabadilla (*Amer, fam*)
tainted *adj* contaminado
take *vt* (*pret* **took**; *pp* **taken**) tomar; **to** — **off** (*clothing, etc.*) quitarse; **Take off your shirt**..Quítese la camisa; **to** — **out** extraer (*form*), extirpar (*form*), sacar; **We have to take out your appendix**..Tenemos que sacarle el apéndice.
talc *n* talco
talcum powder *n* talco, polvos de talco (*Esp*)
talk *vi* hablar
tall *adj* alto; **How tall are you?**.. ¿Cuánto mide Ud?..¿Qué altura tiene Ud?
talus *n* astrágalo
tamoxifen *n* tamoxifeno
tampon *n* tampón *m*
tamponade *n* taponamiento; **cardiac** — taponamiento cardíaco
tamsulosin *n* tamsulosina
tan *adj & n* bronceado; *vi* (*pret & pp* **tanned**; *ger* **tanning**) (*también* **to get a** —) broncearse
tank *n* (*for oxygen*) tanque *m*, cilindro, tubo (*esp. SA*), bombona (*esp. Esp*) (*de oxígeno*)

tannin *n* tanino

tantalum *n* tantalio

tantrum *n* berrinche *m*, rabieta, pataleta

tap *n* (*puncture*) punción *f*; **spinal —** punción lumbar; *vt* (*pret & pp* **tapped**; *ger* **tapping**) hacer una punción

tape *n* cinta, tela; **adhesive —** cinta *or* tela adhesiva, esparadrapo (*esp. Esp*); **measure** *o* **measuring —** cinta métrica

tapeworm *n* tenia, lombriz solitaria

taping *n* vendaje funcional *or* preventivo

tar *n* (*cigarettes, shampoo, etc.*) alquitrán *m*

tarantula *n* tarántula

target *n* diana, blanco (*Amer, inv*); **— organ** órgano diana *or* blanco

tarsal *adj* tarsal

tartar *n* (*dent*) cálculo (*form*), sarro (*dental*)

tartaric acid *n* ácido tartárico

taste *n* sabor *m*, gusto; **— bud** papila gustativa; *vt* (*to try*) probar; **Taste it**..Pruébelo...**Can you taste all right?**..¿Distingue bien los sabores? *vi* saber; **This medicine doesn't taste bad**..Esta medicina no sabe mal; **to — like** saber a

tattoo *n* (*pl* **-toos**) tatuaje *m*

taught *pret & pp de* **teach**

taurine *n* taurina

TB *V.* **tuberculosis**.

tea *n* té *m*; (*medicinal*) infusión *f*

teach *vt* (*pret & pp* **taught**) enseñar

teacher *n* maestro -tra *mf*, profesor -ra *mf*

team *n* equipo; **health care —** equipo de salud, equipo sanitario (*esp. Esp*); **sexual assault response —** equipo multidisciplinario entrenado para tratar la víctima de una agresión sexual y a la vez recolectar evidencia

tear *n* (*muscle, etc.*) desgarro, rotura (*esp. Esp*); *vt, vi* (*pret* **tore**; *pp* **torn**) desgarrar(se), sufrir un desgarro *or* una rotura; **I tore my calf muscle**..Me desgarré el músculo de la pantorrilla.

tear *n* (*from crying*) lágrima

tearful *adj* llorando, que está llorando

tease *vt* (*ped*) molestar, fastidiar

teaspoonful *n* (*pl* **-fuls**) cucharadita

technetium *n* tecnecio

technician *n* técnico -ca *mf*

technique *n* técnica; **relaxation —** técnica de relajación; **sterile** *o* **aseptic —** técnica aséptica *or* estéril

technology *n* (*pl* **-gies**) tecnología

teenage *adj* adolescente, de 13 a 19 años (de edad)

teenager *n* adolescente *mf*, joven *mf* de 13 a 19 años (de edad)

teens *npl* los años 13 a 19 (de edad)

teeth *pl de* **tooth**

teethe *vi* salir(le) (a uno) los dientes; **Is he teething yet?**..¿Ya le están saliendo los dientes?

teething *n* dentición *f* (*form*), erupción *f* dental (*form*), salida de los dientes

telangiectasia *n* telangiectasia; **hereditary hemorrhagic —** telangiectasia hemorrágica hereditaria

telemedicine *n* telemedicina

telemetry *n* telemetría

telephone *n* teléfono; **cellular —, cell phone** (*fam*) teléfono celular, celular *m* (*fam*)

telithromycin *n* telitromicina

temazepam *n* temazepam *m*

temperament *n* temperamento

temperature *n* temperatura; (*fam*) fiebre *f*, calentura; **axillary —** temperatura axilar; **oral —** temperatura oral; **rectal —** temperatura rectal; **room —** temperatura ambiente; **to take** (someone's) **—** tomarle la temperatura (a alguien); **to take your** (own) **temperature** tomarse la temperatura; **Did you take your temperature at home?**..¿Se tomó la temperatura en casa?

temple *n* (*anat*) sien *f*

temporal *adj* temporal

temporary *adj* temporal, provisional; **This bandage is only temporary** ..Este vendaje es solo temporal.

temporomandibular *adj* temporomandibular

tendency *n* (*pl* **-cies**) tendencia

tender *adj* (*sore*) dolorido

tenderness *n* dolor *m* (al tocar)

tendinitis *n* tendinitis *f*; **calcific —** tendinitis calcificante

tendon *n* tendón *m*; **Achilles —** tendón de Aquiles

tendonitis *V.* **tendinitis**.

tenesmus *n* (*form*) tenesmo (*form*), pujo

tennis *n* tenis *m*

tennis elbow *n* epicondilitis *f* (*form*), codo de tenista

tenofovir *n* tenofovir *m*

tenosynovitis *n* tenosinovitis *f*

TENS *abbr* **transcutaneous electrical nerve stimulation**. *V.* **stimulation**.

tense *adj* tenso; *vt* (*one's muscles*) tensar (*los músculos*); *vi* **to — up** ponerse tenso; **Try not to tense up** ..Trate de no ponerse tenso.

tension *n* tensión *f*; **nervous —** tensión nerviosa

tent *n* tienda; **oxygen —** tienda de oxígeno

teratogenic *adj* teratogénico

teratogenicity *n* teratogenicidad *f*

teratoma *n* teratoma *m*

terazosin *n* terazosina

terbinafine *n* terbinafina

terbutaline *n* terbutalina

terfenadine *n* terfenadina

term *n* término; **at —** a término

terminal *adj* terminal

tertiary *adj* de tercer nivel

test *n* prueba, examen *m*, análisis *m*; **Your tests show**..Sus exámenes muestran; **blood —** análisis *or* prueba de sangre; **exercise stress —** prueba de esfuerzo, ergometría (*form*); **eye —** examen oftalmológico, examen de los ojos, examen de la vista; **(oral) glucose tolerance —** prueba de tolerancia (oral) a la glucosa; **hearing —** prueba *or* examen de audición; **HIV —** prueba del VIH; **Pap —** (*fam*) citología cervical (*form*), citología (*fam*), prueba de Papanicolaou; **patch —** prueba de(l) parche; **pregnancy —** prueba de embarazo; **pulmonary function —** prueba de función pulmonar; **screening —** cribado

(*form*), examen *m* de detección; **skin —** prueba cutánea; **TB —** prueba de la tuberculina (*form*), PPD *m&f*, prueba de la tuberculosis (*fam*); **tilt table —** prueba de la mesa basculante; **urine —** análisis *or* examen de orina; *vt* analizar, hacer una prueba (un examen, un análisis), examinar; **I would like to test your urine for opiates.**. Quisiera hacerle un análisis de la orina para detectar opiáceos.

test dose *n* dosis *f* de prueba

testicle *n* testículo; **undescended —** testículo no descendido

testicular *adj* testicular

testing *n* evaluación *f*, valoración *f*, diagnóstico, análisis *m*, realización *f* de análisis *or* pruebas para fines diagnósticos; **exercise stress —** ergometría (*form*), (realización de) pruebas de esfuerzo; **fecal occult blood —** análisis de sangre oculta en heces; **genetic —** diagnóstico genético; **HIV —** (realización de) pruebas del HIV; **random drug —** (realización de) pruebas aleatorias de detección de drogas; **urodynamic —** evaluación *or* valoración urodinámica

testosterone *n* testosterona

test strip *n* tira reactiva (*para sangre*)

test tube *n* tubo de ensayo

tetanus *n* tétanos *m*

tetracycline *n* tetraciclina

tetrahydrocannabinol (THC) *n* tetrahidrocannabinol *m*

tetralogy of Fallot *n* tetralogía de Fallot

thalamus *n* tálamo

thalassemia *n* talasemia

thalidomide *n* talidomida

thallium *n* talio

THC *V.* **tetrahydrocannabinol**.

theophylline *n* teofilina

theory *n* (*pl* **-ries**) teoría

therapeutic *adj* terapéutico

therapist *n* terapeuta *mf*; (*fam, psych*) psicoterapeuta *mf*; **massage —** masajista *mf*; **occupational —** terapeuta ocupacional; **physical —** fisioterapeuta *mf*; **speech —** logopeda *mf* (*form*), fonoaudiólogo -ga *mf*, terapeuta del lenguaje, especialista *mf* en trastornos del lenguaje

therapy *n* (*pl* **-pies**) terapia, tratamiento; **combination** — tratamiento combinado, terapia combinada; **consolidation** — terapia de consolidación; **directly observed** — tratamiento directamente observado; **electroconvulsive** — **(ECT)** terapia electroconvulsiva (TEC); **group** — terapia de grupo *or* grupal; **heat** — termoterapia; **highly active antiretroviral** — **(HAART)** tratamiento *or* terapia antirretroviral de gran actividad (TARGA); **hormonal** — hormonoterapia; **hormone-replacement** — terapia hormonal sustitutiva; **induction** — terapia de inducción; **maintenance** — (*oncology, addiction medicine, etc.*) terapia de mantenimiento; **nicotine-replacement** — terapia de sustitución nicotínica; **occupational** — terapia ocupacional; **physical** — fisioterapia; **radiation** — radioterapia; **respiratory** — fisioterapia respiratoria, terapia respiratoria (*esp. Amer*); **root canal** —, **root canal** (*fam*) endodoncia (*form*), tratamiento de conducto; **salvage** — terapia de rescate; **speech** — logoterapia (*form*), terapia del lenguaje; **ultrasound** — ultrasonoterapia, terapia ultrasónica; **whirlpool** — hidromasaje *m*

thermal *adj* termal

thermometer *n* termómetro; **rectal** — termómetro rectal

thiabendazole *n* tiabendazol *m*

thiamine *n* tiamina

thiazide *n* tiazida

thick *adj* (*dimension*) espeso, grueso; (*consistency*) espeso

thickness *n* (*dimension*) espesor *m*, grosor *m*; (*consistency*) espesor *m*, densidad *f*

thigh *n* muslo

thin *adj* (*comp* **thinner**; *super* **thinnest**) delgado, flaco (*fam*); (*hair*) escaso, ralo, delgado; (*liquid*) poco espeso; (*fam, blood*) anticoagulada; **to become** — adelgazarse, (*esp.*

unintentionally) enflaquecer(se); **to — one's blood** tratar con un anticoagulante, diluirle la sangre (*fam*), adelgazarle la sangre (*Ang*); **We need to thin your blood**..Necesitamos tratarlo con un anticoagulante.

think *vi* (*pret & pp* **thought**) pensar

thioridazine *n* tioridazina

third *n* tercio, tercera parte; **two thirds of a dose**..dos tercios (terceras partes) de una dosis

thirst *n* sed *f*

thirsty *adj* — tener sed; **to make** — dar sed

thoracentesis *n* (*pl* **-ses**) toracocentesis *f*

thoraces *pl de* **thorax**

thoracic *adj* torácico

thoracoscopic *adj* toracoscópico

thoracoscopy *n* toracoscopia, toracoscopía (*Amer, esp. spoken*); **video-assisted** — videotoracoscopia

thoracotomy *n* (*pl* **-mies**) toracotomía

thorax *n* (*pl* **-raxes** *o* **-races**) tórax *m*

thorn *n* espina

thought (*pret & pp de* **think**) *n* pensamiento

threat *n* amenaza

threaten *vt, vi* amenazar

three-day measles *n* (*fam*) rubéola *or* rubeola

threonine *n* treonina

threshold *n* umbral *m*; **auditory** — umbral de audición; **pain** — umbral del dolor

threw *pret de* **throw**

throat *n* garganta; **sore** — dolor *m* de garganta

throb *vi* (*pret & pp* **throbbed**; *ger* **throbbing**) (*pain*) doler con cada latido del corazón

throbbing (*ger de* **throb**) *adj* (*pain*) pulsátil, que duele con cada latido del corazón

thrombectomy *n* (*pl* **-mies**) trombectomía

thrombi *pl de* **thrombus**

thromboangiitis obliterans *n* tromboangeítis *f* obliterante

thrombocytopenia *n* trombocitopenia

thrombocytosis *n* trombocitosis *f*; **essential —** trombocitosis esencial
thromboembolism *n* (*pl* **-li**) tromboembolia
thrombolysis *n* trombolisis *f*
thrombolytic *adj* & *n* trombolítico
thrombophlebitis *n* tromboflebitis *f*
thrombosis *n* (*pl* **-ses**) trombosis *f*; **deep venous — (DVT)** trombosis venosa profunda
thrombus *n* (*pl* **-bi**) trombo
throw *vt* (*pret* **threw**; *pp* **thrown**) **to — one's back out** (*fam*) dislocarse la espalda, lastimarse la espalda (*se refiere al concepto popular de que el dolor repentino de espalda se debe a una dislocación de una vertebra*); *vi* **to — up** (*fam*) *V.* vomit.
thrush *n* candidiasis *f* oral (*form*), algodoncillo (*Mex*), sapo (*PR, SD*), infección *f* por hongos en la boca
thumb *n* pulgar *m*, dedo pulgar
thumbnail *n* uña del pulgar
thumb sucking *n* succión *f* del pulgar (*form*), (el) chuparse el dedo
thump *n* golpe *m*; **precordial —** golpe precordial
thymectomy *n* (*pl* **-mies**) timectomía
thymi *pl de* **thymus**
thymoma *n* timoma *m*
thymus *n* (*pl* **-mi** *o* **-muses**) timo
thyroglobulin *n* tiroglobulina
thyroid *adj* tiroideo; **— storm** crisis tirotóxica, tormenta tiroidea; *n* (*fam, gland*) glándula tiroides, tiroides *m&f* (*fam*)
thyroidectomy *n* (*pl* **-mies**) tiroidectomía
thyroiditis *n* tiroiditis *f*; **Hashimoto's — tiroiditis de Hashimoto; subacute —** tiroiditis subaguda
thyrotoxic *adj* tirotóxico
thyrotoxicosis *n* tirotoxicosis *f*
thyrotropin (*TSH*) *n* tirotropina *or* tirotrofina, hormona estimulante del tiroides
thyroxine *n* tiroxina
TIA *abbr* **transient ischemic attack.** *V.* **attack.**
tiagabine *n* tiagabina
tibia *n* tibia; **— varus** tibia vara
tic *n* tic *m*; **— douloureux** neuralgia del trigémino

tick *n* garrapata
ticker *n* (*fam, heart*) corazón *m*
tickle *n* cosquilleo, (*in the throat*) irritación *f*; *vt* hacer cosquillas; **I don't mean to be tickling you**..No es mi intención hacerle cosquillas.
tickling *n* cosquillas, cosquilleo
ticklish *adj* cosquilloso
tight *adj* apretado; (*control, as of blood sugars*) estricto
time *n* tiempo, vez *f*; (*by the clock*) hora; **in order to save time**..para ahorrar tiempo...**four times a day**..cuatro veces al día...**At what time?** ..¿A qué hora?; **all the —** todo el tiempo; **a long —** mucho tiempo; **a short —** un rato, poco tiempo; **at times** a veces; **each —** *o* **every —** cada vez; **free —** tiempo libre; **from — to —** de vez en cuando; **in — (eventually)** con el tiempo; **leisure —** tiempo de ocio; **partial thromboplastin — (PTT)** tiempo parcial de tromboplastina; **prothrombin — (PT)** tiempo de protrombina; **(PT) the first —** la primera vez; **the last —** la última vez; **the next —** la próxima vez
timid *adj* tímido
timolol *n* timolol *m*
tincture *n* tintura
tinea *n* tiña, tinea (*Latin*), infección *f* por hongos de la piel; **— capitis** tinea capitis, tiña del cuero cabelludo, tiña de la cabeza (*esp. Mex*); **— corporis** tinea corporis, tiña del cuerpo; **— cruris** tinea cruris, tiña inguinal *or* crural; **— pedis** tinea pedis, tiña de los pies; **— versicolor** pitiriasis *f* versicolor
tingle *vi* hormiguear
tingling *n* hormigueo
tinidazole *n* tinidazol *m*
tinnitus *n* tinnitus *m* (*form*), zumbido de oídos (*fam*)
tiotropium *n* tiotropio
tip *n* (*tongue, finger, etc.*) punta; (*recommendation*) consejo
tipranavir *n* tipranavir *m*
TIPS *abbr* **transjugular intrahepatic portosystemic shunt.** *V.* **shunt.**
tiptoes *npl* **to walk on —** caminar de puntillas

tire *vt, vi* (*también* **to — out**) cansarse; **Just walking to the bathroom tires him out**..Con solo caminar al baño se cansa.

tired *adj* (*también* **— out**) cansado; **to get —** cansarse

tiredness *n* cansancio

tiring *adj* cansado, agotador

tirosine *n* tirosina

tissue *n* tejido; (*for blowing one's nose, etc.*) pañuelo (de papel), pañuelo desechable (*esp. Mex*); **connective —** tejido conectivo *or* conjuntivo; **granulation —** tejido de granulación; **scar —** tejido cicatricial; **soft —** partes blandas

tit (*vulg*) *n* (*nipple*) pezón *m*, teta (*vulg*); (*breast*) mama, seno, pecho, teta (*vulg*)

titanium *n* titanio; **— oxide** óxido de titanio

titer *n* título

titrate *vt* titular

titration *n* titulación *f*

toast *n* pan tostado

tobacco *adj* tabáquico; *n* (*pl* **-cos**) tabaco; **chewing —** tabaco de mascar; **— use** tabaquismo

tocolytic *adj & n* tocolítico

tocopherol *n* tocoferol *m*

today *adv* hoy

toe *n* dedo (del pie); **big —** dedo gordo (del pie); **great —** (*form*) dedo gordo (del pie); **little —** dedo chico (del pie)

toenail *n* uña (del pie)

tofu *n* tofu *m*

toilet *n* inodoro, retrete (*esp. Esp*); **— bowl** taza del inodoro *or* retrete; **— paper** papel higiénico, papel sanitario (*Mex, CA, Carib*)

tolazamide *n* tolazamida

tolbutamide *n* tolbutamida

tolerance *n* tolerancia; **(high, low) pain —** (alta, baja) tolerancia al dolor

tolerant *adj* tolerante

tolerate *vt* tolerar, soportar, aguantar

tolteradine *n* tolteradina

toluene *n* tolueno

tomato *n* (*pl* **-toes**) tomate *m*

tomogram *n* tomografía (*estudio imagenológico*)

tomography *n* tomografía (*técnica imagenológica*); **computed — (CT)** tomografía computarizada (TC); **computerized axial — (CAT)** tomografía axial computarizada (TAC); **positron emission — (PET)** tomografía por emisión de positrones (PET *o* TEP); **spiral computed —** tomografía computarizada helicoidal

tomorrow *adv* mañana

tone *n* tono; **heart tones** tonos cardíacos; **muscle —** tono muscular; *vt* (*one's muscles*) tonificar (*los músculos*)

tongue *n* lengua; **— depressor** *o* **blade** depresor *m* (de lengua), bajalenguas *m*, abatelenguas *m* (*Mex*), depresor (lingual) (*Esp*), paleta (*fam*)

tonic *n* tónico, reconstituyente *m*

toning *n* tonificación *f*; **— exercises** ejercicios de tonificación

tonsil *n* amígdala, angina (*fam, usually pl*)

tonsillectomy *n* (*pl* **-mies**) amigdalectomía

tonsillitis *n* amigdalitis *f*

took *pret de* take

tooth *n* (*pl* **teeth**) diente *m*, muela; **baby —** diente de leche; **back —** (*fam*) muela; **canine —** colmillo, (diente) canino; **deciduous —** diente de leche; **false teeth** dentadura postiza, dientes postizos; **front —** incisivo; **permanent —** diente definitivo *or* permanente; **primary —** diente primario; **set of teeth** dentadura; **wisdom —** tercer molar (*form*), muela del juicio

toothache *n* dolor de muelas

toothbrush *n* cepillo de dientes

toothpaste *n* pasta de dientes, dentífrico (*form*), pasta dental *or* dentífrica

tophus *n* (*pl* **-phi**) tofo

topical *adj* tópico

topiramate *n* topiramato

torasemide *n* torasemida

tore *pret de* tear

torn *pp de* tear

torsion *n* torsión *f*; **testicular —** torsión testicular

torso *n* torso
torticollis *n* tortícolis *f*
torture *n* tortura; *vt* torturar
torus *n* torus *m*; — **palatinus** torus palatino
total *adj* & *n* total *m*
touch *n* (*sense*) tacto; *vt* tocar
tough *adj* duro
tourniquet *n* torniquete *m*
towel *n* toalla
To Whom It May Concern A quien corresponda
toxemia *n* toxemia
toxemic *adj* toxémico
toxic *adj* tóxico
toxicity *n* toxicidad *f*
toxicologist *n* toxicólogo -ga *mf*, especialista *mf* en las sustancias tóxicas
toxicology *n* toxicología, estudio de las sustancias tóxicas y sus efectos en el organismo
toxin *n* toxina
toxocariasis *n* toxocariasis *f*
toxoid *n* toxoide *m*; **diphtheria** — toxoide diftérico; **tetanus** — toxoide tetánico
toxoplasmosis *n* toxoplasmosis *f*
tPA *abbr* **tissue plasminogen activator**. *V.* **activator**.
TPN *abbr* **total parenteral nutrition**. *V.* **nutrition**.
trace *n* trazas; **There is a trace of protein in your urine**..Hay trazas de proteínas en su orina.
tracer *n* trazador *m*
trachea *n* (*pl* -cheae *o* -cheas) tráquea
tracheitis *n* traqueítis *f*
tracheobronchitis *n* traqueobronquitis *f*
tracheostomy *n* (*pl* -mies) traqueostomía
tracheotomy *n* (*pl* -mies) traqueotomía
trachoma *n* tracoma *m*
tracing *n* (*ECG, etc.*) registro, trazado
tracks *npl* (*from drug addiction*) marcas de uso de drogas intravenosas
tract *n* tracto, vía; **biliary** — vía biliar (*frec. pl*); **digestive** *o* **gastro-**

intestinal — aparato *or* tubo digestivo; **genital** — aparato genital; **genitourinary** — aparato genitourinario; **(upper, lower) respiratory** — vías respiratorias (altas, bajas), tracto respiratorio (superior, inferior); **urinary** — tracto *or* aparato urinario
traction *n* tracción *f*
train *vi* entrenarse
training *n* entrenamiento, formación *f*; **job** — capacitación *f* laboral (*form*), entrenamiento para ejercer un empleo; **toilet** — (*ped*) entrenamiento para usar el baño
trait *n* rasgo; **thalassemia** — rasgo talasémico
tramadol *n* tramadol *m*
trance *n* trance *m*
tranquilize *vt* (*ant*) tranquilizar
tranquilizer *n* (*ant*) tranquilizante *m*, sedante *m*
transabdominal *adj* transabdominal
transcutaneous *adj* transcutáneo
transdermal *adj* transdérmico
trans fat (*fam*) **trans fatty acid**. *V.* **fatty acid**.
transfer *n* transferencia, (*of a patient*) traslado; **embryo** — transferencia embriónica; **gamete intrafallopian** — **(GIFT)** transferencia intratubárica de gametos; *vt* (*pret* & *pp* -ferred; *ger* -ferring) transferir; (*a patient*) trasladar
transference *n* (*psych, etc.*) transferencia
transferrin *n* transferrina
transformation *n* transformación *f*
transfuse *vt* transfundir (*form*), hacer una transfusión, poner sangre (*fam*)
transfusion *n* transfusión *f*; **Have you ever had a transfusion before?**..¿Ha tenido alguna vez una transfusión? **autologous blood** — autotransfusión *f*; **exchange** — exanguinotransfusión *f*; **to give a** — hacer una transfusión, poner sangre (*fam*); **I need to give you a transfusion**..Tengo que hacerle una transfusión..Tengo que ponerle sangre; — **of red blood cells (platelets, etc.)** transfusión de glóbulos

rojos (plaquetas, etc.)
transgender *adj* transgénero (*inv*); —
woman mujer transgénero
transgenderism *n* transgenerismo
transient *adj* transitorio, pasajero
transition *n* transición *f*
transitional *adj* transicional
translate *vt* traducir
translocation *n* translocación *f*
transmission *n* transmisión *f*
transmit *vt* (*pret & pp* -mitted; *ger*
-mitting) transmitir
transplant *n* trasplante *m*; **bone mar-**
row — trasplante de médula ósea;
hair — trasplante de pelo; **heart** —
trasplante cardíaco *or* de corazón;
kidney — trasplante renal *or* de riñón; **liver** — trasplante hepático *or*
de hígado; **lung** — trasplante pulmonar *or* de pulmón; **organ** —
trasplante de órganos; **renal** —
trasplante renal *or* de riñón; *vt* trasplantar
transport *n* transporte *m*; *vt* transportar
transposition *n* transposición *f*
transrectal *adj* transrectal
transsexual *adj & n* transexual *mf*
transurethral *adj* transuretral
transvaginal *adj* transvaginal
transvestism *n* travestismo
transvestite *n* travesti *mf*
trapeze *n* (*for a hospital bed*) trapecio (*para una cama hospitalaria*)
trapezius *n* (*anat*) trapecio
trauma *n* traumatismo; (*psych*) trauma *m*
traumatic *adj* traumático
traumatize *vt* traumatizar
travel *n* (el) viajar, viajes *mpl*; **for-**
eign — viajes internacionales
tray *n* bandeja, charola (*Mex*)
trazodone *n* trazodona
treadmill *n* caminadora (*Amer*), tapiz
m or cinta rodante (*esp. Esp*)
treat *vt* tratar
treatable *adj* tratable
treatment *n* tratamiento; **breathing**
—nebulización *f*
tremble *vi* temblar
tremor *n* temblor *m*, temblores (*fam*);
essential — temblor esencial
tremulous *adj* tembloroso

trench mouth *n* angina de Vincent,
gingivitis úlceronecrotizante aguda
trend *n* tendencia
tretinoin *n* tretinoína
triage *n* triage *m* (*form*), evaluación *f*
inicial de pacientes de emergencia
para establecer prioridades
trial *n* ensayo, prueba; **clinical** — ensayo clínico; — **and error** ensayo
y error
triamcinolone *n* triamcinolona
triamterene *n* triamtereno
triazolam *n* triazolam *m*
triceps *n* tríceps *m*
trichinosis *n* triquinosis *f*
trichloroacetic acid *n* ácido tricloroacético
trichomoniasis *n* tricomoniasis *f*
tricuspid *adj* tricúspide
tried *pret & pp de* **try**
tries *pl de* **try**
trifluoperazine *n* trifluoperazina
trigeminal *adj* trigémino
trigger *n* — **finger** dedo en resorte;
— **point** punto gatillo; *vt* provocar,
desencadenar
triglyceride *n* triglicérido
trimester *n* trimestre *m*
trimethoprim *n* trimetoprim *m*, tri-
métoprima
trip *vi* (*pret & pp* **tripped**; *ger* **trip-**
ping) tropezar, dar un traspié
triplet *n* trillizo -za *mf*
trismus *n* trismo
trisomy *n* trisomía; — **21** trisomía 21
trivalent *adj* trivalente
trochanter *n* trocánter *m*
trochanteric *adj* trocantérico (*Amer*),
trocantéreo (*Esp*)
troche *n* pastilla para chupar
troglitazone *n* troglitazona
tropical *adj* tropical
trouble *n* molestia (*frec. pl*); **Do you**
have trouble with your back?..
Tiene molestia(s) en la espalda?
true *adj* verdadero
trunk *n* (*anat*) tronco
truss *n* braguero, faja para contener
una hernia
trust *n* confianza; *vt* tener confianza
en, confiar en
try *n* (*pl* **tries**) intento, prueba; *vt*
(*pret & pp* **tried**) tratar de, intentar;

(*a new medication, etc.*) probar
trypanosomiasis *n* tripanosomiasis *f*
trypsin *n* tripsina
tryptophan *n* triptófano
TSH *abbr* **thyroid-stimulating hormone.** *V.* **hormone.**
TTP *abbr* **thrombotic thrombocytopenic purpura.** *V.* **purpura.**
tubal *adj* tubárico
tube *n* tubo, sonda, trompa, manguera; **chest —** tubo de drenaje pleural, tubo torácico; **drainage —** tubo de drenaje; **endotracheal —** tubo endotraqueal; **Eustachian —** conducto auditivo, trompa de Eustaquio; **fallopian —** trompa de Falopio; **feeding —** sonda de alimentación; **gastrostomy —, G-tube** (*fam*) sonda de gastrostomía; **nasogastric —** sonda nasogástrica
tuberculin *n* tuberculina
tuberculoid *adj* tuberculoide
tuberculosis (TB) *n* tuberculosis *f* (TB)
tuberculous *adj* tuberculoso
tuberous *adj* tuberoso
tubing *n* tubería
tubo-ovarian *adj* tubo-ovárico
tubular *adj* tubular
tubule *n* túbulo
tularemia *n* tularemia
tummy *n* (*pl* **-mies**) (*ped*) barriga, panza; **— tuck** (*fam*) *V.* **abdominoplasty.**
tumor *adj* tumoral; *n* tumor *m*; **benign —** tumor benigno; **brain —** tumor cerebral; **desmoid —** tumor desmoide; **malignant —** tumor maligno; **Wilms' —** tumor de Wilms
tuna *n* atún *m*
tuning fork *n* diapasón *m*
tunnel *n* túnel *m*; **carpal —** túnel carpiano
turistas, the (*fam*) traveler's diarrhea. *V.* **diarrhea.**
turn *n* vuelta; *vt* (*a patient in bed*)

cambiar de posición, voltear (*a un encamado*); *vi* darse vuelta; **to — around** darse media vuelta; **to — red (blue, etc.)** ponerse colorado (azul, etc.); **to — out** resultar; **The tests turned out negative.**.Las pruebas resultaron negativas; **to — over** (*on the exam table*) voltearse, darse vuelta
TURP *abbr* **transurethral resection of the prostate.** *V.* **resection.**
turpentine *n* trementina
tweak *vt* (*fam*) usar metanfetamina
tweaker *n* (*fam*) persona que usa metanfetamina
tweezers *npl* pinzas, tenazas (*esp. Mex*)
twice *adv* dos veces; **— daily** dos veces al día
twin *adj & n* gemelo -la *mf*, mellizo *mf*; **conjoined —** gemelo siamés, hermano -na *mf* siamés, gemelo unido; **fraternal —** mellizo, gemelo que no se parece a su hermano; **identical —** gemelo idéntico; **Siamese —** (*ant*) gemelo siamés
twinge *n* punzada, dolor agudo y repentino
twist *vt, vi* (*one's ankle, etc.*) torcerse; **Did you twist your ankle?**..¿Se torció el tobillo?
twitch *n* tic *m*, sacudida (muscular), contracción breve e involuntaria de un músculo
tympanic *adj* timpánico
tympanoplasty *n* (*pl* **-ties**) timpanoplastia
type *n* tipo; **blood —** grupo sanguíneo (*form*), tipo de sangre (*fam*); **tissue —** tipo de tejido
typhoid *adj* tifoideo; *n* fiebre tifoidea, tifoidea
typhus *n* tifus *m*
typical *adj* típico
tyramine *n* tiramina
tyrosine *n* tirosina

U

ugly *adj* feo

ulcer *n* úlcera, llaga; **aphthous** — afta; **decubitus** — úlcera de decúbito (*form*), úlcera por presión, llaga debida a permanecer mucho tiempo sentado o encamado sin cambiar de posición; **duodenal** — úlcera duodenal; **gastric** — úlcera gástrica; **peptic** — úlcera péptica; **stress** — úlcera de estrés

ulcerated *adj* ulcerado

ulceration *n* ulceración *f*

ulna *n* cúbito

ulnar *adj* cubital

ultrafiltration *n* ultrafiltración *f*

ultrasonography *n* ultrasonografía (*técnica imagenológica*)

ultrasound *n* ultrasonografía, ultrasonido

ultraviolet *adj* ultravioleta

umbilical *adj* umbilical

umbilicus *n* (*pl* **-ci**) ombligo

unable *adj* incapaz

unaffected *adj* no afectado

unavoidable *adj* inevitable

unaware *adj* inconsciente, ignorante

unbearable *adj* intolerable, insoportable, inaguantable

unbuckle *vt* desabrochar(se)

unburdening *n* desahogo

unbutton *vt* desabrochar(se), desabotonar; **Can you unbutton your shirt?**..¿Puede desabrocharse la camisa?

uncle *n* tío

uncomfortable *adj* incómodo

uncommon *adj* poco común

uncomplicated *adj* sin complicaciones

unconscious *adj* inconsciente

uncooperative *adj* no colaborador

uncovered *adj* descubierto

underachiever *n* persona que no logra su potencial

underarm *n* axila

undercooked *adj* poco cocido *or* cocinado, mal cocido *or* cocinado

underdeveloped *adj* insuficientemente desarrollado

undergo *vt* (*pret* **-went**; *pp* **-gone**) someterse a; **You underwent an operation?**..¿Se sometió a una operación?

undernourished *adj* desnutrido, mal alimentado

undernourishment *n* desnutrición *f*, subalimentación *f*

underpants *npl* (*men's*) calzoncillos; (*women's*) calzón *m* (*frec. pl*), pantaletas (*esp. Mex*), bloomer *m* (*esp. CA, frec. pl*), panties *mpl* (*esp. Carib*), bragas (*esp. Esp*)

undershirt *n* camiseta

underwater *adj* subacuático, submarino

underwear *n* ropa interior

underwent *pret de* **undergo**

undesirable *adj* indeseable

undetectable *adj* indetectable

undifferentiated *adj* indiferenciado

undigested *adj* indigerido, no digerido

unequal *adj* desigual

unexpected *adj* inesperado

unfavorable *adj* desfavorable

ungual *adj* ungueal

unhappy *adj* infeliz, descontento

unhealthy *adj* poco saludable, no saludable

uniform *adj* uniforme; *n* uniforme *m*

uninsured *adj* sin seguro

union *n* unión *f*

unit *n* unidad *f*; **coronary care** — unidad coronaria; **intensive care** — **(ICU)** unidad de cuidados intensivos (UCI), unidad de terapia intensiva (UTI) (*SA*); **international** — unidad internacional; — **of blood** unidad de sangre

unite *vt, vi* unir(se)

universal *adj* universal

unmarried *adj* soltero

Unna's paste boot *n* bota de pasta de Unna

unpleasant *adj* desagradable

unresectable *adj* irresecable

unresponsive *adj* que no responde

unsanitary *adj* antihigiénico

unsaturated *adj* insaturado

unstable *adj* inestable

unsuitable *adj* inadecuado

untreated *adj* no tratado

unusual *adj* inusual, raro, extraño

unvaccinated *adj* no vacunado

up *adv* hacia arriba, para arriba; (*high*) alto, elevado; **Look up**..Mire hacia arriba...**from the waist up** ..de la cintura para arriba...**Your sugar is up**..Su azúcar está alto (elevado).

uphill *adv* cuesta arriba

upper *adj* (*anat*) superior (*form*), alto, de arriba

upset *adj* molesto, enojado; **to get** *o* **become** — molestarse, enojarse; **to have an** — **stomach** tener dolor de estómago, sentirse mal del estómago; *vt* (*pret & pp* **upset**; *ger* **upsetting**) molestar, enojar

uptake *n* captación *f*

upward *adv* hacia arriba

uranium *n* uranio

urban *adj* urbano

urea *n* urea

uremia *n* uremia

uremic *adj* urémico

ureter *n* uréter *m*

ureteral *adj* ureteral

urethra *n* uretra

urethral *adj* uretral

urethritis *n* uretritis *f*; **non-gonococcal** — uretritis no gonocócica

urgent *adj* urgente

uric acid *n* ácido úrico

urinal *n* (*hand-held*) orinal *m*, pato (*Amer*)

urinalysis *n* (*pl* -ses) análisis *m* de orina

urinary *adj* urinario

urinate *vi* orinar, hacer pis (*fam or*

vulg), hacer pipí (*esp. ped, fam*)

urine *n* orina

urodynamics *n* urodinámica

urogenital *adj* urogenital

urogram *n* urografía (*estudio imagenológico*)

urography *n* urografía (*técnica imagenológica*)

urokinase *n* urokinasa

urologist *n* urólogo -ga *mf*, médico - ca *mf* especialista en el aparato urinario

urology *n* urología, estudio del aparato urinario

urosepsis *n* urosepsis *f*

urticaria *n* urticaria

use *n* uso, empleo; **use of her leg**.. uso de la pierna; **excessive** — uso excesivo; *vt* usar, utilizar, emplear; **to get used to** acostumbrarse a; **to** — **up** usar todo; **Have you used up all your codeine?**..¿Ha usado toda su codeína? **used up** agotado

useless *adj* inútil

user *n* consumidor -ra *mf*, usuario -ria *mf*

usual *adj* usual, habitual; **your usual dose**..su dosis habitual; **as** — como de costumbre, como siempre; **Are you taking your insulin as usual?**..¿Está tomando su insulina como de costumbre? **than** — que de costumbre; **Are you drinking more liquids than usual?**..¿Está tomando más líquidos que de costumbre?

usually *adv* normalmente, en la mayoría de casos

uteri *pl de* **uterus**

uterine *adj* uterino

uterus *n* (*pl* -**ri**) útero, matriz *f*

UTI *abbr* **urinary tract infection.** *V.* **infection.**

utilize *vt* utilizar

uvea *n* úvea

uveitis *n* uveítis *f*

uvula *n* (*pl* -**las** *o* -**lae**) úvula, campanilla (*fam*)

V

vaccinate *vt* vacunar; **Have you been vaccinated against tetanus?** ..¿Ha sido vacunado contra el tétano?

vaccination *n* vacunación *f*

vaccine *n* vacuna; **attenuated** — vacuna atenuada; **BCG** — vacuna BCG; **conjugated** — vacuna conjugada; **DPT** — vacuna DTP; vacuna contra la difteria, el tétanos y la tos ferina; **flu** — vacuna antigripal, vacuna contra la gripe, vacuna contra la influenza (*esp. Mex*); **Haemophilus influenzae type b** — vacuna contra Haemophilus influenzae tipo b; **hepatitis B** — vacuna contra la hepatitis B; **influenza** — *V.* **flu** — *arriba*; **live** — vacuna viva; **meningococcal** — vacuna meningocócica, vacuna contra la meningitis meningocócica; **MMR** — vacuna triple viral; vacuna triple vírica (*Esp*); vacuna contra el sarampión, la rubéola y la parotiditis; **oral polio** — vacuna antipoliomielítica oral, vacuna oral contra el polio; **pneumococcal** — vacuna neumocócica, vacuna contra la neumonía; **rabies** — vacuna contra la rabia; **Sabin** — vacuna Sabin; **Salk** — vacuna Salk; **smallpox** — vacuna contra la viruela; **varicella** — vacuna contra la varicela

vaccinee *n* vacunado -da *mf*

vaccinia *n* vacuna

vagal *adj* vagal

vagina *n* vagina

vaginal *adj* vaginal

vaginitis *n* vaginitis *f*

vaginosis *n* vaginosis *f*; **bacterial** — vaginosis bacteriana

vagotomy *n* (*pl* **-mies**) vagotomía; **selective** — vagotomía selectiva

vagus *n* vago

valacyclovir *n* valaciclovir *m*

valdecoxib *n* valdecoxib *m*

valerian *n* (*bot*) valeriana

valgus *adj* valgo, valgus

valid *adj* válido

validity *n* validez *f*

valine *n* valina

vallecula *n* vallécula

valproate *n* valproato

valproic acid *n* ácido valproico

valsartan *n* valsartán *m*

value *n* valor *m*; **nutritional** — valor nutritivo *or* nutricional

valve *n* válvula; **aortic** — válvula aórtica; **mitral** — válvula mitral; **pulmonic** — válvula pulmonar; **pyloric** — válvula pilórica; **tricuspid** — válvula tricúspide

valvuloplasty *n* (*pl* **-ties**) valvuloplastia

vancomycin *n* vancomicina

vapor *n* vapor *m*

vaporizer *n* vaporizador *m*

vardenafil *n* vardenafil *m*, vardenafilo (*Esp*)

variable *adj* & *n* variable *f*

variant *adj* & *n* variante *f*

variation *n* variación *f*

varicella *n* varicela

varices *pl de* **varix**

varicocele *n* varicocele *m*

varicose *adj* varicoso; — **vein** vena varicosa

varix *n* (*pl* **-ices**) (*frec. pl*) varice *or* várice *f*, variz *f* (*esp. Esp*)

varus *adj* varo, varus

vary *vi* (*pret* & *pp* **-ried**) variar, oscilar

vascular *adj* vascular

vasculitis *n* vasculitis *f*; **hypersensitivity** — vasculitis por hipersensibilidad; **leukocytoclastic** — vasculitis leucocitoclástica; **necrotizing** — vasculitis necrotizante *or* necrosante

vas deferens *n* conducto deferente

vasectomy *n* (*pl* **-mies**) vasectomía

vasoconstriction *n* vasoconstricción

f
vasoconstrictor *n* vasoconstrictor *m*
vasodilation *n* vasodilatación *f*
vasodilator *n* vasodilatador *m*
vasopressin *n* vasopresina
vasospasm *n* vasoespasmo
vasovagal *adj* vasovagal
VD *abbr* **venereal disease**. *V.* **disease**.
vector *n* vector *m*
vegan *adj* & *n* vegano -na *mf*
veganism *n* veganismo
vegetable *adj* vegetal; *n* vegetal *m*, verdura, hortaliza; **to live as a vegetable** (*fam*)..vivir en un estado vegetativo; **leafy green —** verdura de hoja verde
vegetarian *adj* & *n* vegetariano -na *mf*
vegetarianism *n* vegetarianismo
vegetation *n* vegetación *f*
vegetative *adj* vegetativo; **persistent — state** estado vegetativo persistente
veggie (*fam*) *V.* **vegetable**.
vehicle *n* vehículo; (*pharm*) excipiente *m*
vein *n* vena; **antecubital —** vena antecubital; **external jugular —** vena yugular externa; **femoral —** vena femoral; **internal jugular —** vena yugular interna; **portal —** vena porta; **saphenous —** vena safena; **subclavian —** vena subclavia; **varicose —** vena varicosa
vein stripping *n* cirugía de várices
vena cava *n* vena cava; **inferior — —** vena cava inferior; **superior — — —** vena cava superior
venepuncture *n* flebotomía, (el) punzar una vena
venereal *adj* (*ant*) venéreo, de transmisión sexual
venlafaxine *n* venlafaxina
venogram *n* flebografía (*estudio imagenológico*)
venography *n* flebografía (*técnica imagenológica*)
venom *n* veneno
venomous *adj* venenoso
venous *adj* venoso
ventilation *n* ventilación *f*; **mechanical —** ventilación mecánica

ventilator *n* respirador *m*, ventilador *m*
ventral *adj* ventral
ventricle *n* ventrículo
ventricular *adj* ventricular
venule *n* vénula
verapamil *n* verapamilo, verapamil *m*
vertebra *n* (*pl* **-brae**) vértebra
vertebral *adj* vertebral
vertebroplasty *n* vertebroplastia
vertex *n* (*anat*) vértice *m*, parte *f* superior de la cabeza
vertical *adj* vertical
vertigo *n* vértigo
vesicle *n* vesícula, ampolla (*fam*)
vessel *n* vaso; **blood —** vaso sanguíneo
vestibular *adj* vestibular
vestibule *n* vestíbulo
veteran *n* veterano -na *mf*
veterinarian *n* veterinario -ria *mf*
veterinary *adj* veterinario
viable *adj* viable
vial *n* frasco, vial *m*
vibration *n* vibración *f*
vibrator *n* vibrador *m*
victim *n* víctima
vidarabine *n* vidarabina
video *n* video *m* (*Amer*), vídeo (*Esp*)
view *n* (*radiografía, etc.*) vista
vigabatrine *n* vigabatrina
vigor *n* vigor *m*
vigorous *adj* vigoroso
vinblastine *n* vinblastina
vincristine *n* vincristina
vinegar *n* vinagre *m*
violence *n* violencia; **domestic —** violencia doméstica
violent *adj* violento
violin spider (*fam*) **brown recluse spider**. *V.* **spider**.
viper *n* víbora
viral *adj* viral, vírico
viremia *n* viremia
virgin *n* virgen *mf*
virginity *n* virginidad *f*
virility *n* virilidad *f*
virilization *n* virilización *f*
virologic, virological *adj* virológico
virology *n* virología, estudio de los virus
virtual *adj* virtual
virulence *n* virulencia

virulent *adj* virulento

virus *n* (*pl* **viruses**) virus *m*; **attenuated** — virus atenuado; **Epstein-Barr** — **(EBV)** virus de Epstein-Barr; **flu** — virus de la gripe, virus gripal (*form*); **hepatitis B** — **(HBV), hepatitis C** — **(HCV), etc**. virus de la hepatitis B (VHB), virus de la hepatitis C (VHC), etc.; **herpes simplex** — **(HSV)** virus herpes simple (VHS); **human immunodeficiency** — **(HIV)** virus de la inmunodeficiencia humana (VIH); **human T-lymphotrophic** — virus linfotrópico humano (de células T); **influenza** — virus de la influenza; **live** — virus vivo; **Norwalk** — virus Norwalk; **respiratory syncytial** — virus sincitial respiratorio, virus respiratorio sincitial (*esp. Esp*); **varicella-zoster** — virus varicela-zoster; **West Nile** — virus del Nilo Occidental

visceral *adj* visceral

viscosity *n* (*pl* **-ties**) viscosidad *f*

viscous *adj* viscoso

visible *adj* visible

vision *n* visión *f*, vista; **blurred** — visión borrosa; **double** — visión doble; **far** — visión lejana; **near** — visión cercana; **night** — visión nocturna; **peripheral** — visión periférica; **tunnel** — visión (en) túnel

visit *n* visita, consulta; **doctor's** — visita al médico, consulta con el médico; **unscheduled** — visita no programada; *vt* visitar

visitor *n* visitante *mf*

visual *adj* visual

visualization *n* visualización *f*

visualize *vt* visualizar

vital *adj* vital

vitality *n* vitalidad *f*

vitamin *adj* vitamínico; *n* vitamina; **fat-soluble** — vitamina liposoluble; — **A, B$_{12}$, etc.** vitamina A, vitamina B$_{12}$, etc.; — **B complex** vitaminas del complejo B; **water-soluble** — vitamina hidrosoluble

vitiligo *n* vitíligo, vitiligo (*Amer*)

vitreous *adj* vítreo

VLDL *abbr* **very low density lipoprotein**. *V*. **lipoprotein**.

vocal *adj* vocal

voice *n* voz *f*

void *vi* vaciar la vejiga, orinar

volt *n* voltio

volume *n* volumen *m*; **tidal** — volumen tidal

voluntary *adj* voluntario

volunteer *n* voluntario -ria *mf*

volvulus *n* vólvulo

vomit *n* (*frec. pl*) vómito; *vt, vi* vomitar, arrojar (*fam*), devolver (*fam*), deponer (*Mex, fam*); **Did you vomit blood?** ..¿Vomitó sangre?

vomiting *n* vómito (*frec. pl*)

voodoo *n* vudú *m*

voyeurism *n* voyeurismo

VSD *abbr* **ventricular septal defect**. *V*. **defect**.

vulnerable *adj* vulnerable

vulva *n* (*pl* **-vae**) vulva

W

waist *n* cintura
waistline *n* cintura
wait *vi* esperar; **to — for** esperar
waiting list *n* lista de espera
wake *vt, vi* (*pret* **woke**; *pp* **woke** *o* **waked**) (*también* **to — up**) despertar(se)
wake-up call *n* (*fam*) llamada de atención
walk *vi* caminar, andar; **Walk over here**..Camine hacia acá..**Let me see how you walk**..Déjeme ver como camina; **to — in one's sleep** caminar dormido
walker *n* andador *m*, andadera (*Mex*), burrito (*SA*), aparato que se usa como soporte al caminar
wall *n* pared *f*; **abdominal —** pared abdominal
war *n* guerra; **nuclear —** guerra nuclear
ward *n* (*of a hospital*) sala; **maternity —** sala de maternidad; **observation —** sala de observación
warfarin *n* warfarina
warm *adj* tibio, caliente; **to be** *o* **feel —** tener *or* sentir calor; **— water** (*very warm*) agua caliente, (*not very warm*) agua tibia; *vt* (*también* **to — up**) calentar; *vi* **to — up** calentarse; (*sports*) hacer ejercicios de calentamiento, hacer (el) calentamiento
warmth *n* calor *m*
warmup *n* (ejercicios de) calentamiento
warning sign *n* signo *or* señal de alarma
wart *n* verruga; **genital —** verruga genital; **plantar —** verruga plantar
wash *vt* lavar; **to — one's hair (face, hands, etc.)** lavarse el pelo (la cara, las manos, etc.)
washcloth *n* toallita facial, toalla pequeña (para lavarse)

wasp *n* avispa
waste *npl* residuos, desechos; **hazardous —** residuos peligrosos; **metabolic —** desechos metabólicos
wasting *n* desgaste *m*; **muscle —** desgaste muscular
water *n* agua; **distilled —** agua destilada; **drinking —** agua potable; **fresh —** agua dulce; **hard —** agua dura, agua con alto contenido de sales; **mineral —** agua mineral; **purified —** agua purificada; **running —** agua corriente; **salt —** agua salada; **soft —** agua con bajo contenido de sales; **tap —** agua del grifo, agua de la llave (*esp. Mex*), agua de la canilla (*esp. SA*)
waterborne *adj* transmitido por el agua
waterbrash *n* salivación *f* refleja que precede al vómito
watery *adj* acuoso; **— discharge** secreción acuosa
wave *n* onda; **brain —** onda cerebral; **shock —** onda de choque
wavelength *n* longitud *f* de onda
wax *n* cera
weak *adj* débil
weaken *vt, vi* debilitar(se)
weakening *n* debilitamiento, decaimiento
weakness *n* debilidad *f*
wean *vt* destetar
weaning *n* destete *m*; **— from the ventilator** destete del respirador *or* ventilador
weapon *n* arma; **biological —** arma biológica; **chemical —** arma química
wear *vt* (*pret* **wore**; *pp* **worn**) ponerse, usar, llevar; **You should wear a hat**..Debería ponerse (usar) un sombrero..**You need to wear this brace**..Tiene que usar este aparato

ortopédico; *vi* **to — off** pasar; **The numbness will wear off in a couple hours**..El entumecimiento se le va a pasar en un par de horas; **to — out** gastar(se); **This prosthesis will wear out in 10 to 15 years**..Esta prótesis se gastará en 10 a 15 años.

weather *n* tiempo

web *n* membrana; **esophageal —** membrana esofágica

webbed *adj* alado; **— neck** cuello alado

wedge *n* cuña

weed (*fam*) marihuana, mariguana (*Mex*), hierba (*fam*), mota (*Mex, CA; fam*)

week *n* semana

weekend *n* fin *m* de semana

weep *vi* (*pret & pp* **wept**) llorar; (*lesion*) secretar líquido

Wegener's granulomatosis *n* granulomatosis *f* de Wegener

weigh *vt, vi* pesar; **The nurse will weigh you**..La enfermera lo va a pesar...**How much do you weigh?** ..¿Cuánto pesa?

weight *n* peso; (*sports*) pesa; **excess — ** sobrepeso; **ideal —** peso ideal; **lean body —** peso magro

weight lifting *n* levantamiento de pesas, (el) levantar pesas; **— — belt** cinturón de levantamiento, cinturón para levantar pesas

welfare *n* bienestar *m*, bien *m*; (*government program*) asistencia social

well *adj & adv* (*comp* **better**; *super* **best**) bien; **to get —** curarse, recuperarse

well-being *n* bienestar *m*

wellness *n* bienestar *m*

welt *n* verdugón *m*, roncha

went *pret de* **go**

wept *pret & pp de* **weep**

wet *adj* (*comp* **wetter**; *super* **wettest**) mojado; **to get —** mojarse; *vt* (*pret & pp* **wet** *o* **wetted**; *ger* **wetting**) mojar; **to — the bed** mojar la cama

wet dream *n* polución nocturna (*form*), sueño húmedo

wet nurse *n* nodriza

wheal *n* (*hive*) roncha, habón *m* (*esp. Esp*); (*welt*) verdugón *m*, roncha

wheat *n* trigo

wheelchair *n* silla de ruedas; **electric —** silla de ruedas eléctrica; **folding —** silla de ruedas plegable; **manual —** silla de ruedas manual; **motorized —** silla de ruedas motorizada

wheeze *n* sibilancia (*form*), silbido; *vi* tener sibilancias *or* silbidos; **Have you been wheezing?**..¿Ha tenido sibilancias al respirar?..¿Ha tenido silbidos en el pecho?

wheezing *n* sibilancias (*form*), silbidos (en el pecho)

whiplash *n* latigazo cervical

whipworm *n* tricocéfalo

whirlpool *n* bañera de hidromasaje, tina de hidromasaje (*esp. Mex*)

whisper *vt* decir en voz baja; *vi* hablar en voz baja

white *adj* blanco; *n* (*of an egg*) clara

whitener *n* (*dent*) blanqueador *m*

whitening *n* (*dent*) blanqueamiento

white noise *n* ruido blanco

whitish *adj* blanquecino

whitlow *n* panadizo (*debido al herpes en la mayoría de los casos*)

WHO *abbr* **World Health Organization**. *V.* **organization**.

whole *adj* entero, integral; **wholegrain** integral; **whole-grain cereals** cereales integrales; **— wheat** trigo integral

whooping cough *n* tos ferina, coqueluche *m&f* (*fam*)

wick *n* mecha

wide *adj* ancho

widen *vt* ensanchar, hacer más ancho

widow *n* viuda

widowed *adj* viudo

widower *n* viudo

width *n* anchura, ancho

wife *n* (*pl* **wives**) esposa, mujer *f*

wig *n* peluca

wiggle *vt, vi* mover(se); **Wiggle your toes**..Mueva sus dedos del pie.

wild *adj* (*animal*) salvaje, (*plant*) silvestre

will *n* voluntad *f*; **against your —** contra su voluntad; **living —** testamento vital; **of your own free —** por su propia voluntad; **the — to live** la voluntad de vivir; **— power**

fuerza de voluntad

wind *n* viento

windburn *n* resequedad *f* y ardor de la piel producidos por el viento

windpipe *n* (*fam*) tráquea

wine *n* vino; **red** — vino tinto; **white** — vino blanco

wing *n* (*of a hospital*) ala

winged scapula *n* elevación *f* de la escápula

winter *n* invierno; — **itch** resequedad *f* de la piel con comezón que ocurre generalmente en el invierno

wipe *vt* enjugar; **to** — **oneself** (*after moving bowels*) limpiarse

wire *n* alambre *m*

wired *adj* (*fam*) acelerado

wishful thinking *n* (el) creer que algo es verdadero porque se desea intensamente

witchcraft *n* brujería

witch hazel *n* agua de hamamelis

withdrawal *n* síndrome *m* de abstinencia (*form*), síntomas sufridos por el adicto o alcohólico al suspender drogas o alcohol

wives *pl de* **wife**

woke *pret de* **wake**

woman *n* (*pl* **women**) mujer *f*

womb *n* matriz *f*, útero

women *pl de* **woman**

women's room *n* baño de mujeres *or* damas

wool *n* lana

woozy *adj* mareado

word *n* palabra; — **finding difficulty** dificultad *f* para encontrar palabras

wore *pret de* **wear**

work *adj* laboral, del trabajo; *n* trabajo; *vi* (*at a job*) trabajar; (*to function*) funcionar, trabajar; **Your kidneys have stopped working**.. Sus riñones han dejado de funcionar; **to**

— **out** (*exercise*) hacer ejercicio, levantar pesas

worker *n* obrero -ra *mf*, trabajador -ra *mf*; **social** — trabajador social

worker's compensation *n* compensación *f* del trabajador, programa *m* de seguro para compensar heridas relacionadas al trabajo

workout *n* sesión *f* de ejercicio

workplace *n* lugar *m* del trabajo

workshop *n* taller *m*; **parenting** — taller de padres

workup *n* conjunto de exámenes que se realiza para determinar la causa de un síntoma o signo

worm *n* gusano; (*intestinal*) lombriz *f*

worn *pp de* **wear**

worry *n* (*pl* **-ries**) (*frec. pl*) preocupación *f*; *vi* (*pret & pp* **-ried**) preocuparse; **You worry too much**..Se preocupa demasiado.

worse (*comp de* **bad** *y* **poorly**) *adj & adv* peor; **to get** — empeorar, agravarse; **to make** — agravar, empeorar; **Is there anything that makes the pain worse?**..¿Hay algo que le agrave el dolor?

worsening *n* empeoramiento

wound *n* herida; **entrance** — orificio de entrada; **exit** — orificio de salida; **gunshot** — herida de bala, balazo (*fam*); **knife** — cuchillada; **penetrating** — herida penetrante; **puncture** — herida punzante; **stab** — cuchillada, puñalada; *vt* herir

wounded *adj* herido

wrap *vt* (*pret & pp* **wrapped**; *ger* **wrapping**) envolver

wrinkle *n* arruga; *vt, vi* arrugar(se)

wrist *n* muñeca

writer's cramp *n* calambre *m* del escribiente

writhe *vi* retorcerse

X

xanthoma *n* xantoma *m*
x-ray *n* rayo X (*frec. pl*); (*film*) radio-
    grafía, placa (*fam*); **chest x-ray**
    radiografía de tórax; *vt* tomar una
radiografía *or* placa de; **We need to
x-ray your foot**..Tenemos que tomarle una radiografía (placa) del
pie.

Y

yarrow *n* (*bot*) milenrama
yawn *n* bostezo; *vi* bostezar
yaws *n* pian *m*, frambesia
year *n* año
yeast *n* levadura (*frec. pl*), hongos
    (*fam*); **brewer's —** levadura de cer-
    veza
yellow *adj* amarillo
yellowish *adj* amarillento
yellow jacket *n* (tipo de) avispa
yesterday *adv* ayer

yoga *n* yoga *m*
yogurt *n* yogur *m*
yohimbine *n* yohimbina
yolk *n* yema; **egg —** yema de huevo;
    — sac membrana vitelina
young *adj* joven
younger (*comp de* **young**) *adj* más
    joven, menor; **— brother** hermano
    menor
youth *n* juventud *f*
yucca *n* (*bot*) yuca

Z

zafirlukast *n* zafirlukast *m*
zalcitabine *n* zalcitabina
zaleplon *n* zaleplón *m*
zanamivir *n* zanamivir *m*
zen *n* zen *m*
zidovudine *n* zidovudina
zinc *n* zinc *m*; — **oxide** óxido de zinc
zip code *n* código postal
zipper *n* cierre *m*, cremallera (*Esp*),
  ziper *m* (*Ang*)

ziprasidone *n* ziprasidona
zit *n* (*fam*) grano, barro, espinilla
zolmitriptan *n* zolmitriptán *m*
zolpidem *n* zolpidem *m*
zombie *n* zombi *m*; **to feel like a —**
  sentirse como un zombi
zone *n* zona
zoster *V.* **herpes zoster**.
zygote *n* cigoto

SPANISH-ENGLISH

ESPAÑOL-INGLÉS

A

AA *See* **Alcohólicos Anónimos**.
abacavir *m* abacavir
abajo *adv* below; **la parte de abajo**.. the lower part; **de** — lower; **hacia** — downward, down
abandonar *vt* (*una dieta, un tratamiento, etc.*) to give up on
abandono *m* cessation; — **del tabaco** smoking cessation
abastecimiento *m* supply
abatelenguas *m* (*pl* **-guas**) (*Mex*) tongue depressor *o* blade
abdomen *m* abdomen, belly, stomach (*fam*)
abdominal *adj* abdominal; *m* (*ejercicio*) sit-up
abdominoplastia *f* abdominoplasty
abeja *f* bee; — **africanizada** *or* **asesina** Africanized *o* killer bee
abertura *f* opening
abierto -ta (*pp of* **abrir**) *adj* open
ablación *f* ablation
ablandar *vt* to soften
abordaje *m* approach; — **quirúrgico** surgical approach
abortar *vt* to abort; *vi* (*con intención*) to have an abortion; (*sin intención*) to miscarry, to have a miscarriage
abortivo *m* abortifacient
aborto *m* (*provocado*) abortion; (*espontáneo*) miscarriage; — **accidental** accidental abortion; — **de nacimiento parcial** partial birth abortion; — **de repetición** habitual

abortion; — **habitual** habitual abortion; — **incompleto** incomplete abortion; — **parcial** (*fam*) partial birth abortion; — **recurrente** habitual abortion; — **terapéutico** therapeutic abortion; **amenaza de** — threatened abortion; **sufrir un** — to miscarry; **tener un** — to have an abortion
abotagado -da *adj* bloated
abotonar *vt, vr* to button, to button up
abrasión *f* (*form*) abrasion
abrasivo -va *adj* & *m* abrasive
abrazar *vt* to embrace, hug
abrazo *m* embrace, hug
abrigo *m* coat
abrir *vt, vr* (*pp* **abierto**) to open
abrochar *vt, vr* to buckle, to button, to button up
absceso *m* abscess
absentismo *m* (*Esp*) absenteeism
absorbente *adj* absorbent
absorber *vt* to absorb
absorbible *adj* absorbable; **no** — nonabsorbable
absorciometría de rayos X de doble energía *f* dual-energy X-ray absorptiometry (DEXA)
absorción *f* absorption
abstenerse *vr* to abstain; — **del alcohol** to abstain from drinking alcohol
abstinencia *f* abstinence; — **perió-**

dica rhythm method

abuelo -la *m* grandfather, grandparent; *f* grandmother

aburrido -da *adj* bored

aburrir *vt* to bore; *vr* to become bored

abusador -ra *mf* abuser

abusar *vt* to abuse; **Ella abusa de las drogas.**.She abuses drugs.

abusivo -va *adj* abusive

abuso *m* abuse; — **de drogas** drug abuse; — **de sustancias** substance abuse; — **sexual** sexual abuse; **droga de** — drug of abuse

acabar *vi* (*Amer, fam, tener un orgasmo*) to have an orgasm, to come (*fam*); *vr* to run out; **Se me acabaron las pastillas.**.I ran out of pills..My pills ran out.

acalasia *f* achalasia

acantosis nigricans *f* acanthosis nigricans

acarbosa *f* acarbose

acariciar *vt* to caress, to fondle

ácaro *m* mite; (*garrapata*) tick; — **del polvo** dust mite

acaso *adv* **por si** — just in case

acatarrarse *vr* to catch a cold

acatisia *f* akathisia

accesible *adj* accessible

acceso *m* access; (*ataque*) fit, spell; — **a tratamiento** access to treatment; — **para silla(s) de ruedas** wheelchair access; — **venoso** venous access

accidentado -da *adj* injured (*in an accident*); *mf* accident victim

accidental *adj* accidental; **muerte** *f* — accidental death

accidentarse *vr* to have an accident

accidente *m* accident; — **cerebrovascular** cerebrovascular accident, stroke; — **de trabajo** work accident; — **de tráfico** *or* **tránsito** traffic accident; — **isquémico transitorio (AIT)** transient ischemic attack (TIA); — **laboral** work accident

acción *f* action; **de** — **corta** short-acting; **de** — **prolongada** long-acting; **de** — **rápida** fast-acting

acedía *f* heartburn

aceite *m* oil; — **de cacahuate** (*esp.* *Mex*), — **de cacahuete** (*Esp*) peanut oil; — **de cártamo** safflower oil; — **de coco** coconut oil; — **de colza** rapeseed oil; — **de eucalipto** limón lemon eucalyptus oil; — **de geranio** (*bot*) geranium oil; — **de hígado de bacalao** cod-liver oil; — **del árbol del té** tea tree oil; — **de maíz** corn oil; — **de oliva** olive oil; — **de palma** palm oil; — **de pescado** fish oil; — **de ricino** castor oil; — **mineral** mineral oil; — **vegetal** vegetable oil

acelerado -da *adj* (*fam*) hyperactive, nervously energetic, wired (*fam*)

acenocumarol *m* acenocoumarol

acero *m* steel; — **inoxidable** stainless steel

acervo genético *m* gene pool

acetábulo *m* acetabulum

acetaminofén, acetaminofeno *m* acetaminophen

acetato *m* acetate

acetazolamida *f* acetazolamide

acético -ca *adj* acetic

acetona *f* acetone

achacoso -sa *adj* sickly, having many ailments, complaining of many ailments

achaque *m* mild illness, ailment, affliction, complaint

acíbar *m* (*esp. Esp*) aloe

aciclovir *m* acyclovir

acidez *f* acidity; — **estomacal** heartburn, acid stomach (*fam*)

ácido -da *adj* & *m* acid; — **acético** acetic acid; — **acetilsalicílico** acetylsalicylic acid; **ácidos alfa hidróxidos** alpha hydroxy acids; — **ascórbico** ascorbic acid; — **azelaico** azelaic acid; — **bórico** boric acid; — **clorhídrico** hydrochloric acid; — **desoxirribonucleico (ADN)** deoxyribonucleic acid (DNA); — **fólico** folic acid; — **gástrico** gastric acid; — **glutámico** glutamic acid; — **graso** *See* **ácido graso** *as separate entry below*; — **hialurónico** hyaluronic acid — **láctico** lactic acid; — **linoleico** linoleic acid; — **nalidíxico** nalidixic acid; — **nicotínico** nicotinic acid, niacin; — **nítrico** nitric acid; — **paraaminoben-**

zoico **(PABA)** paraaminobenzoic acid (PABA); — **retinoico** retinoic acid; — **ribonucleico (ARN)** ribonucleic acid (RNA); — **salicílico** salicylic acid; — **tartárico** tartaric acid; — **tricloroacético** trichloroacetic acid; — **úrico** uric acid; — **valproico** valproic acid

ácido graso *m* fatty acid; — — **esencial** essential fatty acid; — — **insaturado** unsaturated fatty acid; — — **monoinsaturado** monounsaturated fatty acid; — — **omega-3** omega-3 fatty acid; — — **poliinsaturado** polyunsaturated fatty acid; — — **saturado** saturated fatty acid; — — **trans** trans fatty acid

aclarar *vt* (*la voz* or *la garganta*) to clear (*one's throat*)

aclimatado -da *adj* acclimated

aclimatarse *vr* to become acclimated

acné *m&f* acne; — **quístico** cystic acne; — **rosácea** acne rosacea, rosacea (*fam*)

acojinamiento *m* cushioning

acojinar *vt* to pad, cushion

acolchado -da *adj* padded; *m* padding

acolchar *vt* to pad, cushion

acolchonado *m* padding

acomodar *vt* (*los huesos*) to set (*a bone*), to reduce (*a fracture or dislocation*), to adjust, perform an adjustment on

acompañante *mf* companion

acondicionador *m* conditioner

acondicionamiento *m* conditioning; — **físico** physical conditioning, fitness

acondroplasia *f* achondroplasia

aconsejar *vt, vr* to advise

acordarse *vr* (*also* — **de**) to remember, to recall

acortar *vt* to shorten

acoso *m* harassment; — **sexual** sexual harassment

acostarse *vr* to lie down; (*en la cama, para dormir*) to go to bed

acostumbrarse *vr* to get used to

acrilamida *f* acrylamide

acrílico -ca *adj & m* acrylic

acrofobia *f* acrophobia

acromegalia *f* acromegaly

acropaquia *f* (*form*) clubbing

acta *f* certificate; — **de nacimiento** birth certificate

Actaea racemosa, (*bot*) black cohosh

actínico -ca *adj* actinic

actinomicosis *f* actinomycosis

actitud *f* attitude

activador *m* activator; — **tisular del plasminógeno** tissue plasminogen activator (tPA)

activar *vt* to activate

actividad *f* activity; **actividades de la vida diaria** activities of daily living

activo -va *adj* active, energetic; **sexualmente** — sexually active

acto sexual *m* sexual intercourse, intercourse; **durante el acto sexual..** during sexual intercourse

actual *adj* current

acudir *vt* to seek, to go; — **al médico** to go to the doctor, to seek medical attention

acumulación *f* accumulation, buildup

acumular *vt* to accumulate; *vr* to accumulate, build up; (*blood*) to pool

acumulativo -va *adj* cumulative; **efecto** — cumulative effect

acuoso -sa *adj* aqueous, watery; **secreción** — watery discharge

acupresión *f* acupressure

acupuntura *f* acupuncture

acústico -ca *adj* acoustic

adaptación *f* adaptation

adaptar *vt, vr* to adapt, to adjust; **bien adaptado** well-adjusted

adecuado -da *adj* adequate; appropriate, suitable

adefovir *m* adefovir

adelante *adv* **hacia** — forward

adelgazar *vt* (*la sangre*) (*Ang*) to thin (*one's blood*); *vr* to lose weight, to get thin

adenitis *f* adenitis

adenocarcinoma *m* adenocarcinoma

adenoidectomía *f* adenoidectomy

adenoides *fpl* adenoids

adenoiditis *f* adenoiditis

adenoma *m* adenoma; — **velloso** villous adenoma

adenomatoso -sa *adj* adenomatous

adenovirus *m* (*pl* **-rus**) adenovirus

adentro *adv* inside

adherencia f adhesion; adherence; — **al tratamiento** adherence to treatment

adherido -da adj adherent, attached

adhesivo -va adj & m adhesive

adicción f addiction; — **a la heroína** heroin addiction

adictivo -va adj addictive

adicto -ta adj addicted; **volverse —** to get o become addicted; mf addict; — **a la heroína** heroin addict

adiposo -sa adj fatty; **tejido —** fatty tissue

aditivo -va adj & m additive

administración f administration; **Administración de Alimentos y Drogas** Food and Drug Administration (FDA)

administrar vt to administer (a drug, etc.)

admisión f (Ang, al hospital) admission (to the hospital)

admitir vt (Ang, al hospital) to admit (to the hospital)

ADN abbr **ácido desoxirribonucleico.** See **ácido.**

adolescencia f adolescence

adolescente adj & mf adolescent

adolorido -da (fam) See **dolorido.**

adopción f adoption

adoptar vt to adopt

adoptivo -va adj adoptive; **padres adoptivos** adoptive parents

adormilado -da adj drowsy

adquirido -da adj acquired; — **en la comunidad** community-acquired

adquirir vt to acquire

adrenal adj adrenal; f adrenal gland

adrenalectomía f adrenalectomy

adrenalina f adrenaline

adsorbente adj adsorbent

adulterado -da adj adulterated

adulterar vt to adulterate

adulto -ta adj & mf adult

adverso -sa adj adverse

adyuvante adj (quimioterapia) adjuvant

aeróbic m aerobics; — **de bajo impacto** low impact aerobics

aeróbico -ca adj (metabolismo) aerobic; mpl aerobics; — **de bajo impacto** low impact aerobics

aerobio -bia adj (micro) aerobic

aerosol m aerosol, spray; inhaler; — **de pimienta** pepper spray; — **dosificador** metered dose inhaler; — **nasal** nasal inhaler, nasal spray; **en —** aerosolized

afasia f aphasia

afección f affection; disease, condition, affliction; involvement; — **de los ganglios linfáticos** involvement of the lymph nodes

afectado -da adj affected; — **por** affected by; **no —** unaffected

afectar vt to affect

afectivo -va adj emotional

afecto m affection; (psych) affect

afectuoso -sa adj affectionate

afeitadora f shaver, electric shaver

afeitar vt, vr to shave

afeminado -da adj effeminate

afilado -da adj sharp

afinidad f affinity

aflatoxina f aflatoxin

aflicción f distress; affliction

aflojar vt to loosen; (fam, relajar) to relax; **Afloje el brazo..Relax your arm.**

afónico -ca adj hoarse, having lost one's voice; **estar —** to be hoarse, to have lost one's voice

afrecho m bran

afrodisíaco, afrodisiaco m aphrodisiac

afrontar vt to face, (lidiar con) to cope (with)

afta f aphthous ulcer (form), canker sore; (candidiasis oral) thrush

agachar vt (la cabeza) to bend down (one's head); **Agache la cabeza..** Bend your head down; vr to bend over, bend down, stoop

agammaglobulinemia f agammaglobulinemia

agarrar vt to grasp, grip; (fam, una enfermedad) to catch

agencia f agency

agente m (pharm) agent; — **naranja** Agent Orange

ágil adj agile

agitado -da adj agitated, upset

agitar vt to agitate, to upset; to shake; **Agítese bien antes de usarse..** Shake well before using; vr to become agitated, to become upset

agonía *f* suffering preceding death, period preceding death

agónico -ca *adj* agonal

agorafobia *f* agoraphobia

agotado -da *adj* exhausted, run-down; used up

agotador -ra *adj* tiring

agotamiento *m* extreme fatigue, exhaustion; depletion

agotar *vt* to exhaust, to tire out; to deplete; *vr* to become exhausted, to tire out; to become depleted

agrandar *vt* to enlarge; *vr* to get *o* become bigger

agravar *vt* to aggravate, make worse; *vi, vr* to get worse; **Se agravó**..He got worse.

agregar *vt* to add; **No agregue sal**.. Don't add salt.

agresión *f* aggression; (*asalto*) assault; — **sexual** sexual assault

agresivo -va *adj* aggressive, combative

agrícola *adj* agricultural

agricultor -ra *mf* farmer

agrietado -da *adj* cracked, split, (*labios, piel*) chapped

agrietarse *vr* to crack, to split, (*labios, piel*) to chap, get chapped

agrio -ria *adj* sour

agruras *fpl* (*esp. Mex*) heartburn

agua *f* water; — **corriente** running water; — **de hamamelis** witch hazel; — **del grifo**, — **de la llave** (*esp. Mex*) tap water; — **destilada** distilled water; — **dulce** fresh water; — **dura** hard water; — **en el pulmón (la rodilla, etc.)** water on the lung (the knee, etc.); — **hirviendo** boiling water; — **mineral** mineral water; **aguas negras** sewage, sewer water; — **oxigenada** hydrogen peroxide; — **potable** potable water, drinking water; — **purificada** purified water; **aguas residuales** sewage, sewer water; — **salada** salt water; **aguas termales** hot springs

aguacate *m* avocado

aguamala *f* jellyfish

aguantable *adj* tolerable, bearable

aguantar *vt* to tolerate, endure, stand, bear; — **la respiración** (*fam*) to hold one's breath; **Aguante la res-**

piración..Hold your breath.

agudeza *f* acuity; — **visual** visual acuity

agudización *f* (*form*) exacerbation, flare

agudo -da *adj* (*enfermedad*) acute; (*dolor*) sharp; (*tono*) high-pitched

aguijón *m* stinger

aguja *f* needle; — **con aletas** butterfly needle; — **hipodérmica** hypodermic needle; — **mariposa** butterfly needle

agujero *m* hole

ahogar *vt* to suffocate, smother; to drown; *vr* to suffocate, to smother, to choke (*due to fumes, lack of air, etc.*); to drown; **Siento que me ahogo**..I feel like I'm drowning..I feel short of breath.

ahogo *m* choking sensation, shortness of breath

ahorcar *vt* to hang (*by the neck*); *vr* to hang oneself

AINE *abbr* **antiinflamatorio no esteroideo.** *See* **antiinflamatorio.**

airbag *m* airbag

aire *m* air; — **acondicionado** air conditioning; — **contaminado** air pollution, smog; **al** — **libre** outdoors; **botar aire** (*esp. Carib, SA; fam*), **echar aire** (*Esp*), **sacar aire** (*esp. Mex, CA; fam*) to breathe out; **tener** — (*esp. Mex, fam;en el pecho, abdomen, etc.*) to have air (*in one's chest, abdomen, etc.*) (*refers to a popular belief that pain in the chest or abdomen may be due to trapped air*); **tomar** — to breathe in

aislado -da *adj* isolated; (*emocionalmente*) alienated

aislamiento *m* isolation; — **inverso** reverse isolation; — **protector** protective isolation; — **respiratorio** respiratory isolation

aislar *vt* to isolate

ajo *m* garlic

ajustable *adj* adjustable

ajustador *m* (*Carib*) brassiere

ajustar *vt* to adjust, correct, to fit

ala *f* (*de un hospital*) wing (*of a hospital*)

alacrán *m* scorpion

alado -da *adj* webbed; **cuello —** webbed neck
alambre *m* wire; **— de púas** barbed wire
alanina *f* alanine
albendazol *m* albendazole
albinismo *m* albinism
albino -na *adj & mf* albino
albúmina *f* albumin
albuminuria *f* albuminuria
alcalino -na *adj* alkaline
alcalosis *f* alkalosis
alcance *m* reach; **fuera del — de los niños** out of reach of children
alcanfor *m* camphor
alcanzar *vt, vi* to reach
alcaptonuria *f* alkaptonuria
alcohol *m* alcohol, liquor; **— desnaturalizado** denatured alcohol; **— etílico** ethyl alcohol, ethanol; **— isopropílico** isopropyl alcohol, rubbing alcohol; **— metílico** methyl alcohol, methanol
alcohólico -ca *adj & mf* alcoholic; **— en recuperación** recovering alcoholic
Alcohólicos Anónimos, Alcoholics Anonymous (AA)
alcoholismo *m* alcoholism
aldosterona *f* aldosterone
aldosteronismo *m* aldosteronism
aleatorio -ria *adj* random; **pruebas aleatorias** random testing
alegre *adj* cheerful
alendronato *m* alendronate
alergeno, alérgeno *m* allergen
alergia *f* allergy; **— al polen** allergy to pollen, hay fever; **alergias estacionales** seasonal allergies
alérgico -ca *adj* allergic; **¿Es Ud. alérgico a la penicilina?**..Are you allergic to penicillin?
alergista *mf* allergist
alergología *f* study of allergies
alergólogo -ga *mf* allergist
alerta *adj* alert; *f* alert; **— sanitaria** health alert
aleteo *m* flutter; **— auricular** atrial flutter
alfa *f* alpha; **— feto-proteína** alpha fetoprotein; **— metildopa** alpha methyldopa
alfalfa *f* (*bot*) alfalfa

alfiler *m* pin
algas *fpl* algae
alginato *m* alginate
algodón *m* cotton
algodoncillo *m* (*Mex*) thrush
alheña *f* (*Esp, bot*) henna
alienado -da *adj* alienated
aliento *m* breath; **mal —** bad breath
alimentación *f* feeding, nourishment; diet; **— equilibrada** (*form*) balanced diet; **— por sonda** tube feeding
alimentar *vt* to feed
alimentario -ria *adj* alimentary; (*dietético*) dietary
alimenticio -cia *adj* (*nutricional*) nutritional; (*dietético*) dietary
alimento *m* (*frec. pl*) food; **alimentos enlatados** canned food(s); **alimentos industrializados** processed food(s); **alimentos infantiles** baby food(s); **alimentos naturales** health food(s), natural food(s); **alimentos procesados** processed food(s)
alineación *f* alignment
alineamiento *m* alignment
alinear *vt* to align; *vr* to line up
alitiásico -ca *adj* acalculous
aliviar *vt* to alleviate, soothe, relieve; *vr* (*síntoma*) to resolve, to get better; (*Mex, fam, dar a luz*) to give birth, deliver
alivio *m* relief
almacén *m* store
almacenar *vt* to store, to reserve
almidón *m* starch; **— de maíz** cornstarch
almohada *f* pillow, cushion
almohadilla *f* small pillow, small cushion, pad; **— eléctrica** heating pad
almorrana *f* hemorrhoid
almorzar *vi* to have lunch
almotriptán *m* almotriptan
almuerzo *m* lunch
aloe *m* aloe
alojarse *vr* to lodge
alópata *mf* allopath
alopatía *f* allopathy
alopático -ca *adj* allopathic
alopecia *f* alopecia
alopurinol *m* allopurinol
alovudina *f* alovudine

alpinismo *m* mountaineering

alprazolam *m* alprazolam

alquitrán *m* tar; — de hulla coal tar

alrededor *adv* around; — del brazo around your arm

alsine *m* (*Esp, bot*) chickweed

alta *f* (*del hospital*) discharge (*from the hospital*); dar de — to discharge

alteplasa *f* alteplase

alteración *f* disturbance

alterado -da *adj* (*molesto*) upset

alterar *vt* to upset; *vr* to get *o* become upset

alternar *vt, vi* to alternate

alternativa *f* alternative

alterno -na *adj* alternate; días alternos alternate days

altitud *f* altitude; gran — high altitude

alto -ta *adj* high, tall; upper; Su glucosa está muy alta..Your glucose is very high...¿Es muy alto su papá?..Is your father very tall? vías respiratorias altas upper respiratory tract

altura *f* height; altitude, elevation; ¿Qué altura tiene Ud.?..How tall are you? gran — high altitude

alucinación *f* hallucination

alumbramiento *m* (*form*) delivery of the placenta and fetal membranes; (*fam*) childbirth

alumbre *m* alum

aluminio *m* aluminum

alvéolo, alveolo *m* (*dent*) alveolus, socket (*fam*); (*lung*) alveolus

amable *adj* friendly, kind

ama de casa *f* housewife, homemaker

amalgama *f* (*dent*) amalgam

amamantar *vt* (*form*) to breast-feed, to nurse

amantadina *f* amantadine

amar *vt, vi* to love

amargo -ga *adj* bitter

amargón *m* (*bot*) dandelion

amarillento -ta *adj* yellowish

amarillo -lla *adj* yellow

ambidiestro, ambidextro -tra *adj* ambidextrous

ambiental *adj* environmental

ambiente *m* surroundings, environment

ambliopía *f* amblyopia, lazy eye (*fam*)

ambrosía *f* (*bot*) ragweed

ambulancia *f* ambulance

ambulatorio -ria *adj* ambulatory, outpatient; cirugía — outpatient surgery; paciente *mf* — outpatient; procedimiento — outpatient procedure

ameba *f* ameba

amebiano -na *adj* amebic

amebiasis *f* amebiasis

amenaza *f* threat

amenazar *vt, vi* to threaten

amenorrea *f* amenorrhea

amianto *m* asbestos

amiba *f* (*Mex*) ameba

amibiano -na *adj* (*Mex*) amebic

amibiasis *f* (*Mex*) amebiasis

amígdala *f* tonsil

amigdalectomía *f* tonsillectomy

amigdalitis *f* tonsillitis

amigo -ga *mf* friend

amilasa *f* amylase

amiloidosis *f* amyloidosis

amilorida *f* amiloride

aminoácido *m* amino acid

aminofilina *f* aminophylline

aminoglucósido *m* aminoglycoside

amiodarona *f* amiodarone

amiotrófico -ca *adj* amyotrophic

amistad *f* friendship; *fpl* friends

amitriptilina *f* amitriptyline

amlodipina *f* (*esp. SA*) amlodipine

amlodipino *m* amlodipine

amnesia *f* amnesia

amniocentesis *f* (*pl* -sis) amniocentesis

amnionitis *f* amnionitis

amniótico -ca *adj* amniotic

amoníaco, amoniaco *m* ammonia

amonio *m* ammonium

amor *m* love; hacer el — to make love

amortiguador -ra *adj* buffered; *m* buffer

amoxacilina *f* amoxacillin

ampicilina *f* ampicillin

ampolla *f* blister; — de Vater ampulla of Vater

ampolloso -sa *adj* bullous

amprenavir *m* amprenavir

ámpula *f* (*Mex, Cub*) ampule

amputación *f* amputation; — **por debajo de la rodilla** below-the-knee amputation; — **por encima de la rodilla** above-the-knee amputation

amputado -da *mf* amputee

amputar *vt* to amputate, to cut off (*fam*)

anabólico -ca *adj* anabolic

anacardo *m* cashew

anaeróbico -ca *adj* (*metabolismo*) anaerobic

anaerobio -bia *adj* (*micro*) anaerobic

anafiláctico -ca *adj* anaphylactic

anafilactoide *adj* anaphylactoid

anafilaxia, anafilaxis *f* anaphylaxis

anal *adj* anal

analfabetismo *m* illiteracy

analfabeto -ta *adj* illiterate

analgesia *f* analgesia; — **controlada por el paciente** patient-controlled analgesia

analgésico -ca *adj & m* analgesic

análisis *m* (*pl* **-sis**) analysis, test, laboratory test, assay, testing; (*psych, fam*) psychoanalysis, analysis; — **de heces** stool test; — **de orina** urinalysis, urine test (*fam*); — **de sangre** blood test; — **de semen** semen analysis

analista *mf* (*psych, fam*) psychoanalyst, analyst (*fam*)

analizador *m* analyzer

analizar *vt* to analyze

anastomosis *f* anastomosis

anatomía *f* anatomy; — **patológica** pathology

anatómico -ca *adj* anatomical *o* anatomic

anatomopatólogo -ga *mf* pathologist

ancho -cha *adj* wide; *m* width

anchura *f* width

anciano -na *adj* old, elderly; *m* old man, old person; *f* old woman

andadera *f* (*Mex*) walker

andador *m* walker

andar *vi* to walk

andrógeno *m* androgen

andropausia *f* andropause

anemia *f* anemia; — **aplásica** aplastic anemia; — **de células falciformes** *or* — **falciforme** sickle cell anemia; — **ferropénica** (*form*) iron

deficiency anemia; — **hemolítica** hemolytic anemia; — **perniciosa** pernicious anemia; — **por deficiencia de hierro** iron deficiency anemia; — **sideroblástica** sideroblastic anemia

anémico -ca *adj* anemic

anencefalia *f* anencephaly

anergia *f* anergy

anestesia *f* anesthesia; — **epidural** epidural anesthesia; — **espinal** spinal anesthesia; — **general** general anesthesia; — **local** local anesthesia; — **regional** regional anesthesia

anestesiar *vt* (*local*) to anesthetize, to numb up (*fam*); (*general*) to anesthetize, to put to sleep (*fam*)

anestésico -ca *adj & m* anesthetic; — **general** general anesthetic; — **local** local anesthetic, numbing medicine (*fam*)

anestesiología *f* anesthesiology

anestesiólogo -ga *mf* anesthesiologist

anestesista *mf* anesthesiologist; anesthetist

aneurisma *m* aneurysm; — **de aorta abdominal** abdominal aortic aneurysm; — **disecante** dissecting aneurysm; — **micótico** mycotic aneurysm

anfetamina *f* amphetamine

anfotericina B *f* amphotericin B

angeítis *f* angiitis

angélica *f* (*bot*) angelica

angiitis *f* (*Ang*) angiitis

angina *f* (de pecho) angina; (*frec. pl, amígdala*) tonsil; — **de Prinzmetal** vasospastic *o* Prinzmetal's angina; — **inestable** unstable angina; **tener anginas** (*Mex, fam*) to have tonsillitis; — **vasoespástica** vasospastic angina

anginoso -sa *adj* anginal

angiodisplasia *f* angiodysplasia

angioedema *m* angioedema

angiografía *f* (*técnica imagenológica*) angiography; (*estudio imagenológico*) angiogram

angioma *m* angioma; — **en araña** spider angioma

angiomatosis *f* angiomatosis; — **bacilar** bacillary angiomatosis

angioplastia *f* angioplasty; — **trans-luminal percutánea coronaria** percutaneous transluminal coronary angioplasty

angiosarcoma *m* angiosarcoma

ángulo *m* angle, bend; — **del ojo** angle *o* corner of the eye

angustia *f* anxiety, anguish

anilina *f* aniline

anillo *m* ring; — **vaginal** vaginal ring

animal *adj & m* animal

animalito *m* (*esp. Mex, fam*) bug, insect; parasite

ánimo *m* (*psych*) mood; **estado de —** mood; **oscilación** *f* **del —** mood swing

ano *m* anus

anoche *adv* last night

anomalía *f* anomaly, malformation, abnormality; — **congénita** congenital anomaly, birth defect

anorexia *f* anorexia; — **nerviosa** anorexia nervosa

anorexígeno -na *adj & m* anorexiant

anormal *adj* abnormal

anormalidad *f* abnormality

anovulación *f* anovulation

anovulatorio -ria *adj* anovulatory; *m* (*Esp, form*) oral contraceptive

anquilosis *f* ankylosis

anquilostoma *m* hookworm

anquilostomiasis *f* ancylostomiasis

ansiedad *f* anxiety; — **de desempeño** performance anxiety

ansiolítico -ca *adj* anxiolytic, anti-anxiety; *m* anxiolitic

ansioso -sa *adj* anxious

antagonista *m* antagonist; — **del calcio** calcium antagonist, calcium channel blocker; — **de los receptores de la angiotensina** angiotensin receptor blocker

anteanoche *adv* the night before last

anteayer *adv* the day before yesterday

antebrazo *m* forearm

antecedentes *mpl* past medical history; — **de cáncer (traumatismo, etc.)** history of cancer (trauma, etc.); — **familiares** family history; — **médicos** past medical history

anteojos *mpl* (*esp. Amer*) glasses, eyeglasses; — **bifocales** bifocal glasses *o* eyeglasses, bifocals (*fam*); — **de lectura** reading glasses; — **oscuros** sunglasses

antepasado *m* ancestor

antepié *m* forefoot

anterior *adj* anterior; (*previo*) previous

antes *adv* before; **No tenía dolor antes.**.I didn't have pain before; — **de** before; **antes de las comidas.**. before meals; — **de que** before; **antes de que se vaya.**.before you go

antiácido -da *adj & m* antacid

antialérgico -ca *adj* preventing or treating allergies; **medicamento —** allergy medicine; *m* allergy medicine

antianginoso -sa *adj & m* antianginal

antiarrítmico -ca *adj & m* antiarrhythmic

antiasmático -ca *adj & m* antiasthmatic

antibacteriano -na *adj & m* antibacterial

antibiótico -ca *adj & m* antibiotic; — **de amplio espectro** broad-spectrum antibiotic

anticanceroso -sa *adj* anti-cancer

anticoagulante *adj* anticoagulant; *m* anticoagulant, blood thinner (*fam*); — **lúpico** lupus anticoagulant

anticoagular *vt* to anticoagulate

anticolinérgico -ca *adj & m* anticholinergic

anticoncepción *f* contraception, birth control

anticonceptivo -va *adj & m* contraceptive; — **oral** oral contraceptive, birth control pill

anticongelante *m* antifreeze

anticonvulsivante *adj & m* anticonvulsant, antiepileptic

anticonvulsivo -va *adj & m* anticonvulsant, antiepileptic

anticuerpo *m* antibody; **anticuerpos contra su proprio tejido.**.antibodies against your own tissue; **anticuerpos antifosfolípidos** antiphospholipid antibodies; **anticuerpos antimitocondriales** antimitochondrial antibodies; **anticuerpos antinucleares** antinuclear antibodies

(ANA)

antidepresivo -va *adj & m* antidepressant; — **tricíclico** tricyclic antidepressant

antidiabético -ca *adj* antidiabetic; *m* hypoglycemic agent

antidiarreico -ca *adj & m* antidiarrheal

antídoto *m* antidote

antidroga *adj* antidrug

antiemético -ca *adj & m* antiemetic

antiepiléptico -ca *adj & m* anticonvulsant, antiepileptic

antier *See* **anteayer.**

antiespasmódico -ca *adj & m* antispasmodic

antiespástico -ca *adj & m* antispasmodic

antifúngico -ca *adj & m* antifungal

antígeno *m* antigen; — **carcinoembrionario** carcinoembryonic antigen; — **prostático específico** prostate-specific antigen (PSA)

antigripal *adj* anti-flu

antihelmíntico -ca *adj & m* anthelminthic

antihigiénico -ca *adj* unsanitary

antihipertensivo -va *adj* antihypertensive

antihistamínico -ca *adj & m* antihistamine; — **H₂** H₂ blocker

antiinflamatorio -ria *adj* antiinflammatory; *m* antiinflammatory agent; — **no esteroideo (AINE)** nonsteroidal antiinflammatory drug (NSAID)

antimicótico -ca *adj* antifungal

antimicrobiano -na *adj & m* antimicrobial

antimonial *m* antimonial

antineoplásico -ca *adj* anti-cancer

antioxidante *adj & m* antioxidant

antipalúdico -ca *adj & m* antimalarial

antipático -ca *adj* unfriendly

antipirético -ca *adj & m* antipyretic

antipsicótico -ca *adj & m* antipsychotic

antirreflujo *adj* anti-reflux

antirretroviral, antirretrovírico -ca *adj & m* antiretroviral

antiséptico -ca *adj & m* antiseptic

antisocial *adj* antisocial

antisuero *m* antiserum

antitabaco, antitabáquico -ca *adj* antismoking

antitérmico -ca (*esp. Esp*) *adj & m* antipyretic

antitoxina *f* antitoxin

antitranspirante *adj & m* antiperspirant

antitrombótico -ca *adj* antithrombotic

antiulceroso -sa *adj* preventing or treating ulcers; **medicamento —** ulcer medicine; *m* ulcer medicine

antiviral, antivírico -ca *adj & m* antiviral

antojo *m* craving; (*derm, fam*) birthmark

antracosis *f* anthracosis, black lung (*fam*)

ántrax *m* carbuncle; (*Ang, carbunco*) anthrax

anual *adj* annual

anular *adj* annular

anzuelo *m* fishhook

añadir *vt* to add

año *m* year; **Tengo tres años..**I'm three years old..I'm three.

añoso -sa *adj* older

aorta *f* aorta

aórtico -ca *adj* aortic

apachurrar *vt* to mash, press down

aparato *m* apparatus, device; (*digestivo, etc.*) tract, system; (*obst, fam*) intrauterine device (IUD); — **de ortodoncia** braces, bands (*fam*); — **digestivo** digestive *o* gastrointestinal tract, digestive system; — **extraoral** (*orthodontics*) headgear; — **genital** genital tract; — **genitourinario** genitourinary tract; — **locomotor** musculoskeletal system; — **ortopédico** brace; — **reproductor** reproductive system; — **respiratorio** respiratory system; — **urinario** urinary tract

aparecer *vi, vr* to appear, to develop

apariencia *f* appearance

apatía *f* apathy

apático -ca *adj* apathetic, listless

apellido *m* last name

apenarse *vr* (*tener vergüenza*) to feel embarrassed

apéndice *m* appendix

apendicectomía *f* appendectomy
apendicitis *f* appendicitis
apetito *m* appetite
Apgar *m* (*fam*) Apgar score
apio *m* celery
aplásico -ca *adj* aplastic
aplastamiento *m* crushing; — **ver-tebral** vertebral compression fracture
aplastante *adj* (*dolor*) crushing
aplastar *vt* to crush
aplicación *f* application
aplicador *m* applicator, swab; — **de algodón** cotton applicator, cotton swab
aplicar *vt* to apply
apnea *f* apnea; — **del sueño** sleep apnea
apófisis *f* (*pl* -**sis**) (*anat*) process; — **mastoides** mastoid process; — **xifoides** xiphoid process
apósito *m* dressing
apoyar *vt* to support
apoyo *m* support; — **moral** moral support
apraxia *f* apraxia
aprender *vt, vi* to learn; **aprender a caminar**..to learn to walk
aprendizaje *m* learning
apretado -da *adj* tight
apretar *vt* to squeeze, to constrict; (*ropa, calzado*) to pinch, to be too tight for; — **los dientes** to bite down; *vi* (*ropa, calzado*) to bind, to be too tight
apropiado -da *adj* appropriate, suitable
aproximadamente *adv* approximately
aptitud *f* aptitude; — **física** fitness, physical conditioning
A quien corresponda To Whom It May Concern
araña *f* spider; — **marrón** *or* **parda** brown recluse spider; — **vascular** spider angioma; — **violinista** (*esp. Mex*) brown recluse spider
arañar *vt* to scratch (*esp. with claws*)
arañazo *m* scratch
arcada *f* (*frec. pl*) retching, dry heaves (*fam*)
arco *m* arch; — **del pie** arch of the foot

arder *vi* to burn, to sting; **Esto le va a arder un poco**..This will burn a little bit.
ardiente *adj* burning
ardilla *f* squirrel
ardor *m* (*sensación*) burning, burning sensation; **Siento ardor en los pies**..I feel burning in my feet.
área *f* area, district
arete *m* earring
arginina *f* arginine
argón *m* argon
aripiprazol *m* aripiprazole
arma *f* weapon; — **biológica** biological weapon; — **de fuego** firearm; — **química** chemical weapon
armadillo *m* armadillo
armazón *m&f* (*para lentes*) frames (*for eyeglasses*)
ARN *abbr* **ácido ribonucleico**. *See* **ácido**.
árnica *f* (*bot*) arnica
aromaterapia *f* aromatherapy
arqueado -da *adj* bowed, curved; **con las piernas arqueadas** bow-legged; **piernas arqueadas** genu varum (*form*), bowed legs
arquear *vt* to arch; — **la espalda** to arch one's back
arrastrar *vt* — **las palabras** to slur one's words *o* speech
arreglar *vt* (*fam*) to repair, fix
arremangarse *vr* to roll up (*one's sleeve, pants leg, etc.*)
arriba *adv* — **de 100** (*Amer*) higher than 100; **de** — upper; **hacia** — upward, up
arriesgar *vt* to risk; *vr* to take a risk
arritmia *f* arrhythmia
arrojar *vt, vi* (*fam*) to vomit, to throw up (*fam*); (*Mex, fam*) to cough up
arrollar *vt* (*atropellar*) to run over
arroz *m* rice
arruga *f* wrinkle
arrugar *vt, vr* to wrinkle
arsenal terapéutico *m* armamentarium
arsénico *m* arsenic
artemisinina *f* artemisinine
arteria *f* artery; — **braquial** brachial artery; — **carótida (común)** (common) carotid artery; — **coronaria** coronary artery; — **coronaria cir-**

cunfleja circumflex (coronary) artery; — **coronaria derecha** right coronary artery; — **coronaria descendente anterior** left anterior descending (coronary) artery; — **coronaria izquierda** left (main) coronary artery; — **femoral** femoral artery; — **humeral** brachial artery; — **ilíaca**, — **iliaca** (*esp. Mex*) iliac artery; — **mesentérica** mesenteric artery; — **poplítea** popliteal artery; — **radial** radial artery; — **subclavia** subclavian artery

arterial *adj* arterial

arterioesclerosis *f* arteriosclerosis

arteriografía *f* (*técnica imagenológica*) angiography; (*estudio imagenológico*) angiogram

arteriosclerosis *f* arteriosclerosis

arteriovenoso -sa *adj* arteriovenous

arteritis *f* arteritis; — **de células gigantes** temporal *o* giant cell arteritis; — **de Takayasu** Takayasu's arteritis

articulación *f* joint; — **de la rodilla, — del tobillo, etc.** knee joint, ankle joint, etc.

articular *adj* articular (*form*); **dolor** — joint pain

artificial *adj* artificial

artrítico -ca *adj* arthritic

artritis *f* arthritis; — **juvenil** juvenile arthritis; — **reumatoide** rheumatoid arthritis

artrografía *f* (*técnica imagenológica*) arthrography; (*estudio imagenológico*) arthrogram

artroplastia *f* arthroplasty

artroscopia, artroscopía (*Amer, esp. spoken*) *f* arthroscopy

artroscópico -ca *adj* arthroscopic

artrosis *f* osteoarthritis

asa *f* (*intestinal*) loop (*of bowel*)

asado -da *adj* roasted, grilled; — **a la parrilla** grilled, broiled, barbecued

asaltar *vt* to assault

asalto *m* assault

asar *vt* to roast, to grill; — **a la parrilla** to grill, broil, to barbecue

asbesto *m* asbestos

asbestosis *f* asbestosis

ascariasis, ascaridiasis *f* ascariasis

áscaris *m* (*pl* **-ris**) roundworm

ascendente *adj* ascending

ascitis *f* ascites

asco *m* (*Mex, CA; fam*) nausea

ascórbico -ca *adj* ascorbic

asegurado -da *adj* insured

aseguranza *f* (*Mex*) insurance

asegurarse *vr* to be sure, to make sure

aseo *m* hygiene; — **bucal** oral hygiene

aséptico -ca *adj* aseptic

asertividad *f* assertiveness

asfixia *f* asphyxia, suffocation, choking

asfixiar *vt, vr* to asphyxiate, suffocate, choke

asiento *m* seat; — **infantil (para vehículo)** (*esp. Esp*), — **para bebé (para el coche)** infant car seat

asilo *m* asylum, institution, home; — **de ancianos** rest home

asintomático -ca *adj* asymptomatic

asistencia *f* assistance; — **domiciliaria** home care; — **médica** health care; — **pública** welfare ; — **sanitaria** (*Esp, SA*) health care; — **social** welfare

asistente *mf* assistant, aide; — **de enfermera** nursing assistant, nurse aide; — **médico** medical assistant

asistir *vt* to assist, aid; (*una clínica, clase, etc.*) to attend

asistolia *f* asystole, flatline (*fam*)

asma *f* asthma

asmático -ca *adj* & *mf* asthmatic

asociación *f* association

asociado -da *adj* associated, linked; **asociado con**..associated with.. linked to

asolearse *vr* to get sun

asparagina, asparragina *f* asparagine

aspecto *m* appearance

aspereza *f* roughness

aspergilosis *f* aspergillosis

áspero -ra *adj* (*piel, etc.*) rough

aspiración *f* aspiration; — **articular** joint aspiration; — **con aguja fina** fine needle aspiration

aspirar *vt* to aspirate, to inhale, breathe in; (*por la nariz*) to sniff, (*drogas*) to snort (*fam*)

aspirina *f* aspirin

asqueroso -sa *adj* (*esp. Mex, CA*) nauseating
astemizol *m* astemizole
astenia *f* asthenia
astigmatismo *m* astigmatism
astilla *f* sliver, splinter, chip, fragment
astillar *vt, vr* to chip
astrágalo *m* talus
astringente *adj & m* astringent
asustar *vt* to frighten
atacar *vt* to attack
ataduras *fpl* (*para limitar los movimientos de un paciente agitado*) physcial restraints, restraints
ataque *m* attack, bout, spell, fit; (*fam, crisis epiléptica*) convulsion, seizure; — **cardíaco** *or* **al corazón** (*fam*) heart attack; — **cerebral** stroke; — **de asma** (*fam*) asthma attack; — **de nervios** (*fam*) anxiety attack, panic attack; — **de pánico** panic attack; — **isquémico transitorio (AIT)** transient ischemic attack (TIA)
atarantado -da *adj* dazed, in a daze, stunned
atarantar *vt* to daze, stun; *vr* to become dazed *o* stunned
ataxia *f* ataxia
atáxico -ca *adj* ataxic
atazanavir *m* atazanavir
atención *f* attention; — **(médica) domiciliaria** home (health) care; — **especializada** tertiary care; — **médica** medical attention, health care; — **prenatal** prenatal care; — **primaria** primary care; — **terciaria** tertiary care
atender *vt* (*a un paciente*) to take care of, to treat, to attend; (*un parto*) to deliver; **La Dra. Gomez atendió tres partos anoche**..Dr. Gomez delivered three babies last night...**Atendió a la señora Reid**..She delivered Mrs. Reid...**Atendió a los gemelos**..She delivered the twins.
atenolol *m* atenolol
atenuado -da *adj* attenuated
ateroesclerosis *f* atherosclerosis
ateroma *m* atheroma
aterosclerosis *f* atherosclerosis

atípico -ca *adj* atypical
atleta *mf* athlete
atlético -ca *adj* athletic
atmósfera *f* atmosphere
atomizador nasal *m* nasal inhaler (*esp. for nicotine*)
atópico -ca *adj* atopic
atorvastatina *f* atorvastatin
atovacuona *f* atovaquone
atracón *m* food binge
atragantamiento *m* choking (*on food*)
atragantarse *vr* to choke; — **con** to choke on
atrapamiento *m* entrapment; — **de un nervio** entrapped nerve, nerve entrapment, pinched nerve (*fam*)
atrás *adv* back; ago, earlier; **hacia —** backward; **la parte de —** the back part; **tres días —** three days ago, three days earlier
atrasado -da *adj* behind, delayed
atrofia *f* atrophy
atrofiarse *vr* to atrophy
atropellar *vt* to run over
atropina *f* atropine
atún *m* tuna
aturdido -da *adj* dazed, in a daze, stunned
aturdimiento *m* daze
aturdir *vt* to stun, daze, make dizzy; *vr* to become stunned *o* dazed *o* dizzy
audición *f* sense of hearing, hearing
audífono *m* hearing aid
audiograma *m* audiogram
audiología *f* audiology
audiólogo -ga *mf* audiologist
audiometría *f* audiometry
audiométrico -ca *adj* audiometric
audiómetro *m* audiometer
audioprotesista *mf* (*esp. Esp*) specialist in hearing aids
auditivo -va *adj* auditory
aumentar *vt, vi* to increase; — **de tamaño** to enlarge
aumento *m* increase, gain, rise, augmentation; — **de mamas** breast augmentation
aura *f* aura
aurícula *f* (*del corazón*) atrium
auricular *adj* atrial
auriculoventricular *adj* atrioventri-

cular
ausencia *f* absence
ausente *adj* absent
ausentismo *m* absenteeism
autismo *m* autism
autista *adj* autistic; *mf* autist (*form*), autistic person, person with autism
autístico -ca *adj* autistic
autoayuda *f* self-help
autoclave *f* autoclave
autoconciencia *f* self-awareness
autoconfianza *f* self-confidence
autoconocimiento *m* self-awareness
autocontrol *m* self-control
autodestructivo -va *adj* self-destructive
autodisciplina *f* self-discipline
autoestima *f* self-esteem
autoevaluación *f* self-examination
autoexamen *m* self-examination
autoexploración *f* (*form*) self-examination; — **mamaria** breast self-examination
autoimagen *f* self-image
autoinfligido -da *adj* self-inflicted
autoinmune *adj* autoimmune
autoinmunidad *f* autoimmunity
autolimitado -da *adj* self-limited
autólogo -ga *adj* autologous
automedicarse *vr* to self-medicate
automóvil *m* automobile, car
autonomía *f* autonomy; — **del paciente** patient autonomy
autopsia *f* autopsy
autorrealización *f* self-realization
autorrecetarse *vr* to self-prescribe
autorregulación *f* autoregulation
autorrespeto *m* self-respect
autosómico -ca *adj* autosomal
autosondaje *m* self-catheterization (*of bladder*)
autotransfusión *f* autologous blood transfusion

autotratamiento *m* self-treatment
auxiliar *adj* auxiliary; *mf* assistant, aide; — **de enfermería** nurse aide
auxilio *interj* Help! *m* help, assistance; (*después de un desastre*) aid, relief; **primeros auxilios** first aid
AV *See* **auriculoventricular.**
avance *m* advance, progress
avanzado -da *adj* advanced
ave *f* bird; **aves de corral** poultry, fowl
avena *f* oatmeal
aversión *f* aversion
avisar *vt* to notify
aviso *m* advisory; — **sanitario** health advisory
avispa *f* wasp, yellow jacket
avispón *m* hornet
axila *f* (*fam*) axilla, armpit (*fam*); **Tengo un grano en la axila**..I have a pimple under my arm.
axilar *adj* axillary
ay *interj* Ouch!
ayer *adv* yesterday
ayuda *f* help, assistance, aid, relief
ayudante *mf* assistant, aide
ayudar *vt, vi* to help, assist, aid
ayunar *vi* to fast
ayunas, en fasting; **glucosa en ayunas**..fasting glucose
ayuno *m* fast, fasting
azahar *m* (*bot*) lemon flower
azar *m* **al** — at random
azarcón *m* lead oxide (*toxic Mexican folk remedy*)
azatioprina *f* azathioprine
azitromicina *f* azithromycin
AZT *m* AZT
azúcar *m&f* sugar; **sin** — sugarless
azufre *m* sulfur
azul *adj* blue; — **de metileno** methylene blue
azulado -da *adj* bluish

B

baba *f* drool
babear *vi* to drool
babeo *m* drooling
babero *m* bib
babesiosis *f* babesiosis
bacilo *m* bacillus, rod; — **de Calmette-Guérin (BCG)** bacille Calmette-Guérin (BCG)
bacinica *f* bedpan
bacinilla *f* bedpan
bacitracina *f* bacitracin
baclofeno, baclofen *m* baclofen
bacteria *f* bacterium; [*Nota: en inglés se usa casi siempre el plural:* bacteria]
bacteriano -na *adj* bacterial
bactericida *adj* bactericidal
bacteriemia *f* bacteremia
baja *f* fall, drop
bajada *f* drop; — **de la leche** (*obst*) letdown
bajalenguas *m* (*pl* -**guas**) tongue depressor *o* blade
bajar *vt* to lower, to reduce; *vi, vr* to go down, fall, drop; **Le bajó el potasio**..Your potassium went down; — **de peso** to lose weight; **bajarle la regla** (*fam*) to have one's period, to start one's period; **Me bajó la regla ayer**..My period started yesterday.
bajo -ja *adj* low; (*anat*) lower; (*de estatura*) short; **Su sodio está bajo**.. Your sodium is low...**una dieta baja en fibra**..a low-fiber diet...**la parte baja**..the lower part; **de — grado** (*tumor*) low-grade; **espalda** — lower back; **más — que** lower than; **más — que antes**..lower than before; **parte — del abdomen, parte — de la espalda, etc.** lower abdomen, lower back, etc.
bala *f* bullet
balanceado -da *adj* (*comida, etc.*) balanced
balanitis *f* balanitis
balanza *f* balance scale, scale

balazo *m* gunshot wound
balbucear *vi* (*ped*) to babble
balbuceo *m* (*ped*) babble
balneario *m* health resort, health spa (*with therapeutic baths*)
balneoterapia *f* water therapy, therapeutic bathing
balón *m* (*deportes*) ball; (*de un catéter*) balloon; — **de contrapulsación (intraaórtico)** intraaortic balloon counterpulsation
baloncesto *m* basketball
bálsamo *m* balm, salve; — **labial** (*esp. Esp*) lip balm
banco *m* bank; — **de alimentos** food bank; — **de órganos** organ bank; — **de sangre** blood bank
banda *f* (*ortodoncia, etc.*) band
bandeja *f* tray
bañadera *f* (*Cub, tina*) bathtub
bañar *vt* to wash, bathe; *vr* to wash oneself, bathe, take a bath; (*nadar*) to go swimming
bañera *f* bathtub; — **de hidromasaje** whirlpool
baño *m* bath; bathroom, restroom; — **de asiento** sitz bath; — **de damas** women's room; — **de esponja** sponge bath; — **de hombres** men's room; — **de mujeres** women's room; — **de regadera** (*esp. Mex*) shower; — **de vapor** steam bath; **hacer del** — (*Mex*) to have a bowel movement; **ir al** — (*euph, defecar*) to have a bowel movement, to go to the bathroom (*euph*)
baranda *f* bedrail, side rail
barba *f* beard, whiskers
barbacoa *f* barbecue; **asar a la** — (*esp. Mex*) to barbecue
barbero *m* barber
barbijo *m* (*SA*) mask, surgical mask
barbilla *f* chin
barbitúrico -ca *adj & m* barbiturate
bardana *f* (*bot*) burdock
bariátrico -ca *adj* bariatric
bario *m* barium

barotrauma, barotraumatismo *m* barotrauma

barra *f* (*ortho*) rod; — **de Harrington** Harrington rod

barrera *f* barrier; — **placentaria** placental barrier

barriga *f* belly, stomach (*fam*), tummy (*ped, fam*)

barrigón -na *adj* potbellied

barriguita *f* (*ped*) tummy

barro *m* blackhead, pimple

basal *adj* baseline, basal; **valor** — baseline value

báscula *f* scale (*for weighing*)

base *f* (*chem, pharm, de una úlcera, etc.*) base; **a** — **de aceite, a** — **de agua, etc.** oil-based, water-based, etc.; — **de datos** data base; — **libre** (*cocaína*) freebase (*cocaine*)

básico -ca *adj* basic

basquetbol *m* (*Amer*) basketball

bastón *m* cane; (*del ojo*) rod

bastoncillo de algodón *m* (*Esp*) cotton swab

bata *f* gown

baumanómetro *m* blood pressure cuff

bazo *m* spleen

BCG *abbr* bacilo de Calmette-Guérin. *See* **bacilo.**

bebé *mf* (*pl* bebés) baby

bebedor -ra *mf* drinker

beber *vt, vi* to drink

bebida *f* drink

beclometasona *f* beclomethasone

béisbol *m* baseball

belcho *m* (*bot*) ephedra

belladona *f* (*bot*) belladonna

benazepril *m* benazepril

bencedrina *f* benzedrine

benceno *m* benzene

beneficio *m* benefit; **para su** — for your benefit

beneficioso -sa *adj* beneficial

benigno -na *adj* benign

benzoato *m* benzoate; — **sódico** (*form*) or **de sodio** sodium benzoate

benzodiazepina, benzodiacepina *f* benzodiazepine

benzoína *f* benzoin

beriberi *m* beriberi

berrinche *m* tantrum

besar *vt* to kiss

beso *m* kiss

beta *f* beta; **beta-hemolítico** beta-hemolytic

betabloqueador *m* (*esp. Mex*) beta-blocker

betabloqueante *m* beta-blocker

betametasona *f* betamethasone

bezoar *m* bezoar

biberón *m* baby bottle

bicarbonato *m* bicarbonate; — **sódico** (*form*) or **de sodio** sodium bicarbonate

bíceps *m* (*pl* bíceps) biceps

bicho *m* bug, tiny animal

bicicleta *f* bicycle; — **estática** stationary bicycle; **ir** *or* **montar en** — to ride a bicycle

bicúspide *adj* & *m* bicuspid

bien *adj* & *adv* well, OK *o* okay; **Estoy bien**..I'm well...**Estoy comiendo bien**..I'm eating well; — **parecido** good-looking; *m* good, benefit, welfare; **por su** — for your benefit; **por su propio** — for your own good

bienestar *m* well-being, welfare; wellness

bifenilo policlorado (BPC) *m* polychlorinated biphenyl (PCB)

bifocal *adj* bifocal; *mpl* (*fam*) bifocal glasses *o* eyeglasses, bifocals (*fam*)

bigote *m* moustache

biliar *adj* biliary

bilingüe *adj* bilingual

bilirrubina *f* bilirubin

bilis *f* bile

bioactivo -va *adj* bioactive

biodegradable *adj* biodegradable

bioestadística *f* biostatistics

bioimpedancia *f* bioimpedance

bioingeniería *f* bioengineering

biología *f* biology

biológico -ca *adj* biological

biomecánica *f* biomechanics

biomédico -ca *adj* biomedical

biometría hemática completa *f* complete blood count

bioprótesis *f* (*pl* -sis) bioprosthesis

biopsia *f* biopsy; — **cutánea** (*esp. Esp*) skin biopsy, punch biopsy; — **de hígado** liver biopsy; — **de mama** breast biopsy; — **de médula**

ósea bone marrow biopsy; — **de piel** skin biopsy, punch biopsy; — **de próstata** prostatic biopsy, biopsy of the prostate; — **de riñón** renal biopsy; — **escisional** excisional biopsy; — **estereotáxica** stereotactic biopsy; — **excisional** excisional biopsy; — **hepática** liver biopsy; — **incisional** incisional biopsy; **por aspiración con aguja fina** (*esp. Mex*) fine needle aspiration biopsy; — **por congelación** frozen section; — **prostática** prostatic biopsy; — **renal** renal biopsy

bioquímico -ca *adj* biochemical; *f* biochemistry

biorretroalimentación *f* biofeedback

biotecnología *f* biotechnology

bioterrorismo *m* bioterrorism

bióxido *See* **dióxido.**

biper *m* (*Amer*) beeper, pager

bipolar *adj* bipolar

bisabuelo -la *m* great-grandfather, great-grandparent; *f* great-grandmother

bisel *m* (*de un aguja*) bevel (*of a needle*)

bisexual *adj* bisexual

bisfosfonato *m* bisphosphonate

bismuto *m* bismuth

bisnieto -ta *m* great-grandson, great-grandchild; *f* great-granddaughter

bisoprolol *m* bisoprolol

bistec *m* steak, beefsteak

bisturí *m* (*pl* **-ríes** *or* **-rís**) scalpel

bizco -ca *adj* cross-eyed; *mf* cross-eyed person

blanco -ca *adj* white, (*tez*) fair; (*diana*) target; **órgano** — target organ

blando -da *adj* soft; (*comida*) bland

blanqueador *m* bleach; (*dent*) whitener

blanqueamiento *m* (*dent*) whitening

blanquecino -na *adj* whitish

blanquillo *m* (*Mex*) egg

blastomicosis *f* blastomycosis

blefaritis *f* blepharitis

blefaroplastia *f* blepharoplasty

bleomicina *f* bleomycin

bloomer *m* (*esp. CA, frec. pl*) panties, (women's) underpants

bloqueado -da *adj* blocked

bloqueador *m* (*esp. Mex*) blocker; —

beta beta-blocker; — **neuromuscular** neuromuscular blocker

bloqueante *m* blocker; — **neuromuscular** neuromuscular blocker

bloquear *vt* (*pharm, physio*) to block

bloqueo *m* block; obstruction, blockage; — **cardíaco** heart block; — **de rama** bundle branch block; — **nervioso** nerve block

blot *m* (*pl* **blots**) blot; **Western** —, **Southern** —, **etc.** Western blot, Southern blot, etc.

blusa *f* blouse

boca *f* mouth; — **abajo** prone (*form*), facedown; — **a** — mouth-to-mouth; — **arriba** faceup; — **del estómago** pit of the stomach; **por la** — by mouth

bocadillo *m* snack

bocado *m* mouthful, bite (*of food*)

bochorno *m* (*esp. Mex*) hot flush (*form*), hot flash

bocio *m* goiter; — **multinodular tóxico** toxic multinodular goiter

bola *f* lump, bump

bolita *f* small lump *o* bump

bolo *m* bolus

bolsa *f* bursa; bag; — **de agua caliente** hot-water bottle; — **de aguas,** — **de las aguas** (*esp. Esp*) bag of waters; — **de hielo** ice pack

bomba *f* pump; (*arma*) bomb; — **atómica** atomic bomb; — **de insulina** insulin pump; — **de tiempo** time bomb

bombear *vt* (*sangre*) to pump (*blood*)

bombero -ra *mf* fireman

bombona *f* (*esp. Esp*) — **de oxígeno** oxygen tank

boqueras *fpl* (*fam*) cheilitis

boquilla *f* mouthpiece

borde *m* border, edge, margin

borderline *adj* (*psych, Ang*) borderline

bordón *m* cane

bórico -ca *adj* boric

borrachera *f* drunkenness, (*por varios días seguidos*) binge

borracho -cha *adj & mf* drunk

borrarse *vr* (*la vista*) to blur; **Se me borra la vista.**.My vision blurs.

borreliosis *f* relapsing fever

borroso -sa *adj* blurred, blurry; **vi-**

sión — blurred vision
bostezar *vi* to yawn
bostezo *m* yawn
bota *f* boot
botana *f* (*Mex*) snack
botánico -ca *adj* botanical
botar *vt* (*esp. Carib, fam*) to eliminate, expel, pass; — **aire** to breathe
out; — **una piedra** (*al orinar*) to
pass a stone
bote *m* can
botella *f* bottle
botica *f* pharmacy, drugstore
boticario -ria *mf* pharmacist, druggist (*ant*)
botiquín *m* medicine chest *o* cabinet;
— **de primeros auxilios** first-aid
kit
botón *m* button; — **de llamada** call
button; — **de oro** (*bot*) goldenseal
botulismo *m* botulism
bóveda palatina *f* (*form*) hard palate
bovino -va *adj* bovine
BPC See **bifenilo policlorado.**
brackets *mpl* (*orthodontia*) brackets,
(*fam, aparato de ortodoncia*)
braces, bands (*fam*)
bradicardia *f* bradycardia
bragas *fpl* (*esp. Esp*) panties, (wom-
en's) underpants
braguero *m* truss
bragueta *f* fly (*of trousers*)
braille *m* Braille
brakets See **brackets.**
braquial *adj* brachial
braquiterapia *f* brachytherapy
brassiere *m* (*esp. Mex*) brassiere
brazalete *m* bracelet; — **de alerta
médica** medic alert bracelet; — **de
identificación** ID bracelet
brazo *m* arm
brécol *m* broccoli
breve *adj* (*tiempo*) brief, short
brida *f* (*adherencia*) adhesion
bróculi, brócoli *m* broccoli
bromo *m* bromine
bromocriptina *f* bromocriptine
bromuro de ipratropio *m* ipratropium bromide
bronceado -da *adj* tan; *m* suntan, tan
broncearse *vr* to tan, to get a suntan
broncoalveolar *adj* bronchoalveolar
broncoconstricción *f* bronchocon-

striction
broncodilatador *m* bronchodilator
broncoespasmo *m* bronchospasm
broncogénico -ca *adj* bronchogenic
bronconeumonía *f* bronchopneumo-
nia
broncoscopia, broncoscopía (*Amer,
esp. spoken*) *f* bronchoscopy
broncoscopio *m* bronchoscope
bronquial *adj* bronchial
bronquiectasia *f* bronchiectasis
bronquio *m* bronchus
bronquiolitis *f* bronchiolitis; — **obliterante** bronchiolitis obliterans
bronquiolo *m* bronchiole
bronquitis *f* bronchitis; — **crónica**
chronic bronchitis
brote *m* outbreak
brucelosis *f* brucellosis
brujería *f* witchcraft
brujo *m* (*chamán*) shaman
bruxismo *m* bruxism
bubón *m* bubo
bubónico -ca *adj* bubonic
bucal *adj* oral
buceo *m* (*deporte*) diving
budesonida, budesónida (*OMS*) *f*
budesonide
bueno -na *adj* (buen *before masculine singular nouns*) good; **un buen
médico**..a good doctor
bulbar *adj* bulbar
bulbo *m* bulb; — **raquídeo** medulla
bulimia *f* bulimia
bulímico -ca *adj* bulimic
bulloso -sa *adj* bullous
bulto *m* (*esp. Esp*) large lump *o*
bump, swelling
bumetanida *f* bumetanide
buprenorfina *f* buprenorphin
bupropión *m* bupropion
burbuja *f* bubble
burnout *m* (*Ang*) burnout
burrito *m* (*SA, andador*) walker
bursitis *f* bursitis; — **anserina** anserine bursitis; — **olecraneana**
olecranon bursitis; — **prepatelar,
—prerrotuliana** (*Esp*) prepatellar
bursitis; — **subacromial** subacromial bursitis; — **trocantérica**
(*Amer*), — **trocantérea** (*Esp*) trochanteric bursitis
buscapersonas *m* (*pl* -**nas**) (*Esp, SA*)

beeper, pager
buspirona *f* buspirone
busto *m* bust, female breast
busulfán, busulfano (*OMS*) *m* busulfan
bypass *m* (*Ang*) bypass; — **corona-**

rio *or* **aortocoronario** coronary bypass; — **femoro-poplíteo** femoropopliteal bypass; — **gástrico** gastric bypass; — **triple (cuádruple, etc.)** triple (quadruple, etc.) bypass

C

cabecear *vi* to nod out (*fam*)
cabecera *f* head (*of a bed*); **a la** — at the bedside; **de** — bedside
cabello *m* hair (*head only*)
cabestrillo *m* sling
cabeza *f* head; — **de la familia** head of the family
cabra *f* goat
caca *f* (*fam or vulg*) stool (*form*), bowel movement, poo poo (*ped, fam*); **hacer** — to have a bowel movement, to go poo poo (*ped, fam*)
cacahuate *m* (*esp. Mex*) peanut
cacahuete *m* (*esp. Esp*) peanut
cacaraña *f* pockmark
cactus, cacto *m* (*pl* **-tus, -tos**) cactus
cadáver *m* cadaver, corpse
cadavérico -ca *adj* cadaveric
cadena *f* chain; — **de custodia** chain of custody; — **de frío** chain of cold; — **de supervivencia** chain of survival; — **ligera** light chain; — **pesada** heavy chain; **de** — **larga** long-chain; **de** — **media** medium-chain; **de** — **ramificada** branched-chain
cadera *f* hip
cadmio *m* cadmium
caducado -da *adj* (*medicamento,*

etc.) outdated, out of date
caducidad *f* (*de un medicamento*) expiration; **fecha de** — expiration date
caer *vi* **caer(le) bien (a uno)** to agree with; **No me cae bien**..It doesn't agree with me; *vr* to fall, fall down, collapse; (*los párpados, etc.*) to droop, sag; (*una costra, etc.*) to slough
café *m* coffee; — **molido** ground coffee; **de color** — brown
cafeína *f* caffeine
caído -da *adj* fallen; *f* fall, collapse, loss; — **del cabello** hair loss; — **de mollera** sunken fontanel, (*Mex, CA*) pediatric folk illness manifest by a sunken fontanel and other signs of dehydration and believed to be caused by improper handling of the infant
caja *f* (*de cigarrillos*) pack; — **torácica** rib cage
cajetilla *f* (*de cigarrillos*) pack; **cajetillas diarias** packs per day
calambre *m* cramp; — **del escribiente** writer's cramp
calamina *f* calamine
calcetín *m* sock
calcificar *vr* to calcify

calcio *m* calcium
calcitonina *f* calcitonin
calcitriol *m* calcitriol
cálculo *m* calculus (*form*), stone; (*dent*) calculus (*form*), tartar; — biliar (*form*) gallstone; — renal (*form*) renal calculus (*form*), kidney stone
caldo *m* broth
calefacción *f* heating
calendario *m* — de vacunación (*Esp, SA*), — vacunal (*Esp*) vaccination schedule
calentamiento *m* warmup; hacer ejercicios de — or hacer (el) — to warm up (*before exercise*)
calentar *vt, vr* to warm (up), to heat (up)
calentura *f* fever; (*frec. pl, en los labios*) fever blister, cold sore
calibrar *vt* to calibrate
calibre *m* gauge; aguja de — 21 21 gauge needle
calidad *f* quality; — de vida quality of life
caliente *adj* warm, hot
calistenia *f* calisthenics
callo *m* callus; (*en el pie*) corn (*on the foot*)
callosidad *f* callus, hardened skin
calma *f* calm
calmante *adj & m* sedative
calmar *vt* to calm, soothe; *vr* to calm down, quiet down
calor *m* heat, warmth; — corporal body heat; tener *or* sentir — to be *o* feel hot; Tengo mucho calor..I'm very hot.
caloría *f* calorie
calostro *m* colostrum
calvicie *f* baldness; — del vértice (*form*) vertex baldness; — frontal frontal baldness
calvo -va *adj* bald
calzado *m* footwear; — ortopédico orthopedic shoes
calzón *m* (*frec. pl*) panties, (women's) underpants
calzoncillos *mpl* (men's) underpants
cama *f* bed; — de enfermo sickbed; — hospitalaria hospital bed; guardar — to stay in bed; reposo en — bed rest

cámara *f* chamber; — espaciadora spacer (*for metered dose inhaler*); — hiperbárica hyperbaric chamber
camarón *m* shrimp
cambiar *vt, vi* to change
cambio *m* change, adjustment; — de sexo sex change; — de vendaje bandage change
camedrio *m* (*bot*) germander
camilla *f* stretcher, litter, gurney; (*SA, para consultorio*) exam table
caminadora *f* treadmill
caminar *vi* to walk
caminata *f* long walk, hike
camisa *f* shirt; — de fuerza straitjacket
camiseta *f* undershirt
campanilla *f* uvula
campaña *f* campaign; field; — antitabaco anti-smoking campaign; — de vacunación vaccination campaign; hospital de — field hospital
campo *m* field; rural area, country; — visual visual field
cana *f* gray hair
canadillo *m* (*bot*) ephedra
canal *m* canal; — del parto birth canal
cancelar *vt* to cancel
cáncer *m* cancer, malignancy; — cervical cervical cancer; — colorrectal colorectal cancer; — cutáneo (*form*) skin cancer; — de cabeza y cuello head and neck cancer; — de cérvix cervical cancer; — de colon colon cancer; — de cuello uterino cervical cancer; — de esófago esophageal cancer, cancer of the esophagus; — de estómago gastric cancer (*form*), stomach cancer; — de hígado liver cancer; — de hueso (*fam*) bone cancer; — de laringe laryngeal cancer, cancer of the larynx; — de mama (*form*) breast cancer; — de ovario ovarian cancer; — de páncreas pancreatic cancer; — de pecho (*fam*) breast cancer; — de piel skin cancer; — de próstata prostate cancer; — de pulmón (de células no pequeñas, no microcítico [*esp.*

Esp]; **de células pequeñas, micro-cítico** [*esp. Esp*]) lung cancer (non-small cell; small cell); — **de recto** rectal cancer, cancer of the rectum; — **de riñón** renal (cell) cancer, cancer of the kidney (*fam*); — **de tiroides** thyroid cancer; — **de útero** uterine cancer, cancer of the uterus; — **de vejiga** bladder cancer; — **gástrico** (*form*) gastric cancer (*form*), stomach cancer; — **laríngeo** laryngeal cancer; — **óseo** bone cancer; — **rectal** rectal cancer; — **renal** (*form*) renal (cell) cancer; — **uterino** uterine cancer; — **vesical** (*form*) bladder cancer

cancerígeno -na *adj* carcinogenic, cancer-causing

cancerología *f* (*esp. Mex*) oncology

canceroso -sa *adj* cancerous, having cancer, pertaining to cancer

candesartán *m* candesartan

candidato -ta *mf* candidate; **candidato a trasplante hepático**..candidate for a liver transplant

candidiasis *f* candidiasis

canilla *f* leg, shin

canillera *f* (*CA, SA*) shin guard

canino *m* (*diente*) cuspid, canine tooth

cannabinoide *adj & m* cannabinoid

cannabinol *m* cannabinol

cannabis *m* cannabis

cansado -da *adj* tired; (*agotador*) tiring

cansancio *m* tiredness, fatigue; — **visual** eyestrain

cansar *vt* to tire (out), to make tired; *vr* to tire (out), to get tired

cantidad *f* quantity, amount; — **por porción** amount per serving

canto negro *m* (*PR, fam*) bruise

canturrear *vt, vi* to hum (*a tune, etc.*)

cánula *f* cannula; — **nasal** nasal cannula, nasal prongs

capa *f* coating, layer; **capas de la piel**..layers of the skin

capacidad *f* ability, capacity; — **para manejar** ability to drive; — **vital forzada** forced vital capacity

capacitación laboral *f* job training

capaz *adj* capable, competent

capilar *adj & m* capillary

capiquí *m* (*SA, bot*) chickweed

capitación *f* capitation

capsaicina *f* capsaicin

cápsula *f* capsule, pill; — **endoscópica** capsule endoscopy

capsulitis *f* capsulitis; — **adhesiva** or **retráctil** adhesive capsulitis

captación *f* uptake

captopril *m* captopril

capuchón *m* (*de aguja, etc.*) cap; — **cervical** cervical cap

carabela portuguesa *f* (*Esp*) Portuguese man-of-war, type of jellyfish

caracol *m* snail

carácter *m* characteristic; **caracteres sexuales secundarios** secondary sex *o* sexual characteristics

característico -ca *adj & f* characteristic

caramelo *f* (*dulce*) candy, piece of candy; *fpl* candy, sweets

carbamazepina, carbamacepina *f* carbamazepine

carbidopa *f* carbidopa

carbohidrato *m* carbohydrate

carbón *m* coal, charcoal; — **activado** activated charcoal

carbonatado -da *adj* carbonated

carbonato *m* carbonate; — **cálcico** (*form*), — **de calcio** calcium carbonate; — **de amonio** ammonium carbonate, (*que se utiliza para reanimar a un desmayado*) smelling salts

carbono *m* carbon (*element*)

carbunco *m* anthrax

cárcel *f* jail; prison

carcinógeno -na *adj* carcinogenic; *m* carcinogen

carcinoide *adj* carcinoid; **tumor —** carcinoid tumor

carcinoma *m* carcinoma; — **basocelular** basal cell carcinoma; — **broncogénico** bronchogenic carcinoma; — **de células no pequeñas** non-small cell carcinoma; — **de células pequeñas** small cell carcinoma; — **de células renales** renal cell carcinoma; — **de células transicionales** transitional cell carcinoma; — **ductal in situ** ductal carcinoma in situ; — **escamoso** or

espinocelular squamous cell carcinoma; — **hepatocelular** hepatocellular carcinoma; — **microcítico** (*Esp*) small cell carcinoma; — **no microcítico** (*Esp*) non-small cell carcinoma; — **renal** renal cell carcinoma

carcinomatosis *f* carcinomatosis

cardenal *m* (*Esp*) bruise

cardíaco, cardiaco -ca *adj* cardiac

cardiogénico -ca *adj* cardiogenic

cardiología *f* cardiology

cardiólogo -ga *mf* cardiologist

cardiomiopatía *f* cardiomyopathy; — **hipertrófica** (*esp. Mex*) hypertrophic cardiomyopathy

cardiopatía *f* cardiopathy; — **isquémica** ischemic cardiomyopathy

cardiopulmonar *adj* cardiopulmonary

cardiorrespiratorio -ria *adj* cardiorespiratory

cardiosaludable *adj* heart-healthy

cardiotocógrafo *m* (*form*) fetal heart monitor

cardiovascular *adj* cardiovascular

cardioversión *f* cardioversion

cardioversor *m* cardioverter

carditis *f* carditis

cardo *m* thistle; — **mariano** (*bot*) milk thistle

carecer *vt* — **de** to lack, to be deficient in

carencia *f* lack, deficiency

carga *f* burden, load; — **tumoral** tumor burden; — **viral** viral load

cargo de conciencia *m* guilty conscience

caries *f* (*dent*) caries, tooth decay

cariño *m* affection

cariñoso -sa *adj* affectionate

cariotipo *m* karyotype

carisoprodol *m* carisoprodol

carne *f* flesh; meat; — **de cerdo** pork; — **de cordero** lamb; — **de gallina** goosebumps; — **de puerco** pork; — **de res** (*esp. Amer*), — **de vaca** (*esp. Esp*) beef; — **viva** raw flesh

carnicero -ra *mf* butcher

carnitina *f* carnitine

carnosidad *f* (*en el ojo*) pterygium (*form*), benign growth on the eye

carnoso -sa *adj* fleshy

caroteno *m* carotene; **beta-caroteno** beta-carotene

carotídeo -a *adj* carotid

carótido -da *adj* carotid

carpiano -na *adj* carpal

carpintero -ra *mf* carpenter

carraspear *vi* to clear one's throat

carraspera *f* irritation of the throat, phlegm in the throat

carro *m* cart; (*Amer*) car, automobile; — **de reanimación** crash cart

cartílago *m* cartilage

carvedilol *m* carvedilol

casa *f* home; — **de cuna** (*Mex*) orphanage; — **de reposo** convalescent home; **en** — at home

casado -da *adj* married

cáscara sagrada *f* (*bot*) cascara sagrada

casco *m* helmet; — **de seguridad** hard hat

cascorvo -va *adj* (*CA, SA*) bowlegged

casero -ra *adj* made in the home; **remedio** — home remedy

caso *m* case; **en 9 de 10 casos**..in 9 out of 10 cases

caspa *f* dandruff; (*de animales*) dander

castaño -ña *adj* brown

castración *f* castration

castrar *vt* to castrate

casualidad *f* chance; **por** — by chance

catabólico -ca *adj* catabolic

catalepsia *f* catalepsy

cataplasma *f* medicinal plaster (*ant*), poultice (*ant*)

catarata *f* cataract

catarro *m* cold; runny nose

catarsis *f* (*pl* -**sis**) (*psych*) catharsis

catártico -ca *adj* (*psych*) cathartic

catástrofe *f* catastrophe

catatonía *f* catatonia

catatónico -ca *adj* catatonic

catéter *m* catheter, line; — **central de inserción periférica** peripherally-inserted central catheter (PICC); — **de arteria pulmonar** pulmonary artery catheter; — **de Hickman** Hickman catheter; — **de Swan-Ganz** pulmonary artery *o* Swan-Ganz catheter; — **epidural**

epidural catheter; — **implantable** implantable catheter; — **venoso central** central venous catheter, central line (*fam*)

cateterismo *m* catheterization; — **cardíaco** cardiac catheterization

cateterización *f* catheterization

cateterizar *vt* to catheterize

catgut *m* catgut

caucho *m* (*esp. Esp*) rubber

causa *f* cause

causalgia *f* causalgia

causar *vt* to cause

cáustico -ca *adj* caustic

cauterio *m* cautery

cauterización *f* cauterization

cauterizar *vt* to cauterize

cavidad *f* cavity

cc *abbr* **centímetro cúbico**. *See* **centímetro**.

cebolla *f* onion

cecear *vi* to lisp

ceceo *m* lisp

cedazo *m* sieve

cefaclor *m* cefaclor

cefalea *f* (*form*) headache; — **de tensión** tension headache; — **en racimos** cluster headache; — **tensional** tension headache; — **vascular** vascular headache

cefalexina *f* cephalexin

cefálico -ca *adj* cephalic

cefalorraquídeo -a *adj* cerebrospinal

cefalosporina *f* cephalosporin

ceftriaxona *f* ceftriaxone

ceguera *f* blindness; — **nocturna** night blindness

ceja *f* eyebrow, brow

celecoxib *m* celecoxib

celíaco -ca *adj* celiac

celiaquía *f* celiac disease

célula *f* cell; — **asesina natural** natural killer cell; — **B** B cell; — **CD4** CD4 cell;— **cerebral** brain cell; **células escamosas atípicas de significado indeterminado** atypical squamous cells of undetermined significance (ASCUS); — **madre** stem cell; — **plasmática** plasma cell; — **T citotóxica** cytotoxic T cell; — **T colaboradora** helper T cell; — **transicional** transitional cell; — **T supresora** suppressor T cell

celular *adj* cellular; (*fam, teléfono*) cellular telephone, cell phone (*fam*)

celulitis *f* cellulitis; (*depósitos de grasa*) cellulite

cena *f* dinner, supper

centígrado -da *adj* Centigrade; **37 grados centígrados**..37 degrees Centigrade

centímetro (cm) *m* centimeter (cm); — **cúbico (cc)** cubic centimeter (cc)

central *adj* central; *f* station; — **de enfermeras** (*esp. Mex*) nursing station

centro *m* center; — **ambulatorio** clinic; — **de acogida** (*Esp*) shelter; — **de acogida para mujeres** women's shelter; — **de cirugía** surgical *o* surgery center; — **de salud** medical center; — **de salud rural** rural health center; — **diurno** day center; — **médico** medical center, hospital; — **quirúrgico** surgical *o* surgery center; — **sanitario** (*Esp*) medical center

Centro de Toxicología, Poison Control Center

Centros para Control de Enfermedades, Centers for Disease Control and Prevention (CDC)

cepa *f* (*de una bacteria, etc.*) strain (*of a bacteria, etc.*)

cepillado *m* brushing

cepillar *vt* to brush; *vr* — **el pelo** to brush one's hair; — **los dientes** to brush one's teeth

cepillo *m* brush, (*para el pelo*) hairbrush; — **de dientes** toothbrush

cera *f* wax; — **de los oídos** earwax

cerca de, close to, near

cercano -na *adj* close; **amigo -ga** *mf* — close friend

cerclaje *m* cerclage

cerda *f* bristle; **de — dura** stiff-bristle *o* hard-bristle; **de — suave** soft-bristle

cerdo *m* pork

cereal *m* cereal, grain

cerebelo *m* cerebellum

cerebral *adj* cerebral

cerebro *m* brain; — **medio** midbrain

cerebrovascular *adj* cerebrovascular

cerrado -da *adj* (*traumatismo, etc.*) closed

cerrar *vt* to close; **cuando cierro los ojos**..when I close my eyes; **— la mano** to make a fist; *vi, vr* to close

certificado -da *adj* certified; *m* certificate; **— (médico) de defunción** death certificate; **— de nacimiento** birth certificate

cerumen *m* cerumen, earwax (*fam*)

cerveza *f* beer

cervical *adj* (*obst & ortho*) cervical

cervicitis *f* cervicitis

cervix *f* (*pl* -**vix**) cervix

cerviz *f* (*pl* -**vices**) back of the neck

cesárea *f* cesarean section

cetirizina *f* cetirizine

cetoacidosis *f* ketoacidosis

cetona *f* ketone

cetónico -ca *adj* ketotic

cetósico -ca *adj* **no —** nonketotic

chalazión *m* chalazion

chamaco -ca *m* boy, child; *f* girl

chamán *m* shaman

chamarra *f* (*Mex*) jacket

chamorro *m* (*Mex, fam*) calf (*of leg*)

champú *m* (*pl* -**pús**) shampoo

chancro *m* chancre; **— blando** soft chancre

chancroide *m* chancroid

chaparro -ra *adj* short and stocky

chaqueta *f* jacket; (*Mex, vulg*) masturbation

charola *f* (*Mex*) tray

chasquido *m* (*card*) click

chata *f* bedpan

chequear *vt* to check

chequeo *m* checkup

chichón *m* lump, bump (*due to trauma, esp. about the head*)

chichote *m* (*Nic, fam*) lump, bump (*due to trauma, esp. about the head*)

chicle *m* chewing gum

chico -ca *adj* little, small; *m* boy, child; *f* girl

chile *m* chili pepper

chimpinilla *f* (*CA, fam*) shin

chinche *f* bedbug; (*vector de la enfermedad de Chagas*) kissing bug

chindondo *m* (*El Salv, fam*) lump, bump (*due to trauma, esp. about the head*)

chipote *m* (*Mex, fam*) lump, bump (*due to trauma, esp. about the head*)

chiva *f* (*Mex, fam*) heroin; (*PR*) jaw

chivola *f* (*El Salv*) bump, lump

chocolate *m* chocolate

choque *m* shock; (*fam, accidente de tránsito*) automobile accident; **— anafiláctico** anaphylactic shock; **— cardiogénico** cardiogenic shock; **— hipovolémico** hypovolemic shock; **— neurogénico** neurogenic shock; **— séptico** septic shock

choquezuela *f* (*fam*) kneecap

chorro *m* (*de la orina*) stream (*of urine*); **— miccional** (*form*) urinary stream

chucho *m* (*Amer*) chill (*esp. due to malaria*)

chueco -ca *adj* (*Mex*) crooked

chupar *vt* to suck; *vr* **— el dedo** to suck one's thumb

chupete *m* pacifier; (*marca producida por un beso*) hickey

chupetón *m* (*marca producida por un beso*) hickey

chupón *m* pacifier; (*marca producida por un beso*) hickey

CIA *abbr* **comunicación interauricular**. See **comunicación**.

cianocobalamina *f* cyanocobalamin, vitamin B_{12}

cianosis *f* cyanosis

cianótico -ca *adj* cyanotic

cianuro *m* cyanide

ciático -ca *adj* sciatic; *f* sciatica

cicatriz *f* (*pl* -**trices**) scar; **dejar —** to leave a scar

cicatrización *f* healing; scarring

cicatrizar *vt, vr* to heal (*a wound*)

ciclamato *m* cyclamate

cíclico -ca *adj* cyclic, cyclical

ciclismo *m* (*sport*) cycling

ciclo *m* cycle; **— anovulatorio** anovulatory cycle; **— biológico** life cycle; **— menstrual** menstrual cycle; **— ovulatorio** ovulatory cycle; **— reproductivo** reproductive cycle; **— vital** life cycle

ciclobenzaprina *f* cyclobenzaprine

ciclofosfamida *f* cyclophosphamide

ciclosporina *f* cyclosporine

cicuta *f* (*bot*) hemlock
cidofovir *m* cidofovir
ciego -ga *adj* blind; *mf* blind person; *m* (*anat*) cecum
ciempiés *m* (*pl* -**piés**) centipede
científico -ca *adj* scientific; *mf* scientist
cierre *m* zipper; (*surg*) closure
cifoescoliosis *f* kyphoscoliosis
cifosis *f* kyphosis
cifra *f* number
cigarrillo *m* cigarette
cigarro *m* (*esp. Mex*) cigarette
cigoto *m* zygote
cilindro *m* cylinder; — **de oxígeno** oxygen tank
cilostazol *m* cilostazol
cimetidina *f* cimetidine
Cimicifuga racemosa (*bot*) black cohosh
cinc See **zinc.**
cinesiología *f* kinesiology
cinético -ca *adj* kinetic
cinta *f* band, tape; — **adhesiva** adhesive tape; — **métrica** tape measure *o* measuring tape; — **rodante** (*esp. Esp*) treadmill
cinto *m* belt
cintura *f* waist, waistline; (*anat*) girdle; (*fam, espalda baja*) lower back; **de la cintura hacia arriba..** from the waist up; — **escapular** shoulder girdle; — **pélvica** *or* **pelviana** pelvic girdle
cinturón *m* belt; — **de seguridad** seat belt
ciprofloxacina *f* (*esp. Amer*) ciprofloxacin
ciprofloxacino *m* ciprofloxacin
ciproheptadina *f* cyproheptadine
circadiano -na *adj* circadian
circulación *f* circulation, blood flow; — **colateral** collateral circulation; — **extracorpórea** extracorporeal circulation; — **fetal** fetal circulation; — **pulmonar** pulmonary circulation; — **sistémica** systemic circulation
circular *vi* to circulate, to flow; **estar circulando** (*un virus, etc.*) to be going around
circulatorio -ria *adj* circulatory
círculo *m* circle; — **vicioso** vicious circle
circuncidar *vt* (*pp* -**ciso**) to circumcise
circuncisión *f* circumcision
circunciso -sa (*pp of* **circuncidar**) *adj* circumcised
circundante *adj* surrounding
circunscrito -ta *adj* localized
cirrosis *f* cirrhosis; — **biliar primaria** primary biliary cirrhosis
cirrótico -ca *adj* & *mf* cirrhotic
cirugía *f* surgery; — **a corazón abierto** open heart surgery; — **ambulatoria** ambulatory *o* outpatient surgery; — **bariátrica** bariatric surgery; — **bucal** oral surgery; — **de revascularización coronaria** coronary artery bypass surgery; — **de várices** vein stripping; — **electiva** elective surgery; — **estética** cosmetic surgery; — **general** general surgery; — **laparoscópica** laparoscopic surgery; — **maxilofacial** maxilofacial surgery; — **mayor** major surgery; — **menor** minor surgery; — **oral** oral surgery; — **ortopédica** orthopedic surgery; — **plástica** plastic surgery; — **radical** radical surgery; — **reconstructiva** reconstructive surgery; — **robótica** robotic surgery; — **torácica** thoracic surgery
cirujano -na *mf* surgeon; — **dentista** (*esp. Mex*) dentist; — **general** general surgeon; — **oral** oral surgeon; — **ortopédico** orthopedic surgeon; — **torácico** thoracic surgeon; — **vascular** vascular surgeon
cisplatino *m* cisplatin
cistectomía *f* cystectomy, removal of the bladder
cisteína *f* cysteine
cisticercosis *f* cysticercosis
cístico -ca *adj* cystic (*artery, duct*)
cistinuria *f* cystinuria
cistitis *f* cystitis; — **intersticial** interstitial cystitis
cistocele *m* cystocele
cistoscopia, cistoscopía (*Amer, esp. spoken*) *f* cystoscopy
cistoscopio *m* cystoscope
cita *f* appointment
citalopram *m* citalopram

citología *f* cytology; — **cervical** Papanicolaou smear, Pap smear (*fam*)
citomegalovirus (CMV) *m* cytomegalovirus (CMV)
citometría *f* cytometry; — **de flujo** flow cytometry
citotóxico -ca *adj* cytotoxic
citrato *m* citrate
cítrico -ca *adj* citric; *mpl* citrus fruits
CIV *abbr* comunicación interventricular. *See* comunicación.
clamidia *f* chlamydia
clara *f* — **de huevo** egg white
claritromicina *f* clarithromycin
claro -ra *adj* clear; *f* (*del huevo*) white (*of an egg*)
clase *f* class
clásico -ca *adj* classic
claudicación *f* claudication; — **intermitente** intermittent claudication
claustrofobia *f* claustrophobia
clavícula *f* clavicle, collarbone (*fam*)
clavo *m* nail; (*ortho*) pin
clima *m* climate
climaterio *m* climacteric
clímax *m* (*pl* -max) climax, orgasm
clindamicina *f* clindamycin
clínico -ca *adj* clinical; *mf* clinician, practitioner; *f* clinic; — **ambulatoria** *or* **de consulta externa** outpatient clinic; — **de urgencias** urgent care clinic; — **gratuita** free clinic
clítoris *m* clitoris
cloasma *m* melasma
clofazimina *f* clofazimine
clofibrato *m* clofibrate
clomifeno *m* clomiphene
clon *m* clone
clonazepam *m* clonazepam
clónico -ca *adj* clonic
clonidina *f* clonidine
clonus *m* clonus
clopidogrel *m* clopidogrel
cloración *f* chlorination
clorado -da *adj* chlorinated
clorambucilo *m* chlorambucil
cloranfenicol *m* chloramphenicol
clordano *m* chlordane
clordiazepóxido *m* chlordiazepoxide
clorfeniramina, clorfenamina *f* chlorpheniramine
clorhexidina *f* chlorhexidine

clorhidrato *m* hydrochloride
clorhídrico -ca *adj* hydrochloric
cloro *m* chlorine
cloroformo *m* chloroform
cloroquina *f* chloroquine
clorpromazina, clorpromacina *f* chlorpromazine
clorpropamida *f* chlorpropamide
clortalidona *f* chlorthalidone
cloruro *m* chloride; — **de polivinilo** polyvinyl chloride; — **de potasio** potassium chloride; — **de sodio** sodium chloride; — **potásico** (*form*) potassium chloride; — **sódico** (*form*) sodium chloride
clostridio *m* clostridium
clotrimazol *m* clotrimazole
club *m* club; — **de salud** health club
cm *See* centímetro.
CMV *See* citomegalovirus.
coagulación *f* coagulation; — **intravascular diseminada** disseminated intravascular coagulation (DIC)
coagular *vt, vr* to coagulate, to clot
coágulo *m* clot
coagulopatía *f* coagulopathy
coartación *f* coarctation
cobalamina *See* cianocobalamina.
cobalto *m* cobalt
cobayo -ya *m* guinea pig
cobertura *f* (*seguro*) coverage
cobija *f* (*esp. Mex*) blanket
cobrar *vt, vi* to charge
cobre *m* copper
cobro *m* bill, charge
coca *f* (*bot*) coca; (*fam*) cocaine, coke (*fam*)
cocaína *f* cocaine
cocainómano -na *mf* cocaine addict
coccidioidomicosis *f* coccidioidomycosis, valley fever (*fam*)
cóccix *m* coccyx, tailbone (*fam*)
cocer *vt* (*carne, etc.*) to boil; — **al horno** to bake; — **al vapor** to steam
coche *m* automobile, car
cocido -da *adj* boiled; — **al horno** baked; — **al vapor** steamed
cociente intelectual (CI) *m* intelligence quotient (IQ)
cocinar *vt, vi* to cook
cocinero -ra *mf* cook
cóclea *f* cochlea

coclear *adj* cochlear
coco *m* (*bacteria*) coccus; (*nuez*) coconut
cóctel *m* (*de medicamentos*) cocktail (*of medications*)
codeína *f* codeine
codependencia *f* codependency
código azul *m* (*Ang*) Code Blue
código postal *m* zip code
codo *m* elbow; — **de golfista** golfer's elbow; — **de tenista** tennis elbow
coeficiente intelectual (CI) *m* intelligence quotient (IQ)
coenzima Q *f* coenzyme Q
coger *vt* (*esp. Esp, una enfermedad*) to contract, to catch (*a disease*)
cognitivo -va *adj* cognitive
cohibición *f* inhibition
cohibido -da *adj* inhibited
coinfección *f* coinfection
coito *m* coitus; — **interrumpido** coitus interruptus
coitus interruptus *m* (*form*) coitus interruptus
cojear *vi* to limp
cojera *f* limp
cojín *m* cushion, pad; — **eléctrico** (*esp. Mex*) heating pad
cojo -ja *adj* lame, crippled; *mf* lame person, crippled person
cojón *m* (*vulg, frec. pl*) testicle, ball (*fam, frec. pl*)
colaborador -ra *adj* cooperative; **no — uncooperative**
cola de caballo *f* (*bot*) horsetail, pewterwort
colador *m* sieve
colágeno *m* collagen
colangiocarcinoma *m* cholangiocarcinoma
colangiografía *f* (*técnica imagenológica*) cholangiography; (*estudio imagenológico*) cholangiogram; — **transhepática percutánea** percutaneous transhepatic cholangiography; percutaneous transhepatic cholangiogram
colangiopancreatografía retrógrada endoscópica (CPRE) *f* endoscopic retrograde cholangiopancreatography (ERCP)
colangitis *f* cholangitis
colapsar *vr* (*un pulmón, etc.*) to collapse

colapso *m* collapse; (*crisis*) breakdown; — **nervioso** nervous breakdown
colar *vt* to strain; **Tiene que colar su orina para buscar piedras..**You have to strain your urine for stones.
colateral *adj* collateral
colcha *f* blanket
colchicina *f* colchicine
colchón *m* mattress
colecistectomía *f* cholecystectomy
colecistitis *f* cholecystitis; — **alitiásica** acalculous cholecystitis
colectomía *f* colectomy
colega *mf* colleague
colelitiasis *f* cholelithiasis
cólera *m* cholera; *f* anger, rage
colesevelam *m* colesevelam
colestasis *f* cholestasis; — (**intrahepática**) **del embarazo** cholestasis of pregnancy
colesteatoma *m* cholesteatoma
colesterol *m* cholesterol; — **LDL,** — **HDL, etc.** LDL cholesterol, HDL cholesterol, etc.; — **total** total cholesterol
colestipol *m* colestipol
colestiramina *f* cholestyramine
colgajo *m* (*surg*) flap
colgar *vt* to hang, to dangle
cólico -ca *adj* colonic, pertaining to the colon; *m* (*ped, etc.; frec. pl*) colic; — **menstrual** menstrual cramp(s); **¿Tiene cólicos?..**Does he have colic?
coliflor *f* cauliflower
coliforme *adj* & *m* coliform
colirio *m* eyewash, eye drops
colita *f* (*Amer, fam*) coccyx, tailbone (*fam*)
colitis *f* colitis; — **isquémica** ischemic colitis; — **seudomembranosa** pseudomembranous colitis; — **ulcerosa** ulcerative colitis
collar *m* (*esp. SA, ortho*) collar; — **cervical (rígido, blando)** (hard, soft) cervical collar
collarín *m* collar; — **cervical (rígido, blando)** (hard, soft) cervical collar
colmillo *m* cuspid, canine tooth; (*de un animal*) fang

colocación f placement
colocar vt to position, to place
coloide m colloid
colon m colon, large bowel; — **ascendente** ascending colon; — **derecho** right colon; — **descendente** descending colon; — **espástico** irritable bowel syndrome, spastic colon (ant); — **izquierdo** left colon; — **sigmoide** or **sigmoideo** sigmoid colon; — **transverso** transverse colon
colonización f colonization
colonografía f colonography
colonoscopia, colonoscopía (Amer, esp. spoken) f colonoscopy; — **virtual** virtual colonoscopy
colonoscopio m colonoscope
color m color
coloración f (micro) stain; — **de Gram** Gram's stain
colorado -da adj red
colorante m dye; — **vegetal** or **alimentario** food coloring
colorrectal adj colorectal
colostomía f colostomy; **bolsa de** or **para** — colostomy bag
colposcopia, colposcopía (Amer, esp. spoken) f colposcopy
columna f column; (fam, espina) spinal column, backbone, spine; — **cervical** cervical spine; — **dorsal** thoracic spine; — **lumbar** lumbar spine; — **lumbosacra** lumbosacral spine; — **torácica** thoracic spine; — **vertebral** spinal column, backbone, spine
colutorio m (form) mouthwash
coma m coma; **en** — in a coma
comadrón m male who assists at labor, male midwife
comadrona f midwife
comatoso -sa adj comatose
combinación f combination
comenzar vt, vi to begin
comer vt, vi to eat; (esp. Mex) to have lunch; **dar de** — to feed; vr — **las uñas** to bite o chew one's nails
comestible m food
comezón f itch, itching, itchiness; **sentir** or **tener** — to itch; **Tengo comezón**..I'm itching..I have an itch.

comida f food, meal; (esp. Mex) lunch; — **balanceada** (Amer) balanced meal; — **basura** (esp. Esp) or — **chatarra** junk food; — **enlatada** canned food; — **equilibrada** (Esp) balanced meal; — **para bebés** baby food; — **procesada** processed food; — **rápida** fast food
comienzo m onset, beginning; **de** — **precoz** early-onset
comodidad f comfort
cómodo -da adj comfortable; m (Mex, bacinilla) bedpan
compañero -ra mf companion; — **sentimental** significant other
compartir vt to share; — **agujas** or **jeringas** to share needles
compasión f compassion, sympathy
compasivo -va adj compassionate, sympathetic
compatible adj compatible
compensación f — **del trabajador** worker's compensation
compensar vi to compensate
competente adj competent
complejo m complex; — **de Edipo** Oedipus complex; — **Mycobacterium avium** Mycobacterium avium complex (MAC)
complemento m complement
completo -ta adj complete
complexión f build, constitution
complicación f complication
componente m component
componer vt (pp -puesto) to fix; vr (fam, recuperarse) to get well
comportamiento m behavior
comportarse vr to behave
comprensivo -va adj sympathetic
compresa f compress, pack
compresión f compression, (de un nervio) entrapment; — **medular** or **de la médula espinal** spinal cord compression
comprimido m (form) tablet
comprimir vt to compress
comprometer vt to compromise
compuesto (pp of **componer**) m compound
compulsión f compulsion
compulsivo -va adj compulsive
computadora f computer
común adj common; **un problema**

común..a common problem; **poco — uncommon**

comunicación *f* communication; **— interauricular (CIA)** atrial septal defect (ASD); **— interventricular (CIV)** ventricular septal defect (VSD)

comunicar *vt, vr* to communicate

comunidad *f* community

comunitario -ria *adj* pertaining to the community; **participación —** community involvement

cóncavo -va *adj* concave

concebir *vi* to conceive

concentración *f* concentration

concentrado -da *adj* concentrated; *m* (*pharm*) concentrate

concentrador *m* concentrator; **— de oxígeno** oxygen concentrator

concentrar *vt, vr* to concentrate

concepción *f* (*obst, etc.*) conception

conciencia *f* conscience; (*conocimiento*) consciousness, awareness; **cargo de —** guilty conscience; **— colectiva** collective consciousness; **perder la —** to lose consciousness; **pérdida de —** loss of consciousness

conclusión *f* (*psych*) closure

concusión *f* concussion

condado *m* county (*US*)

condición *f* condition, state; **— física** physical conditioning, fitness; **— preexistente** pre-existing condition

condicionado -da *adj* conditioned

condicionamiento *m* conditioning; **— físico** physical conditioning, fitness

condimentado -da *adj* spicy

condimento *m* spice

condón *m* condom, rubber (*fam*)

condrocalcinosis *f* chondrocalcinosis

condrosarcoma *m* chondrosarcoma

conducción *f* conduction

conducir *vt* (*un vehículo*) to drive

conducta *f* behavior

conducto *m* duct, canal, conduit; **— arterioso persistente** patent ductus arteriosus (PDA); **— auditivo** Eustachian tube; **— biliar** bile duct; **— cístico** cystic duct; **— colédoco** common bile duct; **— de Eustaquio** Eustachian tube; **—**

deferente vas deferens; **— hepático** hepatic duct; **— ileal** ileal conduit; **— lagrimal** lacrimal duct, tear duct (*fam*); **conductos nasales** nasal passages; **— pancreático** pancreatic duct; **— semicircular** semicircular canal

conductor -ra *mf* driver; **— designado** designated driver

conectar *vt* to connect, attach

conectivopatía *f* (*Esp*) connective tissue disease

conejillo de Indias *m* guinea pig (*esp. figuratively*)

conexión *f* connection

confabulación *f* confabulation

confiable *adj* reliable

confianza *f* confidence, trust; **— en uno mismo** self-confidence; **tener — (en)** to trust

confiar *vi* to trust; **Confío en mis hijos**..I trust my children.

confidencial *adj* confidential

confidencialidad *f* confidentiality

confirmar *vt* to confirm

conflicto *m* conflict

confort *m* comfort

confortar *vt* to comfort

confrontar *vt* to confront

confundido -da *adj* confused

confundir *vt* to confuse; *vr* to get *o* become confused

confusión *f* confusion

congelamiento *m* (*daño a los tejidos por el frío*) frostbite

congelar *vt, vr* to freeze

congénito -ta *adj* congenital

congestión *f* congestion; **— nasal** nasal congestion

congestionado -da *adj* congested

congestivo -va *adj* congestive

conización *f* conization; **— con asa diatérmica** loop electrosurgical excision procedure (LEEP)

conjugado -da *adj* conjugated

conjuntiva *f* conjunctiva

conjuntival *adj* conjunctival

conjuntivitis *f* conjunctivitis, pinkeye (*fam*)

conminuta *adj* comminuted

conmoción cerebral *f* concussion

cono *m* (*anat, gyn, ophthalmology, etc.*) cone

conocimiento *m* consciousness; **— de uno mismo** insight; **perder el —** to lose consciousness, to black out; **pérdida de —** loss of consciousness, blackout

consciencia *f* consciousness, awareness; **— colectiva** collective consciousness; **perder la —** to lose consciousness; **pérdida de —** loss of consciousness

consciente *adj* conscious, aware

consecuencia *f* consequence

consecutivo -va *adj* consecutive

consejero -ra *mf* counselor

consejo *m* advice, counseling; (*pauta*) recommendation, tip; **— genético** genetic counseling

consentimiento *m* consent; **— informado** informed consent

consentir *vt* to pamper, spoil; *vi* to consent; **— en** to consent to

conservador -ra *adj* conservative, conserving; **— de mama** breast-conserving; *m* (*esp. Mex, conservante*) preservative

conservante *m* preservative

conservar *vt* to conserve, preserve

consistencia *f* consistency

consolador *m* (*juego sexual*) dildo

consolar *vt* to console, to comfort

consolidación *f* consolidation

constante *adj* constant; *fpl* **— vitales** (*Esp*) vital signs

constipación *f* (*catarro, congestión*) cold, nasal congestion; (*estreñimiento*) constipation

constipado -da *adj* (*congestionado*) having a cold, congested, having nasal congestion; (*estreñido*) constipated; *m* cold, nasal congestion

constiparse *vr* to catch a cold, to become congested; (*estreñirse*) to become constipated

constitución *f* constitution

constricción *f* constriction

consuelda *f* (*bot*) comfrey

consulta *f* visit, doctor's visit; (*con un especialista*) consult; **— externa** clinic; **— subsecuente** (*Mex*) follow-up; **horas de —** office hours; **pasar —** (*Esp*) to round, to visit patients

consultar *vt, vi* to consult

consultorio *m* office (*of a doctor*)

consumidor -ra *mf* user

consumo *m* consumption, intake

contacto *m* contact, exposure; **— cercano** close contact; **— visual** eye contact

contagiar *vt* to infect, to give (*a disease*); *vr* to become infected, to catch (*a disease*)

contagioso -sa *adj* (*una enfermedad*) communicable (*form*), contagious, infectious, catching (*fam*); (*fam, una persona*) capable of infecting others, contagious (*fam*); [*Nota: en principio* contagioso *y* contagioso *se aplican a las enfermedades y no a las personas aún cuando ambos son aplicados a personas en lenguaje familiar.*]

contaminación *f* contamination, pollution; **— ambiental** pollution (*of the environment*); **— atmosférica** air pollution, smog; **— del agua** water pollution; **— del aire** air pollution, smog

contaminado -da *adj* contaminated, polluted

contaminar *vt* to contaminate; *vr* to become contaminated

contar *vt, vi* to count; **— calorías** to count calories

contener *vt* to contain; **— la respiración** to hold one's breath

contenido *m* content (*frec. pl*)

contento -ta *adj* happy

conteo *m* count; **— de bacterias** bacterial count; **— de glóbulos rojos, plaquetas, etc.** red blood cell count, platelet count, etc.

contextura *f* build

continuo -nua *adj* continuous, constant

contorno *m* contour

contracción *f* contraction; **— auricular prematura (CAP)** premature atrial contraction (PAC); **contracciones de Braxton-Hicks** Braxton-Hicks contractions; **— ventricular prematura (CVP)** premature ventricular contraction (PVC)

contracepción *f* contraception

contraceptivo -va *adj & m* contraceptive

contractura f contracture; **— de Du-**
puytren Dupuytren's contracture
contraer vt (una enfermedad) to contract, to catch (fam); vr (un músculo, etc.) to contract
contraindicación f contraindication
contraindicado -da adj contraindicated
contrarrestar vt to counteract
contraste m (fam, medio de contraste) contrast medium, contrast
(fam)
contrato m contract
control m control; **— de la natalidad**
birth control; **— de uno mismo**
self-control; **— estricto** (de la
glucemia) tight control (of blood
sugars); **fuera de —** out of control
controlar vt to control
controvertido -da adj controversial
contusión f contusion
convalecencia f convalescence
convalecerse vr to convalesce
convaleciente adj convalescent
convencional adj conventional
conversión f conversion
convexo -xa adj convex
convivir vi **— con** to live with; **con-**
vivir con (el) dolor crónico..to live
with chronic pain
convulsión f convulsion, seizure
convulsionar vi to seize, to have a
seizure
cónyuge mf spouse
cooperar vi to cooperate
coordinación f coordination
copago m copayment
coprocultivo m stool culture
coqueluche m&f (fam) pertussis
(form), whooping cough
coraje m rage
coral m coral
corazón m heart
corazoncillo m St. John's wort
cordal See **muela cordal**.
cordero m lamb
cordón m cord; **— umbilical** umbilical cord
cordura f sanity
corea m&f chorea; **— de Huntington**
Huntington's chorea
coriocarcinoma m choriocarcinoma
coriorretinitis f chorioretinitis

córnea f cornea
corneal adj corneal
corona f (anat, dent) crown
coronación f (obst) crowning
coronario -ria adj coronary
corporal adj corporal, pertaining to
the body
corpúsculo m corpuscle
correa f strap, belt
corrección f correction, adjustment
correctivo -va adj corrective
correcto -ta adj correct
corrector -ra adj corrective; m **—**
dental (esp. Esp, orthodontia)
braces, bands (fam)
corredor mf (atleta) runner; m (pasillo) hall, hallway
corregir vt to correct
correlación f correlation
correr vi to run, to flow
corriente f current
corrosivo -va adj corrosive
corsé m (pl **-sés**) (ortho) corset, truss
cortado -da adj cut; (labios, piel)
chapped; f cut
cortadura f cut
cortar vt to cut, cut off; vr to cut
oneself; **Me corté**..I cut myself; **—**
el pelo to get a haircut; **— las uñas**
to cut one's nails
cortauñas f nail clippers
corte m incision; **— de pelo** haircut
cortesía f courtesy; **— profesional**
professional courtesy
corteza f bark; (anat) cortex
cortical adj cortical
corticosteroide, corticoesteroide m
corticosteroid
cortisol m cortisol
cortisona f cortisone
corto -ta adj short; **a — plazo** short-
term
cortocircuito m (physiological) shunt
corva f back of the knee; **tendón** m
de la — hamstring
coser vt (una herida) to sew, to suture, to stitch (up) (fam)
cosmético -ca adj cosmetic; m cosmetic, makeup
cosquillas fpl tickling; **¿Siente cos-**
quillas?..Do you feel tickling?..
Does that tickle?...**¿Le hago cos-**
quillas?..Am I tickling you?

cosquilleo *m* tickling
cosquilloso -sa *adj* ticklish
costado *m* (*anat*) side
coste *m* (*Esp*) charge, cost
coste-efectividad *m* (*Esp*) cost-effectiveness
coste-efectivo -va *adj* (*Esp*) cost-effective
costilla *f* rib
costo *m* charge, cost
costo-efectividad *m&f* cost-effectiveness
costo-efectivo -va *adj* cost-effective
costocondritis *f* costochondritis
costra *f* eschar (*form*), scab, crust; — láctea (*form*) or de leche cradle cap
costumbre *f* habit; como de — as usual; ¿Está comiendo tanto como de costumbre?..Are you eating as much as usual; mala — bad habit; que de — than usual; ¿Está orinando más que de costumbre?.. Are you urinating more than usual?
cotidiano -na *adj* daily, everyday
cotilo *m* acetabulum
cotonete *m* cotton-tipped swab; [*Note: cotonete is a brand name which is often used generically.*]
coxis *m* coccyx, tailbone (*fam*)
coyuntura *f* (*fam*) joint
CPRE *See* colangiopancreatografía retrógrada endoscópica.
crack *m* (*Ang*) crack cocaine, crack
craneal *adj* cranial
craneano -na *adj* cranial
cráneo *m* cranium (*form*), skull
craneofaringioma *m* craniopharyngioma
craneotomía *f* craniotomy
creatina *f* creatine
creatinina *f* creatinine
crecer *vi* to grow, to get bigger; (*volverse adulto*) to grow up; cuando crezcas..when you grow up
crecimiento *m* growth; — intrauterino retardado (*Esp*) intrauterine growth retardation
creencia *f* belief
crema *f* cream, balm; — bronceadora suntan lotion; — de afeitar shaving cream; — de cacahuate peanut butter; — dental toothpaste;

— limpiadora cold cream; — para manos hand cream; — para los labios lip balm
cremallera *f* (*Esp*) zipper
cresa *f* maggot
cretinismo *m* cretinism
cretino -na *mf* cretin
criar *vt* (*a un niño*) to raise (*a child*)
criatura *f* (*fam*) infant, baby
cribado *m* (*form*) screening; — del cáncer screening for cancer, cancer screening
cricotiroideo -a *adj* cricothyroid
crío -a *mf* infant, young child
criocirugía *f* cryosurgery
crioconservación *f* cryoconservation
crioglobulina *f* cryoglobulin
crioterapia *f* cryotherapy
criptorquidia *f* cryptorchidism
criptosporidiosis *f* cryptosporidiosis
crisis *f* (*pl* -sis) crisis; breakdown; (epiléptica) seizure; — asmática (*form*) asthma attack; — blástica blast crisis; — convulsiva seizure, epileptic seizure; — convulsiva generalizada generalized seizure; — de angustia or ansiedad anxiety attack, panic attack; — de asma asthma attack; — de ausencia absence seizure; — de gran mal (*ant*) tonic-clonic seizure, gran mal seizure (*ant*); — de identidad identity crisis; — del lóbulo temporal temporal lobe seizure; — de (la) mediana edad midlife crisis; — de pánico panic attack, anxiety attack; — de pequeño mal (*ant*) absence seizure, petit mal seizure (*ant*); — nerviosa nervous breakdown; — parcial partial seizure; — parcial compleja complex partial seizure; — psicomotora (*ant*) complex partial seizure, psychomotor seizure (*ant*); — tirotóxica thyroid storm; — tónico-clónica tonic-clonic seizure
cristal *m* crystal
cristalino *m* lens (*of the eye*)
crítico -ca *adj* critical
cromato *m* chromate
cromo *m* chromium
cromoglicato disódico, cromoglicato de sodio (*esp. Mex*) *m* cromolyn

sodium
cromomicosis *f* chromomycosis
cromosoma *m* chromosome
cromosómico -ca *adj* chromosomal
crónicamente *adv* chronically
crónico -ca *adj* chronic
crudo -da *adj* raw; (*Mex, con resaca*) hungover; *f* (*Mex, resaca*) hangover; **tener una** — to have a hangover, to be hungover
cruel *adj* cruel
crueldad *f* cruelty
crup *m* croup
cruzar *vt* — **los brazos** to fold one's arms
Cruz Roja *f* Red Cross
cuaderno *m* log
cuadrado -da *adj* square; **metro** — square meter
cuadrante *m* quadrant
cuadriceps *m* (*pl* -**ceps**) quadriceps
cuadril *m* hip bone, hip
cuadrillizo -za *mf* quadruplet
cuadriplejía *f* (*esp. SA*) quadriplegia
cuadripléjico -ca *adj & mf* (*esp. SA*) quadriplegic
cuanto *adv* ¿**Cada cuánto (tiempo)?** ..How often?..¿**Cada cuánto (tiempo) se puede donar sangre?**..How often can you donate blood?
cuarentena *f* quarantine; (*Mex, CA; obst*) forty days following childbirth; *vt* **poner en** — to quarantine
cuarto *m* fourth, quarter; (*habitación*) room, bedroom; (*de galón*) quart; — **de baño** bathroom
cuatrillizo -za *mf* quadruplet
cubierta *f* (*de una pastilla*) coating (*of a pill*)
cubierto *pp of* **cubrir**
cubital *adj* ulnar
cúbito *m* ulna
cubreboca *m* (*Mex, surg*) mask
cubrir *vt* (*pp* **cubierto**) to cover; **Su seguro cubre**..Your insurance covers..
cucaracha *f* cockroach
cucharada *f* spoonful, tablespoonful; — **grande** tablespoonful
cucharadita *f* spoonful, teaspoonful
cuchillada *f* knife wound, stab wound, gash
cuchillo *m* knife

cuclillas *fpl* **ponerse en** — to squat
cuello *m* neck; collar; — **uterino** or **de la matriz** cervix
cuenca *f* (*del ojo*) eye socket
cuenta *f* bill
cuentagotas *m* medicine dropper, eyedropper
cuerda *f* cord; — **vocal** vocal cord
cuerdo -da *adj* sane
cuero cabelludo *m* scalp
cuerpo *m* body; — **de bomberos** fire department; — **extraño** foreign body; — **lúteo** corpus luteum; **dar del** — (*Carib*) to have a bowel movement
cuesta arriba *adv* uphill
cuestionario *m* questionnaire
cuidado *m* care; **cuidados de enfermería** nursing care; **cuidados de larga duración** (*Esp*) long-term care; — **del pie, de la piel, etc.** foot care, skin care, etc.; **cuidados intensivos** intensive care; — **médico** health care; **cuidados prolongados** long-term care; **tener** — to be careful; **Tenga cuidado**..Be careful.
cuidador -ra *mf* caregiver
cuidar *vt* take care of, to care for; **Yo lo cuido solo**..I take care of him by myself; *vr* to take care of oneself; (*fam, usar anticoncepción*) to use birth control
culdocentesis *f* (*pl* -**sis**) culdocentesis
culebra *f* snake
culebrilla *f* (*esp. Carib*) shingles
culo (*vulg*) *m* buttocks; (*ano*) anus
culpa *f* guilt; **sentimientos de** — feelings of guilt
cultivar *vt* (*micro*) to culture
cultivo *m* (*micro*) culture; — **de garganta** throat culture; — **de heces** stool culture; — **de orina** urine culture; — **de sangre** blood culture; — **faríngeo** (*form*) throat culture
cultura *f* culture
culturismo *m* bodybuilding
culturista *mf* bodybuilder
cumpleaños *m* (*pl* -**años**) birthday; **¡Feliz cumpleaños!**..Happy birthday!
cumplimiento *m* compliance; — **del**

tratamiento compliance with treatment

cuna f cradle, crib; — **portátil** bassinet

cunnilingus m (form) cunnilingus (form), oral sex, oral stimulation of the vulva and clitoris

cuña f wedge

cuñado -da m brother-in-law; f sister-in-law

cura m priest; f cure; (vendaje) bandage, dressing (often adhesive); — **oclusiva** occlusive dressing

curable adj curable

curación f healing, recovery

curandería f folk o traditional medicine; faith healing

curanderismo m folk o traditional

medicine; faith healing

curandero -ra mf folk o traditional healer; faith healer

curar vt to cure, heal; vr to be cured, heal, get well

curativo -va adj curative

cureta f curette

curetaje m curettage

curita f (Amer) small adhesive bandage

curso m course

curva f curve, bend; — **de aprendizaje** learning curve; — **de crecimiento** growth curve

curvatura f curvature

cutáneo -a adj cutaneous

cutícula f cuticle

cutis m complexion, skin (of the face)

D

dacriocistitis f dacryocystitis

Dacron m Dacron; [Nota: los dos términos son marcas.]

daltoniano -na adj color-blind

daltonismo m color blindness

damiana f (bot) damiana

danazol m danazol

dañado -da adj damaged, impaired

dañar vt to damage, harm

dañino -na adj harmful

daño m damage, harm; — **cerebral** brain damage; **hacer** — to hurt, damage, harm; to be bad for (one), to make (one) sick; **La caída no le hizo ningún daño**..The fall didn't hurt him at all; **¿Le hace daño la medicina?**..Is the medicine making you sick?

dapsona f dapsone

dar vt to give; vi **dar(le) (a uno)** to catch, get; **Me dio un catarro**..I caught (got) a cold; — **a luz** to give birth to, deliver; **La señora Ruiz dio a luz a una niña ayer**..Mrs. Ruiz gave birth to a baby girl yesterday; — **de alta** to discharge (from the hospital); **Le dieron de alta ayer**..They discharged him yesterday; — **de comer** to feed; — **del cuerpo** (Carib) to have a bowel movement; — **de mamar** or — **el pecho** to breast-feed, to nurse; **¿Le va a dar el pecho?**..Are you going to breast-feed him? — **un traspié** to trip; vr — **cuenta** to notice; — **vuelta** to turn; (voltearse) to turn over, roll over

dátil *m* date *(fruit)*

datos *mpl* data

daunorubicina *f* daunorubicin

DCI *abbr* **desfibrilador cardioversor implantable**. *See* **desfibrilador**.

DDT *See* **diclorodifeniltricloroetano**.

DEA *abbr* **desfibrilador externo automático**. *See* **desfibrilador**.

deambulación *(form)* *f* ambulation *(form)*

deambular *(form)* *vi* to ambulate *(form)*, to walk

debajo *adv* **por — de** below, lower than; **por debajo de 40**..below 40.. lower than 40...**por debajo de la rodilla**..below the knee

debido -da a, due to

débil *adj* weak

debilidad *f* weakness

debilitado -da *adj* debilitated, run-down

debilitamiento *m* weakening

debilitante *adj* debilitating

debilitar *vt* to weaken, make weak; *vr* to weaken, become weak

decaer *vi* to weaken, to get worse; to become depressed

decaído -da *adj* weak, run down; depressed

decaimiento *m* weakening, weakness; depression

decibel *m* *(Amer)* decibel

decibelio *m* *(Esp)* decibel

decidir *vt, vr* to decide

decilitro *m* deciliter

decisión *f* decision

declaración *f* **de — obligatoria** reportable

declarar *vt* to report

decúbito -ta *adj* *(form)* recumbent *(form)*, lying down; — **prono** *(form, inv)* prone, facedown

dedo *m* digit, (de la mano) finger; (del pie) toe; — **anular** ring finger; — **chico (del pie)** little toe; — **del corazón** middle finger; — **(del pie) en martillo** hammertoe; **dedos en palillo de tambor** clubbing, clubbed fingers; — **en resorte** trigger finger; — **gordo (del pie)** big toe;

— **índice** index finger, forefinger; — **medio** middle finger; — **meñique** little finger; — **pulgar** thumb

deducible *adj* deductible

defecación *f* *(form)* defecation *(form)*, bowel movement; — **dolorosa** painful bowel movement

defecar *vi* to defecate, to have a bowel movement

defecto *m* defect; — **congénito** congenital defect; — **del tubo neural** neural tube defect; — **de nacimiento** birth defect

defensa *f* defense

defensor -ra *mf* advocate; — **del paciente** patient advocate; — **del pueblo** ombudsman

deficiencia *f* deficiency, deficit

deficiente *adj* deficient

déficit *m* *(pl* **déficits***)* deficit

definitivo -va *adj* definitive

deforme *adj* deformed

deformidad *f* deformity, malformation

defunción *f* death

degeneración *f* degeneration; — **macular** macular degeneration

degenerar *vi* to degenerate

degenerativo -va *adj* degenerative

degradación *f* degradation

dehidroepiandrosterona (DHEA) *f* dehydroepiandrosterone (DHEA)

dejar *vi* — **de** to quit, stop, give up; **¿Cuándo dejó de comer?**..When did you quit eating?...**Debe dejar de fumar**..You should give up smoking.

déjà vu, déjà vu

delantal *m* apron; — **de plomo** lead apron

delavirdina *f* delavirdine

deleción *f* deletion

deletrear *vt* to spell

delgado -da *adj* thin, lean

delicado -da *adj* frail, fagile

delirante *adj* delirious

delirar *vi* to be delirious; **Está delirando**..He is delirious.

delirio *m* delirium; delusion; — **de grandeza** delusions of grandeur

delirium tremens *m* delirium tremens, the d.t.'s *(fam)*

delta *f* delta

deltoides *m* (*pl* **-des**) deltoid
demacrado -da *adj* emaciated
demanda (legal) *f* lawsuit; **presentar una — (contra)** to sue
demandar *vt* (*legal*) to sue
demás *adj* rest of the; **las demás lesiones**..the rest of the lesions
demencia *f* dementia; **— multiinfarto** multi-infarct dementia; **— tipo Alzheimer** Alzheimer's dementia; **— vascular** vascular dementia
demostrar *vt* to demonstrate
dengue *m* dengue
densidad *f* density; (*espesor*) thickness, consistency; **— mineral ósea** bone mineral density
denso -sa *adj* dense
dentadura *f* teeth, set of teeth; **— postiza** denture, false teeth (*fam*)
dental *adj* dental
dentario -ria *adj* dental
dentición *f* (*form*) teething
dentífrico *m* toothpaste
dentina *f* dentin
dentista *mf* dentist
dentro *adv* inside; **dentro de su boca**..inside your mouth
departamento *m* department; **Departamento de Salud Pública** Public Health Department; **Departamento de Vehículos Motorizados,** Department of Motor Vehicles (DMV)
dependencia *f* dependency, dependence; **— de sustancias** chemical dependency; **No quiero crear dependencia**..I don't want to become dependent.
dependiente *adj* dependent
depilatorio *m* depilatory, hair remover (*fam*)
deponer *vt, vi* (*pp* **depuesto**) (*Mex, fam*) to vomit, to throw up (*fam*)
deporte *m* sport; **— de contacto** contact sport; **hacer —** to play sports
deportista *mf* athlete, person who plays sports
deposición *f* (*Esp, SA*) bowel movement
depositar *vt* to deposit
depósito *m* deposit, buildup; **de —** (*pharm*) depot; **— de cadáveres** morgue
depresión *f* depression; **— posparto**

postpartum depression
depresivo -va *adj* depressive
depresor -ra *adj* (*pharm, physio*) depressant; *m* depressant; **— de lengua, — lingual** (*Esp*) tongue depressor *o* blade
deprimido -da *adj* depressed, despondent
deprimirse *vr* to get *o* become depressed
depuesto *pp of* **deponer**
depuración *f* purification
depurado -da *adj* purified
depurador *m* purifier
depurar *vt* to purify
derecho -cha *adj* right; (*recto*) straight; *m* right (*legal, moral*); *f* right, right-hand side
derivación *f* (*surg*) shunt, bypass, diversion; **— cardiopulmonar** cardiopulmonary bypass; **— gástrica** gastric bypass; **— portocava** portacaval shunt; **— portosistémica percutánea intrahepática** transjugular intrahepatic portosystemic shunt (TIPS); **— urinaria** urinary diversion; **— ventriculoperitoneal** ventriculoperitoneal shunt
derivado *m* derivative; **derivados del petróleo** petroleum derivatives; **— proteico purificado** purified protein derivative (PPD)
dermatitis *f* dermatitis; **— atópica** atopic dermatitis; **— del pañal** diaper rash; **— herpetiforme** dermatitis herpetiformis; **— irritativa** irritant dermatitis; **— por cercarias** cercarial dermatitis, swimmer's itch (*fam*); **— por contacto** contact dermatitis; **— por estasis** stasis dermatitis; **— seborreica** seborrheic dermatitis
dermatofibroma *m* dermatofibroma
dermatofito *m* dermatophyte
dermatofitosis *f* dermatophytosis
dermatología *f* dermatology
dermatológico -ca *adj* dermatological, dermatologic
dermatólogo -ga *mf* dermatologist
dermatomiositis *f* dermatomyositis
dérmico -ca *adj* pertaining to the skin
dermoabrasión *f* dermabrasion, peel-

ing
dermografismo *m* dermographism
derrame *m* effusion; (*hemorragia*) hemorrhage, bleed; (*fam, ictus*) stroke; — **cerebral** cerebral hemorrhage, hemorrhagic stroke; — **pericárdico** pericardial effusion; — **pleural** pleural effusion
DES *See* **dietilestilbestrol**.
desabotonar *vt* to unbutton
desabrochar *vt, vr* to unbutton
desafío *m* challenge
desagradable *adj* unpleasant
desahogo *m* (*psych*) unburdening, outlet
desahuciado -da *adj* terminal, hopeless, without possibility of being cured
desalentado -da *adj* discouraged
desanimado -da *adj* discouraged
desaparecer(se) *vi* to disappear
desarrollar *vt* to develop; *vr* to develop, to evolve
desarrollo *m* development; — **físico**, — **sexual, etc.** physical development, sexual development, etc.
desastre *m* disaster
desatender *vt* to neglect
desayunar *vi, vr* to have breakfast
desayuno *m* breakfast
desbridamiento *m* debridement
desbridar *vt* to debride
descafeinado -da *adj* decaffeinated
descalzo -za *adj* barefoot
descamación *f* (*derm, form*) peeling, scaling
descamarse *vr* (*derm, form*) to peel, flake
descansar *vt, vi* to rest
descanso *m* rest, relaxation
descarga eléctrica *f* electric shock
descartable *adj* disposable
descartar *vt* to rule out; **Tenemos que descartar el cáncer**..We need to rule out cancer.
descendente *adj* descending
descendiente *mf* descendant
descenso *m* fall, decline
descompresión *f* decompression
descongestionante *adj & m* decongestant
descongestivo -va *adj & m* decongestant

descontaminar *vt* to decontaminate
descontento -ta *adj* unhappy
descontinuar *vt* to discontinue
describir *vt* to describe
descubierto -ta *adj* uncovered, bare
descuidado -da *adj* careless
descuidar *vt* to neglect
descuido *m* neglect, carelessness
desde *adv* since; **desde que empezó a vomitar**..since you began vomiting; *prep* since; **desde la niñez**.. since childhood
desear *vt* to desire
desechable *adj* disposable
desecho *m* (*frec. pl*) waste; (*secreción*) discharge; **desechos metabólicos** metabolic wastes; **desechos peligrosos** hazardous wastes
desempeño *m* performance
desencadenar *vt* to trigger
desenlace *m* outcome
desensibilización *f* desensitization
desensibilizar *vt* to desensitize
deseo *m* desire; — **sexual** sexual desire, libido
desequilibrio *m* imbalance
desesperación *f* desperation, despair
desesperado -da *adj* hopeless, desperate
desesperarse *vr* to lose hope; to become desperate
desfavorable *adj* unfavorable
desfibrilación *f* defibrillation
desfibrilador *m* defibrillator; — **cardioversor (automático) implantable (DCI)** (automatic) implantable cardioverter defibrillator (ICD); — **externo automático (DEA)** automated external defibrillator (AED)
desfibrilar *vt* to defibrillate
desgarrar *vt* to tear, to lacerate; (*fam, expectorar*) to cough up
desgarre *m* (*Amer, fam*) *See* **desgarro**.
desgarro *m* laceration, tear; (*muscular*) torn muscle, pulled muscle, muscle pull
desgaste *m* wasting; — **muscular** muscle wasting; — **profesional** burnout
desguanzado -da *adj* (*Mex, fam*) tired, run-down

deshabituación *f* cessation; — **tabáquica** smoking cessation
deshidratación *f* dehydration
deshidratado -da *adj* dehydrated
deshidrogenasa láctica *f* lactic dehydrogenase
deshumanizador -ra *adj* dehumanizing
deshumanizante *adj* dehumanizing
deshumedecer *vt* to dehumidify
deshumidificador *m* dehumidifier
desigual *adj* unequal
desinfectante *adj & m* disinfectant
desinfectar *vt* to disinfect
desintoxicación *f* detoxification
desloratadina *f* desloratadine
desmayarse *vr* to faint, pass out, to black out
desmayo *m* faint, blackout
desmielinizante *adj* demyelinating
desmoralizar *vt* to demoralize; *vr* to become demoralized
desnaturalizado -da *adj* denatured
desnudo -da *adj* naked, bare
desnutrición *f* malnutrition
desnutrido -da *adj* malnourished, undernourished
desodorante *m* deodorant
desogestrel *m* desogestrel
desorden *m* disorder
desorientado -da *adj* disoriented
despellejarse *vr* (*fam*) to peel
despersonalización *f* (*psych*) depersonalization
despertar *vt* (*pp* **-tado** *or* **-pierto**) to wake up, rouse; *vr* to wake up
despierto -ta (*pp of* **despertar**) *adj* awake
despigmentación *f* depigmentation
despistaje *m* screening
desplazado -da *adj* displaced
desprenderse *vr* to slough (off)
desprendido -da *adj* detached
desprendimiento *m* detachment; — **de retina** retinal detachment, detached retina
después *adv* after; — **de comer** after eating; *prep* — **de** after; **después de dos días**..after two days
desrealización *f* (*psych*) derealization
destetar *vt* to wean
destete *m* weaning
destilado -da *adj* distilled

destreza *f* skill
destructivo -va *adj* destructive
destruir *vt* to destroy
desvanecerse *vr* to faint
desvelarse *vr* (*Mex*) to go without sleep
desviación septal *f* septal deviation
desviado -da *adj* deviated
detección *f* detection, screening; **examen** *m* **de** — screening test, screen
detectable *adj* detectable
detectar *vt* to detect
detector de humo *m* smoke detector
detergente *adj & m* detergent
deteriorarse *vr* to deteriorate
deterioro *m* deterioration, decline
detrás de *prep* behind
devolver *vt, vi* (*pp* **devuelto**) (*fam*) to vomit, to throw up (*fam*)
dexametasona *f* dexamethasone
dextrometorfano *m* dextromethorphan
dextrosa *f* dextrose
DHEA *See* **dehidroepiandrosterona**.
día *m* day; **cada dos días** every other day; **el — anterior** the day before; **el — siguiente** the day after, the following day; **todos los días** every day
diabetes *f* diabetes; — **gestacional** gestational diabetes; — **insípida** diabetes insipidus; — **mellitus (tipo 1, tipo 2)** (type 1, type 2) diabetes mellitus
diabético -ca *adj & mf* diabetic
diabetológico -ca *adj* diabetic
diacepam *m* diazepam
diafragma *m* (*anat, gyn*) diaphragm
diagnosis *f* (*pl* **-sis**) diagnosis (*process*) (*See also* **diagnóstico**.)
diagnosticar *vt* to diagnose
diagnóstico -ca *adj* diagnostic; *m* diagnosis, testing; — **diferencial** differential diagnosis; — **genético** genetic testing; — **por imagen** diagnostic imaging
diagrama *m* diagram
diálisis *f* dialysis; — **peritoneal** peritoneal dialysis
dializar *vt* to dialyze
diámetro *m* diameter
diana *f* target; **órgano** — target or-

gan
diapasón *m* tuning fork
diariamente *adv* daily
diario -ria *adj* daily; *adv* **a** — daily, every day; *m* log
diarrhea *f* diarrhea; — **del viajero** traveler's diarrhea
diarreico -ca *adj* diarrheal
diastólico -ca *adj* diastolic
diatermia *f* diathermy
diazepam *m* diazepam
diclofenaco *m* diclofenac
diclorodifeniltricloroetano (DDT) *m* dichlorodiphenyltrichloroethane (DDT)
dicloxacilina *f* dicloxacillin
didanosina *f* didanosine
dieldrin *m* dieldrin
diente *m* tooth, front tooth; — **canino** cuspid, canine tooth; — **de conejo** (*fam*) bucktooth; — **definitivo** permanent tooth; — **de leche** primary tooth (*form*), baby tooth; — **impactado** impacted tooth, dental impaction; — **incisivo** incisor, front tooth; — **incluido** (*Esp*) impacted tooth, dental impaction; — **permanente** permanent tooth; **dientes postizos** false teeth; — **primario** primary tooth; — **retenido** impacted tooth, dental impaction; — **salido** bucktooth
diente de león *m* (*bot*) dandelion
diestro -tra *adj* right-handed
dieta *f* diet; — **baja en grasas** low-fat diet; — **balanceada** (*esp. Mex*) balanced diet; — **de adelgazamiento** (*esp. Esp*) weight loss diet; — **equilibrada** balanced diet; — **mediterránea** Mediterranean diet; — **para bajar de peso** weight loss diet; — **para diabéticos** diabetic diet; — **rica en fibra** high-fiber diet; **estar a** — to be on a diet, to diet
dietético -ca *adj* dietary, dietetic; *f* dietetics
dietilamida del ácido lisérgico (LSD) *f* lysergic acid diethylamide (LSD)
dietilestilbestrol (DES) *m* diethylstilbestrol (DES)
dietista *mf* dietitian *o* dietician

difenhidramina *f* diphenhydramine
difenilhidantoína *f* phenytoin
diferenciado -da *adj* differentiated; **bien** — well differentiated; **parcialmente** — partially differentiated; **pobremente** *or* **poco** — poorly differentiated
dificultad *f* difficulty; — **para recordar** difficulty remembering, forgetfulness; — **para respirar** difficulty breathing, shortness of breath
difteria *f* diphtheria
difunto -ta *adj* & *mf* deceased
difusión *f* diffusion
difuso -sa *adj* diffuse
digerible *adj* digestible
digerir *vt* to digest
digestible *adj* digestible
digestión *f* digestion
digestivo -va *adj* digestive
digital *adj* digital; *f* (*pharm*) digitalis
dignidad *f* dignity
digoxina *f* digoxin
dilatación *f* dilation, enlargement; — **y curetaje** *or* — **y legrado** dilation and curettage (D&C)
dilatador *m* dilator
dilatar *vt, vr* to dilate, to expand
diloxanida *f* diloxanide
diltiazem *m* diltiazem
dilución *f* dilution
dilucional *adj* dilutional
diluido -da *adj* dilute
diluir *vt* to dilute
dimensión *f* dimension
dimetil sulfóxido *m* dimethyl sulfoxide (DMSO)
dimetiltriptamina (DMT) *f* dimethyltryptamine (DMT)
dimorfa *adj* (*lepra*) borderline
dióxido *m* dioxide; — **de azufre** sulfur dioxide; — **de carbono** carbon dioxide
dioxina *f* dioxin
diplococo *m* diplococcus
dirección *f* direction; (*domicilio*) address
discapacidad *f* disability; — **física** physical disability; — **intelectual** cognitive disability
discapacitado -da *adj* disabled; — **físico** physically disabled; *mf* dis-

abled person

discapacitante *adj* disabling

discectomía *f* discectomy

discinesia tardía *f* tardive dyskinesia

disciplina *f* discipline

disciplinar *vt* to discipline

disco *m* disc; — **intervertebral** intervertebral disc; — **óptico** optic disc; **hernia de** — herniated disc

discografía *f* discography

discoide *adj* discoid

discrasia *f* dyscrasia

disección *f* dissection; — **aórtica** aortic dissection

diseminación *f* dissemination, spread

diseminado -da *adj* disseminated

diseminar *vt* to spread; *vr* to disseminate, spread, (*cáncer*) to metastasize

disentería *f* dysentery

disfasia *f* dysphasia

disfunción *f* dysfunction; — **eréctil** erectile dysfunction; — **temporomandibular** temporomandibular joint dysfunction

disfuncional *adj* dysfunctional; **familia** — dysfunctional family; **hemorragia uterina** — dysfunctional uterine bleeding

dislexia *f* dyslexia

dislocación *f* dislocation

dislocar *vt* to dislocate; *vr* to become dislocated

disminución *f* reduction, decrease, drop (*in level of something being measured*)

disminuir *vt* to reduce, decrease; *vi, vr* to diminish, decrease

disociación *f* dissociation

disolvente *m* solvent

disolver *vt, vr* (*pp* **disuelto**) to dissolve

disopiramida *f* disopyramide

dispensar *vt* (*pharm*) to dispense

dispepsia *f* dyspepsia

displasia *f* dysplasia

displásico -ca *adj* dysplastic

disponible *adj* available

dispositivo *m* device; — **intrauterino (DIU)** intrauterine device (IUD)

distal *adj* distal

distender *vt* to distend; *vi, vr* to become distended

distendido -da *adj* distended, (*estómago*) bloated

distensión *f* distention *o* dissension; — **abdominal** abdominal distention, bloating; — **muscular** pulled muscle, muscle pull

distinguir *vt* to distinguish

distraído -da *adj* absent-minded, spacey (*fam*), spaced out (*fam*)

distrés *m* distress; — **respiratorio** respiratory distress

distrito *m* district

distrofia *f* dystrophy; — **muscular** muscular dystrophe; — **simpática refleja** reflex sympathetic dystrophy

disuelto *pp of* **disolver**

disulfiram *m* disulfiram

DIU *abbr* dispositivo intrauterino. *See* **dispositivo**.

diuresis *f* diuresis

diurético -ca *adj* diuretic; *m* diuretic, water pill (*fam*)

diverticulitis *f* diverticulitis

divertículo *m* diverticulum; — **de Meckel** Meckel's diverticulum

diverticulosis *f* diverticulosis

dividir *vt* to divide

divieso *m* (*esp. Esp*) abscess, boil

divorciarse *vr* to divorce

divorcio *m* divorce

DMT *See* **dimetiltriptamina**.

doblar *vt* to bend, flex; to double; **Doble el brazo**..Bend your arm; *vr* to bend, bend over, bend down; (*torcerse*) to sprain, twist; **Dóblese** ..Bend over...**Me doblé el tobillo**..I sprained my ankle.

doble *adj* double; **visión** — double vision; *adv* double; **ver** — to see double

doctor -ra *mf* doctor, physician

dolencia *f* ache, pain, ailment

doler *vt, vi* to hurt; **¿Le duele?**..Does it hurt?...**¿Le duele el pie?**..Does your foot hurt?...**¿Dónde le duele?** ..Where does it hurt?

dolor *m* pain, ache; — **de barriga** bellyache, stomachache; — **de caballo** (*Mex, fam*) sideache; — **de cabeza** headache; — **de dientes** toothache; — **de espalda** backache; — **de estómago** stomachache; — **de garganta** sore throat; — **de la espalda baja** low back pain; — **del parto** labor pain; — **de muelas** toothache; — **de oído(s)** earache; — **fantasma** phantom pain; — **lumbar** (*form*) low back pain; — **menstrual** menstrual cramp; **sin** — painless

dolorido -da *adj* sore, tender, painful

doloroso -sa *adj* painful; **muerte** — painful death

domiciliario -ria *adj* home, at home; **fisioterapia** — home physical therapy, physical therapy at home

domicilio *m* home; (*dirección*) address

dominante *adj* dominant; **mano** — dominant hand

donación *f* donation; — **de órganos** organ donation; — **de sangre** blood donation

donante *mf* donor; — **universal** universal donor; — **vivo** living donor; **semen** *m* **de** — donor semen

donar *vt* to donate

dopaje *m* doping

dopamina *f* dopamine

Doppler *m* Doppler (*imaging study*)

dormido -da *adj* asleep; (*adormecido*) numb, asleep; **Tengo dormido el brazo**..My arm is numb..My arm is asleep; **quedarse** — to fall asleep, to go to sleep

dormir *vt* (*a un niño, etc.*) to put to sleep; (*anestesiar*) to anesthetize (*form*), (*local*) to numb (up), (*general*) to put to sleep; **¿Me van a dormir el pie?**..Are you going to numb up my foot? *vi* to sleep; *vr* to go to sleep, to fall asleep; (*adormecerse*) to become numb, to go to sleep, to fall asleep; **Se me duerme el brazo**..My arm gets numb (goes to sleep, falls asleep).

dormitar *vi* to doze

dormitorio *m* bedroom

dorsal *adj* dorsal

dorso *m* (*de la mano*) back (*of the hand*)

dos *m* **hacer del** — (*euph, defecar*) to defecate (*form*), to have a bowel movement, to do number two (*euph*)

dosificación *f* dosage, dosing

dosificador *m* dispenser

dosis *f* (*pl* **dosis**) dose, dosage; **a altas dosis** high-dose; **a bajas dosis** low-dose

doxazocina *f* doxazocin

doxepina *f* doxepin

doxiciclina *f* doxycycline

doxorubicina *f* doxorubicin

drenaje *m* drainage (*material drained*)

drenar *vt* to drain

drepanocitosis *f* sickle cell anemia *o* disease

droga *f* drug; — **blanda** soft drug; — **de diseño** designer drug; — **del amor** (*fam*) methylene dioxyamphetamine (MDA); — **dura** hard drug

drogadicción *f* drug addiction

drogadicto -ta *mf* drug abuser, drug addict

drogado -da *adj* drugged, high (*fam*)

drogar *vt* to drug; *vr* to take drugs, to get high (*fam*)

drogodependencia *f* chemical dependency, dependency on drugs

ducha *f* shower; (*vaginal*) douche; **tomar una** — to take a shower

ducharse *vr* to take a shower, to shower

ductal *adj* ductal

duela *f* (*trematodo*) fluke

duelo *m* (*pena*) grief

dulce *adj* sweet; *m* piece of candy; *mpl* candy, sweets

duloxetina *f* duloxetine

duodenal *adj* duodenal

duodenitis *f* duodenitis

duodeno *m* duodenum

duración *f* duration

duradero -ra *adj* durable

durar *vi* to last; **El dolor me duró toda la noche**..The pain lasted all night.

duro -ra *adj* hard, tough; stiff; **Se me puso duro el brazo**..My arm got stiff; — **de oído** hard of hearing

E

eccema *m* eczema
ECG *See* **electrocardiograma.**
echar *vt* — **de menos** to miss; ¿**Echa de menos a su hija?**..Do you miss your daughter? *vr* — **a perder** to spoil (*food, etc.*)
Echinacea (*bot*) Echinacea
eclampsia *f* eclampsia
ecocardiografía *f* (*técnica imagenológica*) echocardiography; (*estudio imagenológico*) echocardiogram; — **de esfuerzo** stress echocardiography; stress echocardiogram; — **transesofágica** transesophageal echocardiography; transesophageal echocardiogram; — **transtorácica** transthoracic echocardiography; transthoracic echocardiogram
ecocardiograma *m* echocardiogram
ectima *m* ecthyma; — **contagioso** orf
ectópico -ca *adj* ectopic
ectropión *f* ectropion, outward droop of the lower eyelid
eczema *See* **eccema.**
edad *f* age; **de** — **avanzada** elderly; — **fértil** child-bearing age; — **gestacional** gestational age; — **ósea** bone age; **mediana** — middle age; **tercera** — old age
edema *m* edema; — **pulmonar** pulmonary edema
educación *f* education; — **sexual** sex education
educar *vt* to educate
edulcorante *m* sweetener; — **artificial** artificial sweetener
EEG *See* **electroencefalograma.**
efavirenz, efavirenzo (*OMS*) *m* efavirenz
efectividad *f* effectiveness
efectivo -va *adj* effective
efecto *m* effect; — **adverso** adverse effect; — **secundario** side effect; **hacer** *or* **surtir** — to take effect, to have an effect; **No me hizo ningún efecto**..It didn't have any effect (on me).

efedra *f* (*bot*) ephedra
efedrina *f* ephedrine
eficacia *f* efficacy, effectiveness
eficaz *adj* effective
eficiente *adj* efficient
ego *m* ego (*lay sense*)
egocéntrico -ca *adj* egocentric, self-centered
egoísmo *m* egoism
egoísta *adj* egoistic; *mf* egoist
egotismo *m* egotism
egotista *adj* egotistic; *mf* egotist
eje *m* axis
ejercer *vt, vi* (*la medicina*) to practice (*medicine*)
ejercicio *m* exercise; **ejercicios aeróbicos (de bajo impacto)** (low impact) aerobics; **ejercicios de Kegel** Kegel exercises; **hacer** — to exercise
elástico -ca *adj* elastic
eléboro *m* (*bot*) hellebore
elección *f* choice; **medicamento de** — drug of choice; **medicamento de primera (segunda, etc.)** — drug of first (second, etc.) choice
electivo -va *adj* (*surg*) elective
eléctrico -ca *adj* electric, electrical
electrocardiografía *f* electrocardiography
electrocardiograma (ECG) *m* electrocardiogram (ECG)
electrocución *f* electrocution
electrocutar *vt* to electrocute
electrodo *m* electrode
electroencefalograma (EEG) *m* electroencephalogram (EEG)
electroencefalografía *f* electroencephalography
electrofisiología *f* electrophysiology
electrofisiológico -ca *adj* electrophysiological, electrophysio-logic; **estudio** — electrophysiology study (EPS)
electroforesis *f* electrophoresis
electrolítico -ca *adj* pertaining to electrolytes; **desequilibrio** — elec-

trolyte imbalance
electrolito, electrólito *m* electrolyte
electromiografía (EMG) *f* electromyography (EMG)
elefantiasis *f* elephantiasis
elegible *adj* eligible
elemento *m* element
eletriptán *m* eletriptan
elevación *f* elevation, rise; — **de la
escápula** winged scapula
elevar *vt* to elevate, raise; *vi, vr* to
rise
eliminación *f* elimination, removal
eliminar *vt* to eliminate, to pass
elixir, elíxir *m* elixir
ello *m* (*psych*) id
emascular *vt* to emasculate
embarazada *adj* pregnant; **quedarse
—** (*esp. Esp*) to get *o* become pregnant
embarazarse *vr* to get *o* become
pregnant
embarazo *m* pregnancy; **Tengo cuatro meses de embarazo**..I'm four
months pregnant; — **ectópico** ectopic pregnancy; — **tubárico** tubal
pregnancy
embolectomía *f* embolectomy
embolia *f* embolism, (*fam*) stroke; —
cerebral cerebral embolism, embolic stroke; — **pulmonar** pulmonary embolism
embolización *f* embolization; — **de
las arterias uterinas** uterine artery
embolization
émbolo *m* embolus; (*de una jeringa*)
plunger (*of a syringe*)
emborracharse *vr* to get drunk
embriagarse *vr* to get drunk
embriaguez *f* drunkenness
embriología *f* embryology
embrión *m* embryo
emergencia *f* emergency
emergente *adj* emerging; **enfermedad —** emerging disease
emesis *f* emesis
emético -ca *adj & m* emetic
EMG *See* **electromiografía**.
emoción *f* emotion, feeling
emocional *adj* emotional
emoliente *adj & m* emollient
emotivo -va *adj* emotional (*said of a
person*)

empacho *m* (*fam*) indigestion, (*Mex*)
folk illness manifest by abdominal
bloating and other gastrointestinal
complaints believed to be due to
food obstructing the intestine
empañado -da *adj* blurred; **vista —**
blurred vision
empañarse *vr* (*la vista*) to blur, to
become blurred *o* blurry; **Me em-
paña la vista**..My vision blurs..My
vision gets blurred (blurry).
emparentado -da *adj* related; **donante no —** unrelated donor
empastar *vt* (*dent*) to fill (*a cavity*)
empaste *m* (*dent*) filling
empatía *f* empathy
empeine *m* instep, top of foot; (*ingle*)
pubic area; (*tiña*) ringworm
empendible *m* (*PR*) safety pin
empeoramiento *m* worsening, deterioration
empeorar *vt* to make worse; *vi* to get
worse, deteriorate
empezar *vt, vi* to begin
empiema *m* empyema
emplasto *m* (medicinal) plaster
empleador -ra *mf* employer
emplear *vt* to employ; (*utilizar*) to
employ, use
empleo *m* employment, occupation,
job; (*uso*) use
emtricitabina *f* emtricitabine
enalapril *m* enalapril
enamorado -da *adj* — **de** in love
with; *m* boyfriend; *f* girlfriend
enamorarse *vr* — **de** to fall in love
with
enanismo *m* dwarfism
enano -na *mf* dwarf, little person
(*euph*); *mfpl* little people (*euph*)
encajado -da *adj* (*uña, etc.*) ingrown
encamado -da *adj* bedridden, in bed,
in a bed
encarnado -da *adj* (*uña, etc.*) ingrown
encefalitis *f* encephalitis
encefalomielitis *f* encephalomyelitis
encefalopatía *f* encephalopathy; —
de Wernicke Wernicke's encephalopathy; — **espongiforme bovina**
bovine spongiform encephalopathy,
mad cow disease (*fam*)
enchufe *m* electrical outlet

encía f gingiva (form), gum
encima adv above; — de above; encima de su corazón..above your heart; por — de above, over; por encima de 140..above 140..over 140
encinta adj (fam) pregnant
encogerse vr — de hombros to shrug one's shoulders
encorvado -da adj stooped, bent over
encorvamiento m curvature (of the spine)
encorvarse vr to become stooped (as with age); to stoop, bend over; to slouch
endarterectomía f endarterectomy; — carotídea carotid endarterectomy
endémico -ca adj endemic
enderezar vt, vi, vr to straighten
endocardio m endocardium
endocarditis f endocarditis; — infecciosa infectious endocarditis
endocervical adj endocervical
endocérvix m endocervix
endocraneal adj intracranial
endocrino -na adj endocrine
endocrinología f endocrinology
endocrinólogo -ga mf endocrinologist
endodoncia f root canal therapy, root canal (fam)
endometrio m endometrium
endometriosis f endometriosis
endometritis f endometritis
endorfina f endorphin
endoscopia, endoscopía (Amer, esp. spoken) f endoscopy; — digestiva alta esophagogastroduodenoscopy (EGD), upper endoscopy
endoscópico -ca adj endoscopic
endoscopio m endoscope
endotraqueal adj endotracheal
endovenoso -sa adj intravenous (IV)
endurecer vt to harden, make hard; vr to harden, become hard
endurecimiento m hardening
enema m enema; — de bario barium enema; — de retención retention enema; — opaco (Esp) barium enema
energía f energy
ENET abbr estimulación nerviosa

eléctrica transcutánea. See estimulación.
enfadarse vr (esp. Esp) to get o become angry, to get mad
enfermarse vr to become ill, to get sick
enfermedad f disease, sickness, illness; — actual present illness; — cardíaca heart disease; — celíaca celiac disease; — coronaria coronary artery disease; — de Addison Addison's disease; — de Alzheimer Alzheimer's disease; — de células falciformes sickle cell disease; — de Chagas Chagas' disease; — de Crohn Crohn's disease, regional enteritis; — de Cushing Cushing's disease; — de Gaucher Gaucher's disease; — de Graves Graves' disease; — de Hansen Hansen's disease, leprosy; — de Hirschsprung Hirschsprung's disease; — de Hodgkin Hodgkin's disease; — de Huntington Huntington's disease; — de Kawasaki Kawasaki's disease; — de las vacas locas mad cow disease; — del corazón heart disease; — del hígado liver disease; — del injerto contra el huésped graft-versus-host disease; — de los legionarios Legionnaire's disease; — del sueño sleeping sickness; — del suero serum sickness; — del tejido conectivo or conjuntivo connective tissue disease; — de Lyme Lyme disease; — de manos, pies y boca hand-foot-and-mouth disease; — de membrana hialina hyaline membrane disease; — de Ménière Ménière's syndrome; — de neurona motora motor neuron disease; — de Osgood-Schlatter Osgood-Schlatter disease; — de Paget Paget's disease; — de Parkinson Parkinson's disease; — de Raynaud Raynaud's disease; — de Rendu-Osler-Weber Rendu-Osler-Weber syndrome; — de transmisión sexual (ETS) sexually transmitted disease (STD); — de von Willebrand von Willebrand's disease; — de Whipple Whipple's disease; —

de Wilson Wilson's disease; — **diverticular** diverticular disease; — **fibroquística de la mama** fibrocystic disease of the breast; — **hepática** (*form*) liver disease; — **inflamatoria intestinal** inflammatory bowel disease; — **inflamatoria pélvica** pelvic inflammatory disease (PID); — **intersticial pulmonar** interstitial lung disease; — **laboral** occupational illness; — **mamaria benigna** benign breast disease; — **mental** mental illness; — **mixta del tejido conectivo** mixed connective tissue disease; — **ósea de Paget** Paget's disease of bone; — **por arañazo de gato** cat-scratch disease; — **por descompresión** decompression sickness, the bends (*fam*); — **por reflujo gastroesofágico (ERGE)** gastroesophageal reflux disease (GERD); — **profesional** occupational illness; — **pulmonar obstructiva crónica (EPOC)** chronic obstructive pulmonary disease (COPD); — **vascular periférica** peripheral vascular disease; — **venérea** sexually transmitted disease (STD), venereal disease (*ant*); **quinta** — fifth disease

enfermería *f* nursing; (*local para enfermos*) infirmary

enfermero -ra *mf* nurse; — **de turno** *or* **de cargo** charge nurse

enfermizo -za *adj* sickly

enfermo -ma *adj* sick, ill; *mf* sick person, patient

enfisema *m* emphysema

enflaquecer *vi* to become thin

enfocar *vt* to focus

enfrentar *vt* to confront, face

enfrente *adv* **de** — front; **la parte de enfrente de**..the front of

enfuvirtida *f* enfuvirtide

engordar *vi, vr* to get fat

engrosamiento *m* enlargement, thickening

enhorabuena (*Esp; obst, etc.*) *interj* Congratulations!

enjuagar *vt* to rinse, to swish; — **y escupir** swish and spit; — **y tragar** swish and swallow

enjuage *m* rinse; — **bucal** mouthwash

enjugar *vt* to wipe

enlace *m* (*obst, psych*) bond

enloquecerse *vr* to go crazy

enmascarar *vt* (*signos, síntomas*) to mask

enojado -da *adj* angry, mad

enojarse *vr* to become angry, to get mad

enojo *m* rage, anger

enriquecer *vt* to enrich, fortify

enrojecimiento *m* redness, flush, flushing

ensalada *f* salad

ensayo *m* trial; — **clínico** clinical trial; — **y error** trial and error

enseñar *vt* to teach; to show

ensimismado -da *adj* self-absorbed, lost in thought

ensordecimiento *m* hearing loss

ensuciar *vt* to soil, to get (something) dirty; *vi, vr* to soil oneself, to get dirty

entablillar *vt* to splint

enteral *adj* enteral

entérico -ca *adj* enteric; **con capa** — (*esp. Mex*) enteric-coated; **con cubierta** — enteric-coated

enteritis *f* enteritis; — **eosinofílica** eosinophilic enteritis; — **regional** regional enteritis, Crohn's disease

entero -ra *adj* whole

enterococo *m* enterococcus

enterocolitis *f* enterocolitis

enteropatía *f* enteropathy; — **perdedora de proteínas, — pierde-proteínas** (*Esp*) protein-losing enteropathy

enterotoxina *f* enterotoxin

enterrado -da *adj* (*uña, etc.*) ingrown

entornar los ojos, to squint, to squint one's eyes

entorno *m* environment (*immediate surroundings*); — **social** social environment

entrada *f* entry; **portal de** — portal of entry; *fpl* receding hairline

entre *prep* between; — **los dientes** between your teeth

entrecejo *m* space between one's eyebrows

entrecerrar los ojos, to squint

entrenamiento *m* training; — **para usar el baño** (*ped*) toilet training

entrenar *vt, vr* to train

entrepierna *f* (*frec. pl*) pubic area

entristecerse *vr* to become sad

entropión *m* entropion, inward droop of the lower eyelid

entuertos *mpl* postpartum cramps

entumecerse *vr* to become numb, to become numb and swollen

entumecido -da *adj* numb, numb and swollen

entumecimiento *m* numbness, numbness and swelling

entumido -da (*fam*) *See* **entumecido**.

enuresis *f* enuresis, bedwetting (*fam*)

envase *m* container

envejecer *vi* to grow old

envejecimiento *m* aging

envenenamiento *m* poisoning

envenenar *vt* to poison

envolver *vt* to wrap

enzima *m&f* enzyme; — **de conversión de la angiotensina** angiotensin converting enzyme

eosinofilia *f* eosinophilia

eosinófilo *m* eosinophil

epicondilitis *f* lateral epicondylitis, tennis elbow (*fam*)

epicóndilo *m* (*del codo*) lateral epicondyle (*of the elbow*)

epidemia *f* epidemic

epidémico -ca *adj* epidemic

epidemiología *f* epidemiology

epididimitis *f* epididymitis

epidídimo *m* epididymis

epidural *adj* epidural

epifisario -ria *adj* epiphyseal

epífisis *f* (*pl* -**sis**) epiphysis

epigástrico -ca *adj* epigastric

epiglotis *f* epiglottis

epiglotitis *f* epiglottitis

epilepsia *f* epilepsy

epiléptico -ca *adj & mf* epileptic

epinefrina *f* epinephrine

epiplón *m* omentum

episiotomía *f* episiotomy

episodio *m* episode

epispadias *m* epispadias

epitróclea *f* (*del codo*) medial epicondyle (*of the elbow*)

epitrocleítis *f* medial epicondylitis,

golfer's elbow (*fam*)

EPOC *abbr* **enfermedad pulmonar obstructiva crónica**. *See* **enfermedad**.

epoetina alfa *f* epoetin alfa

épulis *m* (*pl* -**lis**) epulis

equilibrado -da *adj* balanced

equilibrio *m* equilibrium, balance

equinococosis *f* echinococcosis

equipo *m* equipment; (*grupo*) team; — **de salud**, — **sanitario** (*esp. Esp*) health care team

equivalente *adj & m* equivalent

erección *f* erection

eréctil *adj* erectile

erecto -ta *adj* erect

ergocalciferol *m* ergocalciferol

ergometría *f* (*form*) (*técnica*) exercise stress testing, (*prueba*) exercise stress test

ergonomía *f* ergonomics

ergonómico -ca *adj* ergonomic

ergotamina *f* ergotamine

erisipela *f* erysipelas

eritema *m* erythema; — **crónico migratorio** erythema chronicum migrans; — **infeccioso** erythema infectiosum, fifth disease; — **marginado** erythema marginatum; — **multiforme** erythema multiforme; — **nodoso** *or* **nudoso** erythema nodosum

eritrocito *m* erythrocyte

eritromicina *f* erythromycin

eritropoyetina *f* erythropoetin, epoetin alfa

erizo de mar *m* sea urchin

erógeno -na *adj* erogenous

erosión *f* erosion

erosionar *vt, vr* to erode

erosivo -va *adj* erosive

erótico -ca *adj* erotic

erradicación *f* eradication

erradicar *vt* to eradicate

error *m* error; — **congénito del metabolismo** inborn error of metabolism; — **de laboratorio** laboratory error; — **de medicación** medication error

eructar *vi* to burp, belch; **hacer** — (*a un bebé*) to burp (*a baby*)

erupción *f* (*derm, form*) eruption, rash, outbreak; (*dent, form*) teething; — **fija (medicamentosa)** fixed drug eruption; — **polimorfa lumínica** polymorphous light eruption

escabiasis *f* (*esp. Mex, form*) scabies

escabiosis *f* (*form*) scabies

escala *f* scale (*of measurement*); — **del dolor** pain scale; — **móvil** sliding scale

escalada *f* rock climbing

escaldadura *f* scalding, scald

escaldar *vt* to scald; *vr* to scald oneself

escalofrío *m* chill

escalpelo *m* scalpel

escama *f* (*derm*) scale, flake

escamoso -sa *adj* (*form*) squamous; (*fam*) flaky, scaly

escán *m* (*Ang*) scan

escanear *vt* (*Ang*) to scan

escáner *m* (*Ang*) scanner

escápula *f* scapula

escara *f* (*form*) eschar (*form*), scab, crust

escarlatina *f* scarlatina (*form*), scarlet fever

escaso -sa *adj* scarce, (*el pelo*) thin

escayola *f* (*Esp, ortho*) plaster; cast

escisión *f* excision

escisional *adj* excisional

escitalopram *m* escitalopram

esclera *See* **esclerótica**.

escleritis *f* scleritis

esclerodermia *f* scleroderma; — **localizada** morphea

esclerosante *adj* sclerosing

esclerosis *f* sclerosis; — **en placas** multiple sclerosis; — **lateral amiotrófica** amyotrophic lateral sclerosis; — **múltiple** multiple sclerosis; — **sistémica progresiva** progressive systemic sclerosis; — **tuberosa** tuberous sclerosis

escleroterapia *f* sclerotherapy

esclerótica *f* sclera

escoliosis *f* scoliosis

escopolamina *f* scopolamine

escorbuto *m* scurvy

escorpión *m* (*esp. Esp*) scorpion

escozor *m* burning, smarting

escritura *f* handwriting

escrófula *f* scrofula

escrotal *adj* scrotal

escroto *m* scrotum

escuchar *vt* to listen to; *vi* to listen

escudo facial *m* face shield

escuela *f* school; — **de medicina** medical school

escupir *vt, vi* to spit

escurrimiento *m* (*esp. Mex*) drainage; **tener — nasal** to have a runny nose

escutelaria *f* (*bot*) skullcap

esencial *adj* essential

esferocitosis *f* spherocytosis; — **hereditaria** hereditary spherocytosis

esfigmomanómetro *m* blood pressure monitor

esfínter *m* sphincter

esfinterotomía *f* sphincterotomy

esforzarse *vr* to exert oneself, to strain oneself; — **demasiado** to overexert oneself

esfuerzo *m* effort, exertion; — **físico** physical exertion

esguince *m* (*form*) sprain

esmalte *m* enamel; — **para uñas,** — **de uñas** (*Esp*) nail polish

esmegma *m* smegma

esnifar *vt* (*Esp, fam*) to sniff, snort (*cocaine, glue, etc.*)

esofágico -ca *adj* esophageal

esofagitis *f* esophagitis; — **erosiva** erosive esophagitis; — **por reflujo** reflux esophagitis

esófago *m* esophagus; — **de Barrett** Barrett's esophagus

esomeprazol *m* esomeprazole

espaciador *m* spacer

espacio *m* space, gap

espalda *f* back; — **baja** low back

esparadrapo *m* (*esp. Esp*) adhesive tape

esparfloxacina *f* (*esp. Amer*) sparfloxacin

esparfloxacino *m* sparfloxacin

espárrago *m* asparagus

espasmo *m* spasm

espasmódico -ca *adj* spasmodic

espasticidad *f* spasticity

espástico -ca *adj* spastic

especia *f* spice

especialidad *f* specialty

especialista *mf* specialist; — **del pulmón,** — **del riñón, etc.** lung specialist, kidney specialist, etc.; — **en alergias,** — **en enfermedades in-**

fecciosas, etc. specialist in allergies, specialist in infectious diseases, etc.

especie f species

específico -ca adj specific; **un análisis específico para..** a laboratory test specific for

espécimen m (pl **-címenes**) specimen

espectinomicina f spectinomycin

espectro m spectrum

espéculo m speculum

espejo m mirror

espejuelos mpl (esp. Carib) glasses, eyeglasses

esperando adj (fam, embarazada) pregnant, expecting (fam)

esperanza f hope; **— de vida** life expectancy; **perder la —** to lose hope; **sin —** hopeless; **tener esperanzas de** to hope for

esperar vt (desear) to hope for; (aguardar) to wait for; (contar con) to expect; vi to hope; to wait

esperma m sperm, semen

espermaticida adj spermicidal; m spermicide

espermatocele m spermatocele

espermatozoide m sperm, spermatozoon

espermicida adj spermicidal; m spermicide

espeso -sa adj thick

espesor m thickness

espina f spine, thorn, sticker; (de un pescado) bone, fishbone; **— bífida** spina bifida; **— dorsal** spinal column, spine, backbone

espinaca f (frec. pl) spinach

espinal adj spinal

espinilla f (anat) shin; (derm) blackhead, pimple

espinillera f shin guard

espino m (bot) hawthorn

espiración f expiration (breathing out)

espirar vt, vi to expire, exhale

espiratorio -ria adj expiratory

espirometría f spirometry; **— incentivada** incentive spirometry

espirómetro m spirometer

espironolactona f spironolactone

espiroqueta f spirochete

esplenectomía f splenectomy

esplénico -ca adj splenic

espolón m (ortho) spur, bone spur

espondilitis anquilosante f ankylosing spondylitis

espondilolistesis f spondylolysthesis

espondilosis f spondylosis

esponja f sponge

espontáneo -a adj spontaneous

espora f spore

esporádico -ca adj sporadic

esporotricosis f sporotrichosis

esposo -sa mf spouse; m husband; f wife

esprue m&f sprue; **— celiaco** or **no tropical** celiac o nontropical sprue; **— tropical** tropical sprue

espuma f foam

espundia f mucocutaneous leishmaniasis

esputo m sputum

esquelético -ca adj skeletal

esqueleto m skeleton

esquema f (de vacunación, etc.) schedule; **— corporal** body image

esquí m skiing

esquirla f sliver, shaving

esquistosomiasis f schistosomiasis

esquizoafectivo -va adj schizoaffective

esquizofrenia f schizophrenia; **— paranoide** paranoid schizophrenia

esquizofrénico -ca adj & mf schizophrenic

esquizoide adj schizoid

estabilidad f stability

estabilización f stabilization

estabilizador m stabilizer; **— del ánimo** or **humor** mood stabilizer

estabilizar vt, vr to stabilize

estable adj stable

estación f station; (del año) season; **— de enfermería** nursing station

estacional adj seasonal

estadía f (esp. SA) stay; **— hospitalaria** hospital stay

estadificación f (de tumores) staging

estadio, estadío m stage (disease, cancer, puberty)

estadística f (dato) statistic; (ciencia) statistics

estado m status, state, condition, shape; **en buen — físico** in shape, fit; **— asmático** status asthmaticus;

— **crítico** critical condition; — **de ánimo** mood; — **de hipercoagulabilidad** hypercoagulable state; — **del arte** state of the art; — **epiléptico** status epilepticus; — **mental** mental state; — **vegetativo** vegetative state

estafilococo *m* Staphylococcus

estancarse *vr* (*la sangre*) to pool

estancia *f* stay; — **hospitalaria** hospital stay

estándar *adj & m* standard

estapedectomía *f* stapedectomy

estasis *m&f* stasis; — **venosa,** — **venoso** (*esp. Esp*) venous stasis

estatina *f* statin

estatura *f* height (*of a person*)

estavudina *f* stavudine

estenosis *f* (*pl* -**sis**) stenosis, stricture; — **aórtica,** — **mitral, etc.** aortic stenosis, mitral stenosis, etc.

estenótico -ca *adj* stenotic

estereotipia *f* stereotypy

estéril *adj* sterile; (*obst*) sterile, infertile

esterilidad *f* sterility; (*obst*) sterility, infertility

esterilización *f* sterilization

esterilizar *vt* to sterilize

esternal *adj* sternal

esternón *m* sternum, breastbone (*fam*)

esteroide *m* steroid; **esteroides inhalados** inhaled steroids

esteroideo -a *adj* steroid

esteticista *mf* cosmetologist

estético -ca *adj* esthetic

estetoscopio *m* stethoscope

estibogluconato, estibamina glucósido (*OMS*) *m* stibogluconate, stibamine glucoside (*OMS*)

estilo de vida *m* lifestyle

estimulación *f* stimulation; — **digital** digital stimulation; — **nerviosa eléctrica transcutánea (ENET)** transcutaneous electrical nerve stimulation (TENS)

estimulante *adj* stimulating, stimulant; *m* stimulant

estimular *vt* to stimulate

estímulo *m* stimulus

estiramiento *m* stretching; **ejercicios de** — stretching exercises; — **facial** face-lift

estirar *vt, vr* to stretch

estirón *m* (*crecimiento rápido*) growth spurt

estirpe *f* lineage; — **mieloide,** — **B, etc.** myeloid lineage, B lineage, etc.

estítico -ca *adj* (*esp. CA*) constipated

estoma *m* stoma

estomacal *adj* pertaining to the stomach; **acidez** — acid stomach (*fam*), heartburn

estómago *m* stomach; (*fam*) abdomen, belly; **ácido del** — stomach acid; **boca del** — pit of the stomach; **dolor** *m* **de** — stomachache

estomaguito *m* (*ped*) tummy

estomatitis *f* stomatitis

estornudar *vi* to sneeze

estornudo *m* sneeze

estrabismo *m* strabismus

estradiol *m* estradiol

estrangulación *f* strangulation

estrangulado -da *adj* strangulated

estrangular *vt, vr* to strangle, choke

estrechez *f* stricture, narrowing

estrecho -cha *adj* narrow

estreñimiento *m* constipation

estreñir *vt* to constipate; *vr* to become constipated

estreptococo *m* Streptococcus

estreptomicina *f* streptomycin

estreptoquinasa, estreptocinasa *f* streptokinase

estrés *m* (*pl* **estreses**) stress; **bajo** — under stress; — **laboral** *or* **del trabajo** job stress

estresado -da *adj* stressed

estresante *adj* stressful

estresar *vt* to stress, to put stress on; *vr* to stress out

estresor *m* stressor

estría *f* stretch mark

estribo *m* (*anat, gyn, etc.*) stirrup

estricnina *f* strychnine

estricto -ta *adj* strict

estriol *m* estriol

estrógeno *m* estrogen; **estrógenos conjugados** conjugated estrogens

estrongiloidiasis *f* strongyloidiasis

estructural *adj* structural

estudiante *mf* student; — **de medicina** medical student

estudio *m* study; — **del sueño** sleep

study; — **doble ciego** double-blind study; — **por imagen** imaging study

estupor *m* stupor
eszopiclona *f* eszopiclone
etambutol *m* ethambutol
etanercept *m* etanercept
etanol *m* ethanol, ethyl alcohol
etapa *f* stage (*disease, sleep*)
éter *m* ether
ético -ca *adj* ethical
etilenglicol *m* ethylene glycol
etinilestradiol *m* ethinylestradiol
etionamida *f* ethionamide
etiqueta *f* label
etmoidal *adj* ethmoid
étnico -ca *adj* ethnic
etosuximida *f* ethosuximide
etretinato *m* etretinate
ETS *abbr* **enfermedad de transmisión sexual.** *See* **enfermedad.**
eucalipto *m* (*bot*) eucalyptus
euforia *f* euphoria
eufrasia *f* (*bot*) eyebright
eunuco *m* eunuch
eutanasia *f* euthanasia, mercy killing
evacuación *f* evacuation; (*del intestino*) bowel movement; — **dolorosa** painful bowel movement
evacuar *vt* to evacuate; (*el intestino*) to have a bowel movement
evaluación *f* evaluation, assessment, testing; — **urodinámica** urodynamic testing
evaluar *vt* to evaluate
evaporación *f* evaporation
evaporarse *vr* to evaporate
eventración *f* incisional hernia
evidencia *f* evidence; **basado en la** — evidence-based; — **científica** scientific evidence
evitación *f* avoidance
evitar *vt* to avoid, prevent; **Evite comer comidas grasosas.**.Avoid eating fatty foods.
evolución *f* evolution; — **natural** natural history (*of a disease*)
evolucionar *vi* evolve
ex *pref* ex-, former; — **esposa** ex-wife, former wife; — **fumador -ra** *mf* ex-smoker, former smoker
exacerbación *f* exacerbation
exactitud *f* accuracy

exacto -ta *adj* exact, accurate
examen *m* examination, exam (*fam*), test; — **de la vista** (*esp. Mex*) vision test, eye exam *o* test; — **de mamas** breast examination; — **de orina** urinalysis (*form*), urine test; — **de senos** breast examination; — **físico** physical examination, physical (*fam*); — **mamario** (*form*) breast examination, — **oftalmológico** (*form*) eye examination, eye exam (*fam*), — **pélvico** pelvic examination, pelvic (*fam*)
examinador -ra *mf* examiner
examinar *vt* to examine, to test
exantema súbito *m* roseola infantum
excederse *vr* to overdo it; **Puede caminar, pero no se exceda.**.You can walk, but don't overdo it.
excesivo -va *adj* excessive
exceso *m* excess
excipiente *m* excipient
excisión *f* excision
excisional *adj* excisional
excitación *f* (*sexual*) (sexual) arousal,
 • (sexual) stimulation
excitar *vt* to arouse (*sexually*); *vr* to become aroused (*sexually*)
excoriación *f* excoriation
excoriado -da *adj* excoriated, raw (*fam*)
excoriar *vt* to excoriate
excremento *m* excrement, stool
excretar *vt* to excrete
excretor -ra *adj* excretory
excusa *f* excuse
exfoliación *f* exfoliation; — **profunda** *or* **por láser** resurfacing, peeling
exfoliativo -va *adj* exfoliative
exhalar *vt, vi* to exhale
exhausto -ta *adj* exhausted, run-down
expandir *vt, vi* to expand
expectativa de vida *f* life expectancy
expectorante *adj & m* expectorant
expectorar *vt* (*form*) to cough up (and spit out)
expediente (clínico) *m* (*Mex, CA*) chart, medical record, file
expeler *vt* to expel
experimental *adj* experimental
experimentar *vi* to experiment

experimento *m* experiment

experto -ta *adj & mf* expert

expirar (*esp. Mex*) *See* **espirar**.

exploración *f* (*form, examen*) examination; — **física** physical examination, physical (*fam*)

explorador -ra *adj* (*surg*) exploratory

explorar *vt* (*form, examinar*) to examine; (*surg*) to explore

exponer *vt* (*pp* **expuesto**) to expose; *vr* to be exposed, to expose oneself; **No se exponga al humo**..Don't expose yourself to the smoke.

exposición *f* exposure

expresar *vt* to express; *vr* to express oneself

exprimir *vt* (*pus, etc.*) to express

expuesto -ta (*pp of* **exponer**) *adj* exposed; **Ella ha estado expuesta a él**..She has been exposed to him.

expulsar *vt* to expel, to pass (*fam*)

expulsión *f* expulsion

éxtasis *m* (*fam*) methylene dioxymethamphetamine (MDMA), ecstacy (*fam*); — **líquido** (*fam*) gamma-hydroxybutyrate (GHB), liquid ecstacy (*fam*)

extender *vt, vr* to extend; (*el brazo, la pierna*) to extend (*form*), to straighten

extensión *f* extension

extensivo -va *adj* extensive

extenso -sa *adj* extensive

extensor *adj & m* extensor

exterior *adj* outer, exterior, outside; *m* exterior, outside

externo -na *adj* external, outer, outside; (*anat*) lateral

extinguidor de incendios *m* (*Amer*) fire extinguisher

extintor de incendios *m* fire extinguisher

extirpar *vt* to excise, to resect

extra *adj* extra

extracción *f* extraction, removal

extracto *m* (*pharm*) extract

extractor de leche *m* (*esp. Mex*) breast pump

extraer *vt* to extract, remove, take out

extrañar *vt* to miss; **Extraño a mis hijos**..I miss my children.

extraño -ña *adj* unusual, foreign; **cuerpo** — foreign body

extravertido -da *See* **extrovertido**.

extremaunción *f* extreme unction

extremidad *f* extremity, limb

extrovertido -da *adj* extroverted; *mf* extrovert

extubación *f* extubation

extubar *vt* to extubate

eyaculación *f* ejaculation; — **precoz** premature ejaculation

eyaculado *m* ejaculate

eyacular *vi* to ejaculate

ezetimiba *f* ezetimibe

F

fabulación *f* confabulation

facciones *fpl* features

facial *adj* facial

facticio -cia *adj* factitious

factor *m* factor; — **V de Leiden** factor V Leiden; — **de protección solar (FPS)** sun protection factor (SPF); — **de riesgo** risk factor; —

intrínseco intrinsic factor; — **reumatoide, — reumatoideo** (*SA*) rheumatoid factor; — **Rh** Rh factor

facultad *f* faculty, ability; — **de medicina** medical school; *fpl* faculties

Fahrenheit *adj* Fahrenheit

faja *f* band (*around waist*); (*para contener una hernia*) truss

falda *f* skirt

fálico -ca *adj* phallic

falla *f* (*Amer, fallo*) failure; — **orgánica múltiple** (*esp. Mex*) multi-system organ failure

fallar *vi* to fail

fallecer *vi* to expire, die, to pass away (*euph*), to pass (*euph*)

fallecimiento *m* death (*esp. for statistics*)

fallo *m* failure; — **del tratamiento** treatment failure; — **de medro** (*Esp*) failure to thrive; — **multiorgánico** multi-system organ failure

falo *m* phallus

faloplastia *f* phalloplasty

falso -sa *adj* false

falta *f* lack, absence, deficit, deficiency; — **de aire** shortness of breath; **hacer(le) — (a uno)** to need; **No le hace falta..**You don't need it.

faltar *vi* **faltar(le) (a uno)** to be low, to need, to lack; **Le falta potasio..**Your potassium is low.. You need potassium; **faltar(le) el aire (a uno)..**to be short of breath; **¿Le falta el aire?..**Are you short of breath? — **a** (*una cita, el trabajo, etc.*) to miss (*an appointment, work, etc.*)

famciclovir *m* famciclovir

familia *f* family; — **extendida** extended family

familiar *adj* familial; *m* relative, family member

famotidina *f* famotidine

fantasía *f* fantasy

farfallota *f* (*Carib*) mumps

fárfara *f* (*bot*) coltsfoot

faringe *f* pharynx

faríngeo -a *adj* pharyngeal

faringitis *f* pharyngitis

farmacéutico -ca *adj* pharmaceutical; *mf* pharmacist

farmacia *f* pharmacy, drugstore

fármaco -ca *adj* pharmaceutical; *m* pharmaceutical, medication

farmacodependencia *f* prescription drug dependency *o* dependence

farmacodependiente *mf* person dependent on prescription drugs

farmacología *f* pharmacology

farmacológico -ca *adj* pharmacological, pharmacologic

farmacólogo -ga *mf* pharmacologist

farmacopea *f* pharmacopoeia

fascia *f* fascia

fascículo *m* tract

fascioliasis *f* fascioliasis

fasciotomía *f* fasciotomy

fascitis *f* fasciitis; — **necrotizante** *or* **necrosante** necrotizing fasciitis

fase *f* phase

fastidiar *vt* (*ped*) to tease

fastidioso -sa *adj* annoying, irritating

fatal *adj* fatal

fatiga *f* fatigue; — **visual** eyestrain

fatigar *vt* to tire, tire out; *vr* to tire, get tired, tire out

fatigoso -sa *adj* tiring

favorable *adj* favorable

febrícula *f* fever (*esp. low-grade and prolonged*)

febril *adj* febrile

fecal *adj* fecal

fecha *f* date; — **de caducidad** expiration date; — **de nacimiento** birth date; — **de vencimiento** expiration date; — **probable de parto** estimated date of delivery, due date (*fam*)

fecundación *f* fertilization; — **in vitro (FIV)** in vitro fertilization (IVF)

fecundar *vt* (*obst*) to fertilize

felación *f* (*form*) fellatio (*form*), oral sex, oral stimulation of the penis

felicidad *f* happiness; **¡Felicidades!** (*obst*) Congratulations!

feliz *adj* happy

felodipina *f* (*esp. SA*) felodipine

felodipino *m* felodipine

femenino -na *adj* feminine, female

feminización *f* feminization

femoral *adj* femoral

fémur *m* femur

fenacetina *f* phenacetin

fenazopiridina *f* phenazopyridine
fenciclidina (PCP) *f* phencyclidine (PCP)
fenilalanina *f* phenylalanine
fenilbutazona *f* phenylbutazone
fenilcetonuria *f* phenylketonuria (PKU)
fenilefrina *f* phenylephrine
fenilpropanolamina *f* phenylpropanolamine
fenitoína *f* phenytoin
fenobarbital *m* phenobarbital
fenofibrato *m* fenofibrate
fenol *m* phenol
fenómeno *m* phenomenon; — **de Raynaud** Raynaud's phenomenon
fenoprofeno *m* fenoprofen
fenotiazina, fenotiacina *f* phenothiazine
fenotipo *m* phenotype
fentanilo *m* fentanyl
fentermina *f* phentermine
feo -a *adj* ugly; (*fam*) bad, awful; **Sabe feo.**.It tastes bad (awful).
feocromocitoma *m* pheochromocytoma
férrico -ca *adj* ferric
ferritina *f* ferritin
ferroso -sa *adj* ferrous
fértil *adj* fertile
fertilización *f* fertilization; — **in vitro (FIV)** in vitro fertilization (IVF)
fertilizar *vt* to fertilize
férula *f* (*form*) splint, removable cast
fetal *adj* fetal
fetiche *m* fetish
fetichismo *m* fetishism
feto *m* fetus
fexofenadina *f* fexofenadine
fiabilidad *f* reliability
fiable *adj* reliable
fibra *f* fiber; — **dietética** dietary fiber; — **insoluble** insoluble fiber; — **muscular** muscle fiber; — **nerviosa** nerve fiber; — **soluble** soluble fiber
fibrilación *f* fibrillation; — **auricular** atrial fibrillation; — **ventricular** ventricular fibrillation
fibrina *f* fibrin
fibrinógeno *m* fibrinogen
fibrinólisis *f* fibrinolysis

fibrinolítico -ca *adj* fibrinolytic
fibroadenoma *m* fibroadenoma
fibroma *m* fibroma
fibromialgia *f* fibromyalgia
fibroquístico -ca *adj* fibrocystic
fibrosis *f* fibrosis; — **quística** cystic fibrosis
fibrositis *f* fibrositis
fibrótico -ca *adj* fibrotic
fiebre *f* fever; — **amarilla** yellow fever; — **botonosa mediterránea** Mediterranean spotted fever; — **del heno** hay fever; — **hemorrágica** hemorrhagic fever; — **maculosa de las Montañas Rocosas** Rocky Mountain spotted fever; — **Q** Q fever; — **reumática** rheumatic fever; — **tifoidea** typhoid fever
figura *f* (*de una persona*) figure
fijación *f* fixation
fijar *vt* — **la vista** to stare; *vr* — **en** to notice
fijo -ja *adj* fixed
filariasis *f* filariasis
filgrastim *m* filgrastim
filoso -sa *adj* sharp
filtración *f* filtration
filtrar *vt, vr* to filter
filtro *m* filter; **cigarillo con** — , **cigarro con** — (*esp. Mex*) filter-tipped cigarette; — **solar** sunscreen
fimosis *f* phimosis
fin *m* end; — **de semana** weekend
final *adj* final
finasterida *f* finasteride
fingido -da *adj* factitious
firma *f* signature
firmar *vt, vi* to sign (*one's name*)
firme *adj* firm
fisiatra *mf* physiatrist, specialist in physical medicine and rehabilitation
fisiatría *f* physiatry, physical medicine and rehabilitation
físico -ca *adj* physical; *m* physique, build
fisicoculturismo *m* bodybuilding
fisicoculturista *mf* bodybuilder
fisiología *f* physiology
fisiológico -ca *adj* physiological, physiologic
fisiólogo -ga *mf* physiologist
fisioterapeuta *mf* physical therapist,

physiotherapist

fisioterapia f physical therapy, physiotherapy

fisioterapista mf physical therapist, physiotherapist

fisostigmina f physostigmine

fístula f fistula, sinus tract; — **anal** anal fistula; — **arteriovenosa** arteriovenous fistula; — **de ano** anal fistula

fisura f fissure, crack, split, hairline fracture; — **anal** anal fissure; — **palatina** cleft palate

fitoterapia f herbal medicine, herbalism

flácido, fláccido -da adj flaccid, flabby, limp

flaco -ca adj (fam) thin, lean

flanco m flank

flato m (form) gas (expelled from rectum)

flatulencia f flatulence

flatulento -ta adj flatulent

flavonoide m flavonoid

flebitis f phlebitis

flebografía f (técnica imagenológica) venography; (estudio imagenológico) venogram

flebotomía f phlebotomy, venepuncture, blood drawing; — **terapéutica** therapeutic phlebotomy

flebotomiano mf phlebotomist

flebotomiano -na mf (esp. Esp) phlebotomist

flebótomo m sandfly

flema f (frec. pl) phlegm, mucus

flemón m phlegmon

flexible adj flexible

flexión (de brazo) f push-up

flexionar vt (form) to flex

flexor adj & m flexor

flictena f (esp. Esp) blister

flojo -ja adj (suelto) loose, lax; (relajado) relaxed, limp; (flácido) flabby

flora f flora

fluconazol m fluconazole

fluctuar vi to fluctuate

fludrocortisona f fludrocortisone

flufenazina f fluphenazine

fluido m fluid; — **corporal** body fluid

fluir vi to flow, to run

flujo m flow, drainage; (fam) vaginal discharge; — **espiratorio máximo** peak (expiratory) flow; — **menstrual** menstrual flow; — **sanguíneo** blood flow; **tener — nasal** to have a runny nose

flumetasona f flumetasone

flunisolida f flunisolide

flúor m fluorine

fluoración f fluoridation

fluorescente adj fluorescent

fluorización f fluoridation

fluoroscopia, fluoroscopía (Amer, esp. spoken) f fluoroscopy

fluorouracilo m fluorouracil

fluoruro m fluoride; — **sódico** (form) or **de sodio** sodium fluoride

fluoxetina f fluoxetine

flurazepam m flurazepam

flúter m (Ang) flutter; — **auricular** atrial flutter

fluticasona f fluticasone

fluvastatina f fluvastatin

fobia f phobia; — **social** social phobia

focal adj focal

foco m focus

fogaje m (Carib, fam) hot flash, flush

fólico -ca adj folic

foliculitis f folliculitis

folículo m follicle; — **ovárico** ovarian follicle; — **piloso** hair follicle

folitropina f follicle-stimulating hormone (FSH)

folleto m booklet, pamphlet, handout

fondillos mpl (Carib, CA; fam) buttocks

fondo m bottom; (de una úlcera) base; — **de ojo** eyeground

fonoaudiólogo -ga mf speech therapist

fontanela f fontanelle o fontanel

foramen oval m foramen ovale; — **— permeable** patent foramen ovale

fórceps m (pl -ceps) (obst) forceps

forense adj forensic

forma f form, shape; **en —** fit, in shape

formación f formation; (entrenamiento) training

formalina See **formol**.

formar vt, vr to form

formol m formalin

formoterol *m* formoterol
fórmula *f* (*math, ped, pharm, etc.*) formula
formulario *m* (*pharm*) formulary; (*cuestionario, etc.*) form
fornido -da *adj* stocky
fortalecer *vt* to strengthen, build up
fortificar *vt* to fortify
forúnculo *m* furuncle
forzar *vt* (*la vista, la voz*) to strain (*one's eyes, one's voice*)
fosa *f* fossa; — **nasal** nostril
fosamprenavir *m* fosamprenavir
fosfatasa alcalina *f* alkaline phosphatase
fosfato *m* phosphate
fósforo *m* phosphorus
fosinopril *m* fosinopril
fotoalergia *f* photoallergy
fotocoagulación *f* photocoagulation
fotosensibilidad *f* photosensitivity
fotosensible *adj* photosensitive
fototerapia *f* phototherapy
fototóxico -ca *adj* phototoxic
FPS *abbr* **factor de protección solar.** *See* **factor.**
fracasar *vi* to fail
fracaso *m* failure; — **del tratamiento** treatment failure; — **multiorgánico** (*Esp*) multi-system organ failure; — **renal agudo** (*Esp*) acute renal failure; — **terapéutico** treatment failure
fracción *f* fraction; — **de eyección** ejection fraction
fractura *f* fracture, break; — **abierta** open *o* compound fracture; — **cerrada** closed fracture; — **conminuta** comminuted fracture; — **craneal** *or* **de cráneo** cranial *o* skull fracture; — **de estrés** stress fracture; — **espiroidea** spiral fracture; — **por aplastamiento vertebral** vertebral compression fracture; — **vertebral** vertebral fracture, (*debida a la osteoporosis*) vertebral compression fracture
fracturar *vt, vr* to fracture, break
fragata portuguesa *f* Portuguese man-of-war, type of jellyfish
frágil *adj* fragile, brittle, frail, delicate
fragmento *m* fragment

frambesia *f* frambesia, yaws
frasco *m* bottle, pill bottle, vial
fraterno -na *adj* fraternal
frazada *f* (*Amer*) blanket
frecuencia *f* frequency, rate; **¿Con qué frecuencia?**..How often? — **cardíaca** heart rate; — **respiratoria** respiratory rate
frecuente *adj* frequent
frecuentemente *adv* frequently, often
freír *vt* to fry
frénico -ca *adj* phrenic
frenos, frenillos *mpl* (*Amer, orthodontia, fam*) braces, bands (*fam*)
frente *f* forehead, brow
fresa *f* strawberry
fresco -ca *adj* fresh; cool
fricción *f* friction
friccionar *vt* to rub; (*masajear*) to massage
frigidez *f* low sexual desire, inability to respond sexually (*said of a woman*)
frígida *adj* having low sexual desire, unresponsive sexually
frigorífico *m* refrigerator
frijoles *mpl* (*Amer*) beans
frío -a *adj* cold; *m* cold; **hacer** — to be cold (*the weather*); **Me duele más cuando hace frío**..It hurts more when the weather is cold; **tener** *or* **sentir** — to be o feel cold; **Tengo frío**..I'm cold.
friolento -ta *adj* sensitive to cold
frito -ta *adj* fried
friza *f* (*PR, SD*) blanket
frontal *adj* frontal
frotar *vt* to rub
frotis *m* (*pl* **-tis**) (*micro*) smear; — **de Papanicolaou** Papanicolaou smear
frovatriptán *m* frovatriptan
fructosa *f* fructose
fruncir *vt* — **el ceño** *or* **entrecejo** to frown; — **los labios** to purse one's lips
fruta *f* fruit; — **cítrica** citrus fruit; — **seca** dried fruit
fuego *m* fire; (*llaga en los labios*) cold sore, fever blister
fuente *f* source; (*obst*) bag of waters; — **de infección** source of infection; — **de proteína** source of protein
fuera *adv* — **de** outside, outside of;

— **de sí** crazy, out of it (*fam*)
fuerte *adj* strong, powerful, severe
fuerza *f* force, (*frec. pl*) strength; **la fuerza de su pierna**..the strength of your leg...**sus fuerzas**..your strength; **de doble** — double-strength; **de** — **extra** extra-strength; — **de cizallamiento** *or* **cizalla** shear force; — **de voluntad** will power
fulminante *adj* fulminant
fumador -ra *mf* smoker
fumar *vt, vi* to smoke; **Prohibido fumar**..No smoking.

fumigar *vt* fumigate; — **con avioneta** to crop-dust
función *f* function
funcionamiento *m* performance
funcionar *vi* to function, to work
funda de almohada *f* pillowcase
funeraria *f* funeral home, mortuary
fúngico -ca *adj* fungal
furia *f* rage
furosemida *f* furosemide
fusil *m* rifle, gun
fusión *f* fusion
fusionar *vi, vr* (*ortho*) to fuse
fútbol *m* soccer; (*americano*) football

G

gabapentina *f* gabapentin
gabinete *m* office (*esp. of a dentist or orthodontist*)
gadolinio *m* gadolinium
gafas *fpl* glasses, eyeglasses, goggles; — **bifocales** bifocal glasses *o* eyeglasses, bifocals (*fam*); — **de lectura** (*Esp*) reading glasses; — **de natación** swimming goggles; — **de seguridad** safety glasses *o* goggles; — **de sol** (*esp. Esp*) sunglasses; — **para nadar** swimming goggles; — **protectoras** safety glasses *o* goggles
gago -ga *mf* (*fam*) stutterer, stammerer
gaguear *vi* (*fam*) to stutter, stammer
galactosa *f* galactose
galactosemia *f* galactosemia
galeno *m* (*fam*) doctor
galio *m* gallium
galleta *f* cookie, (*salada*) cracker
galope *m* (*card*) gallop

gamma *f* gamma
gammaglobulina *f* gamma globulin
gammagrafía *f* (*técnica imagenológica*) nuclear scanning, nuclear medicine; (*estudio imagenológico*) nuclear scan; — **con galio** gallium scanning; gallium scan; — **con talio** thallium scanning; thallium scan; — **ósea** bone scan
gammagrama *m* (*Mex*) nuclear scan
gammahidroxibutirato *m* gamma-hydroxybutyrate (GHB), liquid ecstacy (*fam*)
gammapatía *f* gammopathy; — **monoclonal de significado incierto** monoclonal gammopathy of undetermined significance
ganancia *f* gain; — **de peso** weight gain
ganar *vt* to gain; — **peso** to gain weight
gancho *m* (*de pañal*) safety pin
ganciclovir *m* gancyclovir

ganglio *m* node; (*neuro*) ganglion; **ganglios basales** basal ganglia; — **centinela** sentinel node; — **linfático** lymph node
ganglión *m* (*quiste*) ganglion cyst, (*neuro*) ganglion
ganglioneuroma *m* ganglioneuroma
gangoso -sa *adj* nasal (*voice*)
gangrena *f* gangrene; — **gaseosa** gas gangrene; — **seca** dry gangrene
gargajear *vi* (*fam*) to cough up phlegm
garganta *f* throat
gárgaras *fpl* **hacer —** to gargle
garra *f* claw
garrapata *f* tick
gas *m* gas; **expulsar gases** to pass gas; **gases arteriales** arterial blood gas; — **de la risa** *or* **hilarante** laughing gas; — **lacrimógeno** tear gas; — **natural** natural gas; — **nervioso** nerve gas; **tener gases** to have gas
gasa *f* gauze
gasolina *f* gasoline, gas (*fam*)
gasometría arterial *f* arterial blood gas
gastar *vi, vr* to wear out
gasto *m* output; — **cardíaco** cardiac output; — **energético de reposo** basal metabolic rate; — **urinario** urine output
gastrectomía *f* gastrectomy
gástrico -ca *adj* gastric
gastrina *f* gastrin
gastrinoma *m* gastrinoma
gastritis *f* gastritis
gastrocnemio *m* gastrocnemius
gastroenteritis *f* gastroenteritis
gastroenterología *f* gastroenterology
gastroenterólogo -ga *mf* gastroenterologist
gastroesofágico -ca *adj* gastroesophageal
gastrointestinal *adj* gastrointestinal (GI)
gastroparesia *f* gastroparesis
gastrostomía *f* gastrostomy; — **endoscópica percutánea** percutaneous endoscopic gastrostomy (PEG)
gatear *vi* (*ped*) to crawl
gato *m* cat
gay *adj* gay

gel *m* gel
gelatina *f* gelatin, jelly
gemelo -la *adj & mf* twin; — **idéntico** identical twin; — **siamés** *or* **unido** conjoined twin
gemfibrozilo *m* gemfibrozil
gemido *m* groan, moan
gemir *vi* to groan, moan
gen *m* gene
generación *f* generation; **primera —, segunda —, tercera —, etc.** first generation, second generation, third generation, etc.
generador *m* (*de un marcapasos, etc.*) generator
general *adj* general
generalizado -da *adj* generalized
genérico -ca *adj & m* (*pharm*) generic
género *m* gender
genético -ca *adj* genetic; *f* genetics
genetista *mf* geneticist
genio *m* genius
genital *adj* genital; *mpl* genitals
genoma *m* genome; — **humano** human genome
genotipo *m* genotype
gentamicina *f* gentamicin
gente *f* persons, people
genu valgo, genu valgum
genu varo, genu varum
geriatra *mf* geriatrician
geriatría *f* geriatrics
geriátrico -ca *adj* geriatric; *m* home for the elderly, skilled nursing facility (*for the elderly*)
germen *m* (*pl* **gérmenes**) germ
germinoma *m* germinoma
gerontología *f* gerontology
gerontólogo -ga *mf* gerontologist
gestación *f* gestation
gestacional *adj* gestational
gesto *m* gesture; — **suicida** suicide gesture
giardiasis *f* giardiasis
giba *f* humpback, hunchback, hump
gigante *adj* giant
gigantismo *m* gigantism
gimnasia *f* gymnastics
gimnasio *m* gymnasium, health club, fitness center
ginecología *f* gynecology
ginecológico -ca *adj* gynecologic,

gynecological

ginecólogo -ga *mf* gynecologist

gingivitis *f* gingivitis; — **úlceronecrotizante aguda** acute necrotizing ulcerative gingivitis

ginkgo biloba *m* (*bot*) ginkgo biloba

ginseng *m* (*bot*) ginseng

glande *m* glans

glándula *f* gland; — **adrenal** adrenal gland, adrenal (*fam*); — **endocrina** endocrine gland; — **lagrimal** lacrimal gland; — **mamaria** mammary gland; — **paratiroides** or **paratiroidea** parathyroid gland, parathyroid (*fam*); — **parótida** parotid gland, parotid (*fam*); — **pineal** pineal gland; — **pituitaria** pituitary gland; — **prostática** prostate gland, prostate (*fam*); — **salival** or **salivar** salivary gland; — **sudorípara** sweat gland; — **suprarrenal** adrenal gland, adrenal (*fam*); — **tiroides** or **tiroidea** thyroid gland, thyroid (*fam*)

glaucoma *m* glaucoma

glibenclamida *f* glyburide

glicerina *f* glycerol, glycerin

glicerol *m* glycerol, glycerin

glicina *f* glycine

glimepirida *f* glimepiride

glioblastoma *m* glioblastoma; — **multiforme** glioblastoma multiforme

glioma *m* glioma

glipizida *f* glipizide

global *adj* global

globo *m* — **ocular** or **del ojo** eyeball

globulina *f* globulin

glóbulo *m* — **blanco** leukocyte (*form*), white blood cell; — **rojo** erythrocyte (*form*), red blood cell

glomerulonefritis *f* glomerulonephritis

glositis *f* glossitis

glotis *f* glottis

glucagón *m* glucagon

glucagonoma *m* glucagonoma

glucemia capilar *f* (*form*) fingerstick glucose

glucocorticoide *adj* & *m* glucocorticoid

glucómetro *m* (blood) glucose meter o monitor

gluconato *m* gluconate; — **cálcico** (*form*) or **de calcio** calcium gluconate

glucosa *f* glucose

glucosamina *f* glucosamine

glutamato monosódico *m* monosodium glutamate (MSG)

glutámico -ca *adj* glutamic

glutamina *f* glutamine

glutaraldehído *m* glutaraldehyde

gluten *m* gluten

glúteo -a *adj* gluteal; *m* buttock

gogles *mpl* (*Mex*) goggles

golf *m* golf

golondrino *m* hidradenitis suppurativa (*form*), boils under the arms

golosina *f* candy, piece of candy; *fpl* candy, sweets

goloso -sa *adj* **ser** — (*esp. Esp*) to have a sweet tooth

golpe *m* blow, stroke; — **de calor** heatstroke; — **precordial** precordial thump; — **psicológico** psychological blow

golpeado -da *adj* battered; **refugio para mujeres golpeadas** battered women's shelter

golpear *vt* to strike, hit; **Me golpeó aquí.**.It struck (hit) me here.

goma *m&f* (*de la sífilis*) gumma; *f* rubber; gum; (*CA, resaca*) hangover; **estar de** — (*CA*) to have a hangover; — **de mascar** chewing gum; — **espuma** foam rubber

gónada *f* gonad

gonadorelina *f* gonadorelin

gonadotropina, gonadotrofina (*OMS*) *f* gonadotropin; — **coriónica humana** human chorionic gonadotropin (HCG)

gonce *m* (*CA, fam, articulación*) joint

gonococo *m* gonococcus

gonorrea *f* gonorrhea

gordo -da *adj* fat

gordolobo *m* (*bot*) mullein

gorgoteo *m* gurgle, gurgling

gorra See **gorro**.

gorro *m* cap; — **de baño** bathing o shower cap; — **quirúrgico** or **de cirugía** scrub o surgical cap

goserelina *f* goserelin

gota f drop; (*enfermedad*) gout; **gotas óticas** or **para los oídos** ear drops; **gotas oftálmicas** or **para los ojos** eye drops

gotear vi to drip; **gotearle la nariz** to have a runny nose

goteo m drip; — **postnasal** or **posnasal** postnasal drip

gotero m (*Amer*) medicine dropper, eyedropper

gotoso -sa adj gouty

grado m grade; (*temperatura*) degree; **Está en el séptimo grado**..She's in the seventh grade...**37 grados centígrados**..37 degrees Centigrade; **de bajo** — low-grade; **de alto** — high-grade

graduado -da adj graduated

gradual adj gradual

gradualmente adv gradually

gráfica f graph

gragea f coated pill

Gram negativo -va adj Gram-negative

gramo m gram

Gram positivo -va adj Gram-positive

grande adj big, large; **ponerse más grande**..to get bigger...**¿Qué tan grande era?**..How big was it?... **Cuando seas grande**..When you grow up

grandioso -sa adj grandiose

granito m small pimple; *mpl* rash, fine rash

granjero -ra mf farmer

grano m grain, cereal; (*derm*) pimple; **de** — **entero** whole-grain

granulación f granulation

gránulo m granule

granulocito m granulocyte

granuloma m granuloma; — **piógeno** pyogenic granuloma

granulomatosis f granulomatosis; — **de Wegener** Wegener's granulomatosis

grapa f (*surg*) staple, clip

grasiento -ta adj (*Esp*) greasy, oily

graso -sa adj fatty, oily, greasy; **cabello** — oily hair; **comida** — greasy food; **cutis** m — oily skin, oily complexion; **hígado** — fatty liver; f fat, grease; — **animal** animal fat; — **de leche** milk fat; — **saturada** saturated fat

grasoso -sa adj fatty, oily, greasy

gratificación f gratification

grave adj (*condición*) serious, grave; (*tono*) low-pitched; **Ella está grave** ..She is seriously ill.

gravedad f severity

gray m (*radiology*) gray

greta f toxic Mexican folk remedy containing lead

grieta f crack, split

grima f (*Mex, fam*) nausea

gripa (*Amer, fam*) See **gripe**.

gripal adj pertaining to influenza; **temporada** — flu season

gripe f influenza (*form*), flu; — **asiática** Asian flu; — **aviar** avian influenza o flu, bird flu (*fam*)

gris adj gray

grisáceo -a adj grayish

griseofulvina f griseofulvin

gritar vi to cry, to call out

grito m cry; — **de auxilio** cry for help

grosor m thickness

grueso -sa adj thick

gruñido m grunt

gruñir vi to grunt, (*el estómago*) to growl

grupo m group; — **de apoyo** support group; — **de iguales** or **pares** peer group; — **sanguíneo (A, B, etc.)** blood type (A, B, etc.)

guabucho m (*PR, SD; fam*) lump, bump (*due to trauma*)

guaifenesina f guaifenesin

guante m glove

guapo -pa adj (*fam*) good-looking

guardar cama vt to stay in bed

guardería infantil f nursery, daycare center

guardia f **de** — on call

güero -ra (*Mex*) m blond; f blond o blonde

guerra f war; — **nuclear** nuclear war

guía f guideline; (*orientación*) guidance

gusano m worm; — **plano** flatworm; — **redondo** roundworm

gusto m taste, flavor

H

habilidad *f* skill, ability; **habilidades comunicativas** communication skills; **habilidades parentales** parenting skills; **habilidades sociales** social skills

habitación *f* room, bedroom

hábito *m* habit; **hábitos alimenticios** (*form*) *or* **de comer** eating habits; **mal —** bad habit;

habituación *f* habituation

habitual *adj* habitual, usual; **la hora habitual**..the usual time

habla *f* speech; **desarrollo del —** speech development

hablar *vt, vi* to speak, to talk

habón *m* (*esp. Esp*) hive, wheal

hacer *vt* **hace tres años**..three years ago...**¿Hace cuánto que tiene artritis?**..How long have you had arthritis? **— caca** (*fam or vulg*) to have a bowel movement, to go poo poo (*ped, fam*); **hacer(le) caso** to mind; **— daño** to hurt, to harm; **— efecto** to take effect; **— pipí** (*esp. ped, fam*) to urinate, to pee (*esp. ped, fam*); **— pis** (*fam or vulg*) to urinate, to pee (*esp. ped, fam*); **— popó** *or* **pupú** (*fam*) to have a bowel movement, to go poo poo (*ped, fam*); *vi* **— del baño** (*Mex, fam*), **— del cuerpo** (*Carib*), **— de(l) vientre** (*Esp*) to have a bowel movement; *vr* **— la paja** (*vulg*) *or* **— una paja** (*Esp, vulg*) to masturbate, to jack off (*vulg*)

haces *pl of* **haz**

hachís *m* hashish

halitosis *f* halitosis

hallazgo *m* finding

hallux valgus *m* hallux valgus

hallux varus *m* hallux varus

halo *m* halo

haloperidol *m* haloperidol

halotano *m* halothane

hamartoma *m* hamartoma

hambre *f* hunger; **tener —** to be hungry; **¿Tiene hambre?**..Are you hungry?

hantavirus *m* (*pl* **-rus**) hantavirus

harina *f* flour

haz *m* (*pl* **haces**) (*luz, rayos X, etc.*) beam

hebilla *f* buckle

heces (fecales) *fpl* (*form*) feces (*form*), stool(s), bowel movement(s)

hechicero -ra *mf* shaman

hecho -cha *adj* **— a la medida** custom-fitted

helado -da *adj* frozen, cold; *m* ice cream

hélice *f* helix; **doble —** double helix

helicoidal *adj* helical

helio *m* helium

hemangioma *m* hemangioma; **— cavernoso** cavernous hemangioma

hematocele *m* hematocele

hematocrito *m* hematocrit

hematología *f* hematology

hematólogo -ga *mf* hematologist

hematoma *m* hematoma; **— subdural** subdural hematoma

hembra (*fam*) *adj & f* female

hemiplejía, hemiplejia *f* hemiplegia

hemisferio *m* hemisphere

hemocromatosis *f* hemochromatosis

hemocultivo *m* (*form*) blood culture

hemodiálisis *f* hemodialysis

hemofilia *f* hemophilia

hemofílico -ca *mf* hemophiliac

hemoglobina *f* hemoglobin; **— glicosilada** glycosylated hemoglobin

hemoglobinuria *f* hemoglobinuria; **— paroxística nocturna** paroxysmal nocturnal hemoglobinuria

hemograma completo *m* complete blood count

hemólisis *f* hemolysis

hemolítico -ca *adj* hemolytic

hemorragia *f* hemorrhage, bleeding, bleed; **— digestiva (alta, baja)** (upper, lower) GI bleed; **— nasal** nosebleed, bloody nose (*fam*); **— subaracnoidea** subarachnoid hemorrhage

hemorrágico -ca *adj* hemorrhagic

hemorroide *f* hemorrhoid

hemorroidectomía *f* hemorrhoidectomy

hemosiderosis *f* hemosiderosis

hendidura *f* crack, gap, split

henna *f* (*bot*) henna

heno *m* hay

heparina *f* heparin; **— de bajo peso molecular** low-molecular-weight heparin

hepático -ca *adj* hepatic

hepatitis *f* hepatitis; **— A — B**, etc. hepatitis A, hepatitis B, etc.

hepatología *f* hepatology

hepatólogo -ga *mf* hepatologist

hepatoma *m* hepatoma

hepatorrenal *adj* hepatorenal

herbal *adj* herbal

herbario -ria *adj* herbal

herbicida *m* herbicide

herbolario -ria *mf* herbalist, person who sells herbs; *m* herb shop; *f* herbalism

herborista *mf* herbalist, person who sells herbs

herboristería *f* herb shop

heredar *vt* to inherit

hereditario -ria *adj* hereditary, heritable

herencia *f* heredity

herido -da *adj* injured, wounded; *mf* wounded person; *f* injury, wound, cut, sore; **— de bala** gunshot wound; **— penetrante** penetrating wound; **— punzante** puncture wound

herir *vt* to injure, to wound

hermafrodita *adj & mf* hermaphrodite

hermafroditismo *m* hermaphroditism

hermanastro -tra *m* stepbrother; *f* stepsister

hermano -na *m* brother, sibling; *f* sister; **— siames** conjoined twin, Siamese twin (*ant*)

hernia *f* hernia; **— crural** femoral hernia; **— de hiato** hiatal hernia; **— estrangulada** strangulated hernia; **— femoral** femoral hernia; **— hiatal** hiatal hernia; **— incarcerada** incarcerated hernia; **— inci**-sional incisional hernia; **— inguinal** inguinal hernia; **— reducible** reducible hernia; **— umbilical** umbilical hernia

herniorrafia *f* herniorrhaphy

heroína *f* heroin

herpangina *f* herpangina

herpes *m* herpes; **— labial** labial herpes, cold sore (*fam*), fever blister (*fam*); **— simple** herpes simplex; **— zoster** herpes zoster, shingles (*fam*)

herpesvirus *m* (*pl* **-rus**) herpesvirus; **— humano 6, — humano 8**, etc. human herpesvirus 6, human herpesvirus 8, etc.

herpético -ca *adj* herpetic

hervido -da *adj* boiled; **agua —** boiled water

hervir *vt* (*also* **hacer —**) to boil; *vi* to boil

heterosexual *adj & mf* heterosexual

hidatídico -ca *adj* hydatid

hidatiforme *adj* (*obst*) hydatidiform

hidradenitis supurativa *f* hidradenitis suppurativa

hidralazina, hidralacina *f* hydralazine

hidratante *adj* moisturizing

hidratar *vt* to hydrate, (*la piel*) to moisturize

hidrato *m* hydrate; **— de** carbono carbohydrate; **— de cloral** chloral hydrate

hidrocarburo *m* hydrocarbon

hidrocefalia *f* hydrocephalus; **— normotensiva** normal pressure hydrocephalus

hidrocele *m* hydrocele

hidroclorotiazida *f* hydrochlorothiazide

hidrocodona *f* hydrocodone

hidrocoloide *m* hydrocolloid

hidrocortisona *f* hydrocortisone

hidrofobia *f* hydrophobia

hidrogel *m* hydrogel

hidrogenado -da *adj* hydrogenated

hidronefrosis *f* hydronephrosis

hidroquinona *f* hydroquinone

hidroterapia *f* hydrotherapy; **— del colon** colonic

hidroxicina, hidroxizina (*OMS*) *f* hydroxyzine

hidroxicloroquina f hydroxychloroquine

hidróxido m hydroxide; — **de aluminio** aluminum hydroxide; — **de potasio** potassium hydroxide; — **de sodio** sodium hydroxide; — **potásico** (form) potassium hydroxide; — **sódico** (form) sodium hydroxide

hidroxiurea f hydroxyurea

hiedra venenosa f poison ivy

hielo m ice; **pedacitos** or **trocitos de** — ice chips

hierba f grass; (planta medicinal) herb; (fam, marihuana) marijuana, pot (fam), grass (fam); — **de san Juan** (bot) St. John's wort

hierbabuena f (bot) spearmint, peppermint, mint

hierbatero -ra mf (Mex) herbalist

hierbero -ra mf (Amer) herbalist

hierro m iron

hifema See **hipema**.

hígado m liver; — **graso** fatty liver

higiene f hygiene; — **bucal** oral hygiene

higiénico -ca adj hygienic, sanitary

higienista mf hygienist; — **dental** dental hygienist

hijastro -tra m stepson, stepchild; f stepdaughter

hijo -ja m son, child; — **único** only child; f daughter

hilo dental m dental floss

himen m hymen; — **imperforado** imperforate hymen

hinchado -da adj swollen, puffy, bloated

hincharse vr to swell, swell up

hinchazón f swelling

hioides m hyoid bone

hipar vi to hiccup

hipema m hyphema

hiperactividad f hyperactivity

hiperactivo -va adj hyperactive

hiperalimentación f hyperalimentation

hiperbárico -ca adj hyperbaric

hipercalcemia f hypercalcemia

hiperemesis gravídica f (obst) hyperemesis gravidarum

hiperextensible adj double-jointed

hiperglucemia f hyperglycemia

hiperhidrosis f hyperhidrosis

hipérico m (bot) St. John's wort

hiperlipemia, hiperlipidemia f hyperlipidemia

hipermétrope adj (form) farsighted

hipermetropía f (form) farsightedness

hipermóvil adj hypermobile

hipernatremia f hypernatremia

hipernefroma m nephroma

hiperosmolar adj hyperosmolar

hiperparatiroideo -a adj hyperparathyroid

hiperparatiroidismo m hyperparathyroidism

hiperpigmentación f hyperpigmentation

hiperplasia f hyperplasia; — **prostática benigna** benign prostatic hyperplasia; — **suprarrenal congénita** congenital adrenal hyperplasia

hiperprolactinemia f hyperprolactinemia

hipersensibilidad f hypersensitivity

hipersensible adj hypersensitive

hipertensión f (also — **arterial**) hypertension, high blood pressure (fam); — **de bata blanca** whitecoat hypertension; — **endocraneal benigna** benign intracranial hypertension; — **(arterial) esencial** essential hypertension; — **(arterial) maligna** malignant hypertension; — **portal** portal hypertension; — **pulmonar** pulmonary hypertension; — **renovascular** renovascular hypertension

hipertermia f hyperthermia

hipertiroideo -a adj hyperthyroid

hipertiroidismo m hyperthyroidism

hipertrofia f hypertrophy, enlargement

hipertrófico -ca adj hypertrophic

hiperuricemia f hyperuricemia

hiperventilación f hyperventilation

hiperventilar vi to hyperventilate

hipnosis f hypnosis

hipnótico -ca adj & m hypnotic

hipnotismo m hypnotism

hipnotista mf hypnotist

hipnotizador -ra mf hypnotist

hipnotizar vt to hypnotize

hipo m hiccup; **tener** — to have the hiccups, to hiccup

hipoalergénico -ca *adj* hypoallergen-ic

hipocalcemia *f* hypocalcemia

hipocondría *f* hypochondriasis

hipocondríaco, hipocondriaco -ca *mf* person who worries excessively about his or her health, hypochondriac (*ant*)

hipocratismo digital *m* clubbing

hipodérmico -ca *adj* hypodermic

hipofisario -ria *adj* pituitary

hipófisis *f* pituitary gland

hipoglucemia *f* hypoglycemia

hipoglucemiante *adj* hypoglycemic (*causing hypoglycemia*); *m* hypoglycemic agent; — **oral** oral hypoglycemic agent

hipoglucémico -ca *adj* hypoglycemic (*pertaining to hypoglycemia*); **reacción** — hypoglycemic reaction

hiponatremia *f* hyponatremia

hipoparatiroideo -a *adj* hypoparathyroid

hipoparatiroidismo *m* hypoparathyroidism

hipopigmentación *f* hypopigmentation

hipopituitarismo *m* hypopituitarism

hipopotasemia *f* hypokalemia

hipospadias *m* hypospadias

hipotálamo *m* hypothalamus

hipotensión *f* hypotension; — **ortostática** orthostatic hypotension

hipotensivo -va *adj* hypotensive

hipotensor -ra *adj* hypotensive

hipotermia *f* hypothermia

hipotiroideo -a *adj* hypothyroid

hipotiroidismo *m* hypothyroidism

hipovolémico -ca *adj* hypovolemic

hirsutismo *m* hirsutism

hirsuto -ta *adj* hirsute

hirviendo -da *adj* boiling; **agua** — boiling water

hisopo *m* swab

histamina *f* histamine

histerectomía *f* hysterectomy; — **total abdominal** total abdominal hysterectomy; — **vaginal** vaginal hysterectomy

histeria *f* anxiety attack, severe anxiety, hysteria (*ant*); — **de conversión** conversion reaction

histérico -ca *adj* severely anxious, anxiety-related, hysterical (*ant*)

histidina *f* histidine

histiocitosis *f* histiocytosis; — **X** histiocytosis X

histología *f* histology

histoplasmosis *f* histoplasmosis

historia *f* history; — **clínica** medical record, chart; medical history; — **clínica y examen físico** history and physical

historial médico *m* medical record, chart; medical history

histriónico -ca *adj* histrionic

hito del desarrollo *m* developmental milestone

hogar *m* home; **sin** — homeless

hoja *f* (*de cuchillo, etc.*) blade; — **de afeitar** razor blade

holístico -ca *adj* holistic

Holter *m* Holter monitor

hombre *m* man, male

hombro *m* shoulder; — **congelado** (*fam*) adhesive capsulitis (*form*), frozen shoulder (*fam*)

homeópata *mf* homeopath

homeopatía *f* homeopathy

homeopático -ca *adj* homeopathic

homofobia *f* homophobia

homofóbico -ca *adj* homophobic

homosexual *adj* homosexual, gay; *m* homosexual man, gay man; *f* homosexual woman, lesbian, gay woman

hondo -da *adj* deep

hongo *m* fungus, yeast, mushroom; **infección** *f* **por hongos** fungal infection, yeast infection

honorarios *mpl* fee, bill

hora *f* hour, time; **¿A qué hora comió?**..What time did you eat?.. When did you eat?

horario *m* schedule; — **de consulta** office hours; — **de visita** visiting hours

horizontal *adj* horizontal

hormiga *f* ant; — **de fuego** fire ant

hormiguear *vi* to tingle

hormigueo *m* tingling

hormiguicida *m* ant poison

hormona *f* hormone; — **adrenocorticotrópica** adrenocorticotropic *o* adrenocortical hormone (ACTH); — **antidiurética** antidiuretic hormone; — **de(l) crecimiento** growth hormone (GH); — **de(l) crecimiento bovina** bovine growth hormone; — **estimulante de la tiroides** thyroid-stimulating hormone (TSH); — **folículo estimulante** follicle-stimulating hormone (FSH); — **liberadora de gonadotropinas** gonadotropin-releasing hormone (GnRH); — **luteinizante** luteinizing hormone (LH); — **paratiroidea** parathyroid hormone (PTH); — **tiroidea** thyroid hormone; — **tirotrópica** thyroid-stimulating hormone (TSH)

hormonal *adj* hormonal

horneado -da *adj* baked

hornear *vt* to bake

horno *m* al — baked

hortaliza *f* vegetable

hortensia *f* (*bot*) hydrangea

hospital *m* hospital; — **comunitario** community hospital; — **de enseñanza** teaching hospital; — **del condado** county hospital (US); — **de tercer nivel** tertiary care hospital; — **de veteranos** Veterans Administration (VA) hospital; — **general** general hospital; — **privado** private hospital; — **psiquiátrico** psychiatric hospital, mental institution; — **público** public hospital

hospitalario -ria *adj* pertaining to a hospital

hospitalizar *vt* to hospitalize

hostil *adj* hostile

hostilidad *f* hostility

hoy *adv* today

hoyo *m* hole

hoyuelo *m* dimple

hueco -ca *adj* hollow; *m* hollow, hole; — **de la mano** hollow of the hand

huérfano -na *mf* orphan

huesecillo *m* (*del oído*) ossicle (*of the ear*)

huesero -ra *mf* (*esp. Mex, fam*) person who treats disorders of bones and joints

hueso *m* bone; — **de la cadera** hipbone; — **del pecho** breastbone; — **del tobillo** anklebone; — **ilíaco**, — **iliaco** (*esp. Mex*) ilium; *mpl* (*Mex, CA; fam; articulaciones*) joints; **Se me hinchan los huesos..**My joints swell.

huevecillo *m* small egg (*of a parasite, etc.*)

huevo *m* egg; (*fam, óvulo*) ovum, egg (*fam*); (*esp. Mex, fam*) testicle, ball (*fam*)

hule *m* (*esp. Mex, CA*) rubber; — **espuma** foam rubber

humanitario -ria *adj* humanitarian

humano -na *adj & m* human; **ser** — human being

humectador *m* humidifier

humectante *adj* (*esp. Amer*) moisturizing

humedad *f* humidity, dampness, moisture

humedecer *vt* to humidify, moisturize, moisten

húmedo -da *adj* humid, damp, moist

humeral *adj* brachial

húmero *m* humerus

humidificador *m* humidifier

humidificar *vt* to humidify

humo *m* smoke, fumes; — **ambiental del tabaco** secondhand tobacco smoke

humor *m* humor; (*psych*) mood; (*anat*) humor; **El humor es la mejor terapia..**Humor is the best therapy; **estar de buen** — to be in a good mood; **estar de mal** — to be in a bad mood; — **acuoso** aqueous humor; — **vítreo** vitreous humor; **oscilación** *f* **del** — mood swing

huracán *m* hurricane

hurgarse *vt* — **la nariz** (*Esp*) to pick one's nose

I

ibandronato *m* ibandronate
ibuprofeno, ibuprofen, ibuprofén *m* ibuprofen
ictericia *f (form)* jaundice
ictiosis *f* ichthyosis
ictus *m (pl* **ictus**) *(form)* cerebrovascular accident *(form)*, stroke
ideal *adj* ideal
idéntico -ca *adj* identical
identidad *f* identity; **— de género** gender identity
identificación *f* identification
identificar *vt* to identify; *vr (psych)* **— con** to identify with
idiopático -ca *adj* idiopathic
ido -da *adj* absent-minded, spacey *(fam)*, spaced out *(fam)*
idóneo -a *adj* suitable
ignorante *adj (inconsciente)* unaware
ileal *adj* ileal
ileítis *f* ileitis
íleo *m* ileus
íleon *m* ileum
ileostomía *f* ileostomy
ilíaco, iliaco -ca *(esp. Mex) adj* iliac; **hueso —** ilium *(form)*, hipbone *(fam)*
ilion *m* ilium, hipbone *(fam)*
IM *See* **intramuscular.**
imagen *f (pl* **imágenes**) image; **diagnóstico por —** diagnostic imaging; **estudio por —** imaging study; **— corporal** body image
imagenología *f* imaging
IMC *abbr* **índice de masa corporal.** *See* **índice.**
imipenem *m* imipenem
imipramina *f* imipramine
imiquimod *m* imiquimod
imitar *vt* to mimic
impactación *f* impaction; **— fecal** fecal impaction
impactado -da *adj (dent, etc.)* impacted
impacto *m* impact; **bajo —** low impact
impedimento *m* impediment

imperdible *m* safety pin
imperforación de himen *f* imperforate hymen
imperforado -da *adj* imperforate
impétigo *m* impetigo
implantación *f* implantation
implantar *vt* to implant
implante *m* implant; **— mamario** breast implant
imposible *adj* impossible
impotencia (sexual) *f* erectile dysfunction, (sexual) impotence *(ant)*
impotente *adj* impotent
impresión *f (dent, etc.)* impression
imprevisto -ta *adj* unexpected
impulsar *vt (sangre)* to pump *(blood)*
impulsivo -va *adj* impulsive
impulso *m (sexual, etc.)* drive
impureza *f* impurity
inactividad *f* inactivity
inactivo -va *adj* inactive
inadecuado -da *adj* unsuitable, inappropriate
inaguantable *adj* unbearable
inanición *f* starvation
inapropiado -da *adj* inappropriate
incapacidad *f* inability, disability
incapacitado -da *adj* disabled
incapacitante *adj* incapacitating, disabling
incapaz *adj* incapable, unable
incarcerado -da *adj* incarcerated
incendio *m* fire
incesto *m* incest
incestuoso -sa *adj* incestuous
incidencia *f* incidence
incidentaloma *m (Ang)* incidentaloma
incisión *f* incision; **— y drenaje** incision and drainage (I&D)
incisivo *m* incisor, front tooth
inclinar *vt* **— la cabeza** to nod; *vr* to lean, lean forward; **Inclínese hacia adelante.** .Lean forward.
incluido -da *adj (Esp, dent)* impacted
inclusión dentaria *f (Esp)* dental impaction

incoherente *adj* incoherent

incoloro -ra *adj* colorless

incombustible *adj* nonflammable

incomodidad *f* discomfort

incómodo -da *adj* uncomfortable

incompatible *adj* incompatible

incompetencia *f* incompetence; — **cervical** cervical incompetence

incompetente *adj* incompetent

incompleto -ta *adj* incomplete

inconsciente, inconiente *adj* unconscious, unaware

incontinencia *f* incontinence; — **de esfuerzo** stress incontinence; — **(urinaria) de urgencia** urge incontinence; — **fecal** fecal incontinence; — **por rebosamiento** overflow incontinence; — **urinaria** urinary incontinence

incontinente *adj* incontinent

incrementar *vt* to increase

incrustación *f* (*dent*) inlay

incubadora *f* incubator

incurable *adj* incurable

independiente *adj* independent

independizarse *vr* to become independent

indeseable *adj* undesirable

indetectable *adj* undetectable

indicación *f* indication; (*orden*) order

indicar *vt* to order

índice *m* index, score; — **de Apgar** Apgar score; — **de masa corporal (IMC)** body mass index (BMI)

indiferencia *f* indifference

indiferenciado -da *adj* undifferentiated

indigerido -da *adj* undigested

indigestión *f* indigestion

indinavir *m* indinavir

indistinto -ta *adj* indistinct

individuo *m* individual, person

indoloro -ra *adj* painless

indometacina *f* indomethacin

inducción *f* induction

inducido -da *adj* induced; — **por (el) ejercicio** exercise-induced

inducir *vt* to induce

industrializado -da *adj* (*alimento*) processed

ineficaz *adj* ineffective

inerte *adj* inert

inespecífico -ca *adj* nonspecific

inesperado -da *adj* unexpected

inestable *adj* unstable

inevitable *adj* unavoidable

infancia *f* childhood

infante *m* young child, child less than 7 years old

infantil *adj* infantile

infarto *m* infarct, infarction; — **cerebral** (non-hemorrhagic) stroke; — **de miocardio** myocardial infarction, heart attack (*fam*)

infección *f* infection; — **del tracto urinario (ITU)** urinary tract infection (UTI); — **de transmisión sexual (ITS)** sexually transmitted disease (STD); — **fúngica** (*form*) fungal infection; — **pélvica** pelvic inflammatory disease (PID); — **por hongos** fungal infection; — **respiratoria alta** upper respiratory tract infection; — **urinaria** urinary tract infection (UTI)

infeccioso -sa *adj* infectious; **enfermedad** — infectious disease

infectado -da *adj* infected; — **por** *or* **con** infected with

infectar *vt* to infect; *vr* to become infected

infectólogo -ga *mf* (*Amer*) infectious disease specialist

infeliz *adj* unhappy

inferior *adj* (*anat*) inferior, lower; — **a** lower than, below; **inferior a 70**..lower than 70..below 70

infertilidad *f* infertility

infestación *f* infestation

infestado -da *adj* infested; — **de** infested with

infestar *vt* to infest; *vr* — **con** *or* **de** to become infested with

infiltración *f* infiltration

infiltrante *adj* infiltrating

infiltrar *vt, vr* to infiltrate

inflado -da (del estómago) *adj* bloated

inflamable *adj* flammable, inflammable; **no** — nonflammable

inflamación *f* inflammation

inflamar *vt* to inflame; *vr* to become inflamed

inflamatorio -ria *adj* inflammatory

infliximab *m* infliximab

influenza *f* influenza, flu; — **porcina**

swine flu

información *f* information, data

infraorbitario -ria *adj* infraorbital

infrarrojo -ja *adj* infrared

infundir *vt* to infuse

infusión *f* infusion; (*de hierbas*) infusion, herbal tea

ingeniería genética *f* genetic engineering

ingerir *vt* to ingest

ingesta *f* intake; **— diaria admisible** tolerable daily intake

ingestión *f* ingestion

ingle *f* pubic area, groin

ingrediente *m* ingredient

ingresar *vt* to admit (*to the hospital*); *vr* to be admitted

ingreso *m* admission; **Ingresos** (*área del hospital*) Admitting

inguinal *adj* inguinal

inhalación *f* inhalation; **— de humo** smoke inhalation

inhalador *m* inhaler; **— de polvo seco** dry powder inhaler; **— dosificador** metered dose inhaler; **— nasal** nasal inhaler

inhalar *vt, vi* to inhale, breathe in; (*cocaína, etc.*) to sniff, to snort (*fam*) (*cocaine, etc.*)

inhibición *f* inhibition

inhibido -da *adj* inhibited

inhibidor -ra *adj* inhibiting; *m* inhibitor; **— de conversión de la angiotensina** angiotensin converting enzyme inhibitor; **— de fusión** fusion inhibitor; **— de la bomba de protones** proton pump inhibitor; **— de la colinesterasa** cholinesterase inhibitor; **— de la enzima convertidora de la angiotensina** angiotensin converting enzyme inhibitor; **— de la integrasa** integrase inhibitor; **— de la monoaminooxidasa** monoamine oxidase inhibitor; **— de la proteasa** protease inhibitor; **— no nucleósido de la transcriptasa inversa, — no nucleósido de la transcriptasa reversa** (*esp. Amer*) non-nucleoside reverse transcriptase inhibitor; **— nucleósido de la transcriptasa inversa, — nucleósido de la transcriptasa reversa** (*esp. Amer*) nucleoside re-

verse transcriptase inhibitor; **— selectivo de la recaptación de serotonina** selective serotonin reuptake inhibitor

inhibir *vt* to inhibit, (*el apetito, un deseo, etc.*) to curb

inicial *adj* initial; *fpl* initials

inicio *m* onset; **de — juvenil** juvenile-onset; **de — precoz** early-onset; **de — tardío** late-onset; **edad** *f* **de — age** at onset

injertar *vt* (*pp* **injertado** *or* **injerto**) to graft

injerto (*pp of* **injertar**) *m* graft; **— coronario** coronary artery bypass graft; **— cutáneo** skin graft; **— óseo** bone graft

inmadurez *f* immaturity

inmaduro -ra *adj* immature; (*fruta*) green, not yet ripe

inmediatamente *adv* immediately

inmediato -ta *adj* immediate

inmersión *f* immersion

inmóvil *adj* immobile

inmovilización *f* immobilization

inmovilizador *m* immobilizer; **— de hombro** shoulder immobilizer

inmovilizar *vt* to immobilize

inmune *adj* immune; **— a** immune to

inmunidad *f* immunity; **— colectiva** herd immunity; **— de grupo** *or* **de rebaño** herd immunity; **— frente a** immunity to

inmunitario -ria *adj* immune-related, immune

inmunización *f* immunization

inmunizador -ra *adj* immunizing

inmunizante *adj* immunizing

inmunizar *vt* to immunize

inmunocompetente *adj* immunocompetent

inmunocomprometido -da *adj* immunocompromised

inmunodeficiencia *f* immunodeficiency; **— variable común** common variable immunodeficiency

inmunodeficiente *adj* immunodeficient

inmunodepresión *f* immunodepression

inmunodepresor -ra *adj* immunodepressive

inmunodeprimido -da *adj* immunodepressed

inmunoglobulina *f* (*endógena*) immunoglobulin; (*exógena*) immune globulin

inmunología *f* immunology

inmunológico -ca *adj* immunological, immunologic, immune

inmunólogo -ga *mf* immunologist

inmunosupresión *f* immunosuppression

inmunosupresor *m* immunosuppressant

inmunosuprimido -da *adj* immunosuppressed

inmunoterapia *f* immunotherapy

inoculación *f* inoculation

inocular *vt* to inoculate

inodoro -ra *adj* odorless; *m* toilet, potty (*ped, fam*); **taza del —** toilet bowl

inofensivo -va *adj* (*que no hace daño*) harmless

inoperable *adj* inoperable

inorgánico -ca *adj* inorganic

inquieto -ta *adj* restless

INR *See* **razón internacional normalizada** *under* **razón**.

insaturado -da *adj* unsaturated

insecticida *m* insecticide

insecto *m* insect

inseguridad *f* insecurity

inseguro -ra *adj* insecure

inseminación *f* insemination; **— artificial** artificial insemination

inseminar *vt* to inseminate

insertar *vt* to insert

in situ, in situ

insolación *f* sunstroke, heatstroke

insoluble *adj* insoluble

insomnio *m* insomnia

insoportable *adj* unbearable

inspirar *vt, vi* to inhale, breathe in

instinto *m* instinct; **— maternal** maternal instinct

instrucción *f* instruction; *fpl* (*de un medicamento*) package insert

instructivo impreso *m* (*Mex, CA; pharm*) package insert

instrumental *m* equipment

instrumento *m* instrument

insuficiencia *f* insufficiency, failure; **— aórtica (mitral, etc.)** aortic (mitral, etc.) insufficiency *o* regur-

gitation; **— cardíaca congestiva** congestive heart failure; **— cervical** incompetent cervix; **— hepática** liver failure; **— renal (aguda)** (acute) renal insufficiency *o* failure; **— respiratoria** respiratory failure; **— suprarrenal** adrenal failure; **— venosa** venous insufficiency

insuficiente *adj* insufficient

insulina *f* insulin; **análogo de — de acción rápida** rapid-acting insulin analog; **— aspart, — asparta** (*OMS*) insulin aspart; **— de acción intermedia** intermediate-acting insulin; **— de acción prolongada** long-acting insulin; **— de acción rápida** rapid-acting insulin; **— glargina** insulin glargine; **— humana** human insulin; **— lenta** lente insulin; **— lispro** insulin lispro; **— NPH** NPH insulin; **— recombinante** recombinant insulin; **— regular** regular insulin; **— ultralenta** ultralente insulin; **— ultrarrápida** rapid-acting insulin analog; **ponerse —** (*fam*) to take insulin, to give oneself an insulin injection

insulinoma *m* insulinoma

insumos médicos *mpl* medical supplies

intacto -ta *adj* intact

integral *adj* (*holístico*) holistic; (*entero*) whole, whole-grain; **trigo —** whole wheat

intelecto *m* intellect

intelectual *adj* intellectual

intelectualizar *vi* (*psych*) to intellectualize

inteligencia *f* intelligence

inteligente *adj* intelligent

intensidad *f* intensity

intensificar *vt* to intensify

intensivista *mf* intensivist

intensivo -va *adj* intensive

intenso -sa *adj* intense

intentar *vt, vi* to try

intento *m* try

interacción *f* interaction; **— de drogas** drug interaction

interactuar *vi* to interact

intercambio *m* exchange; **— de agujas** needle exchange

interconsulta *f (form)* consult

intercostal *adj* intercostal

interferir *vi* to interfere

interferón *m* interferon; — **alfa,** — **beta, etc.** alpha interferon, beta interferon, etc.; — **pegilado** pegylated interferon

interior *adj* inner, interior, inside; *m* interior, inside

interiorizar *vt (psych)* to internalize

intermedio -dia *adj* intermediate

intermitente *adj* intermittent

internar *vt* to admit *(to the hospital)*, to hospitalize; *vr* to be admitted, to be hospitalized

internet *m&f* internet; **en** — on the internet

internista *mf* internist

interno -na *adj* internal, inner, inside; *(anat)* medial; *mf* intern

interpersonal *adj* interpersonal

interpretar *vt, vi* to interpret

intérprete *mf* interpreter

interrupción *f* interruption; — **voluntaria del embarazo** *(form)* (elective) abortion

intersticial *adj* interstitial

intertrocantéreo -a *adj (Esp)* intertrochanteric

intertrocantérico -ca *adj (Amer)* intertrochanteric

intervalo *m* interval

intervención *f* intervention

intervencionista *adj* interventional

interventricular *adj* interventricular

intervertebral *adj* intervertebral

intestinal *adj* intestinal

intestino *m* intestine, bowel, gut; — **delgado** small intestine *o* bowel; — **grueso** large intestine *o* bowel, colon

intimidad *f* intimacy, privacy, confidentiality

íntimo -ma *adj* intimate, private

intolerable *adj* intolerable, unbearable

intolerancia *f* intolerance

intolerante *adj* intolerant; — **a** intolerant of *o* to

intoxicación *f* intoxication, poisoning; — **alimentaria** food poisoning

intraabdominal *adj* intraabdominal

intraarticular *adj* intraarticular

intracraneal *adj* intracranial

intracraneano -na *adj* intracranial

intracutáneo -a *adj* intradermal

intradérmico -ca *adj* intradermal

intramuscular (IM) *adj* intramuscular (IM)

intranasal *adj* intranasal

intranquilo -la *adj* restless

intraocular *adj* intraocular

intraoperatorio -ria *adj* intraoperative

intrauterino -na *adj* intrauterine

intravenoso -sa (IV) *adj* intravenous (IV)

introducir *vt (insertar)* to insert

introspección *f* introspection

introvertido -da *adj* introverted; *mf* introvert

intubación *f* intubation

intubar *vt* to intubate

intususcepción *f* intussusception

inundación *f* flood

inusual *adj* unusual

inútil *adj* useless

invadir *vt* to invade

invaginación intestinal *f* intussusception

invalidante *adj (incapacitante)* disabling

invalidez *f (discapacidad)* disability

inválido -da *adj (discapacitado)* disabled; *mf* disabled person

invasivo -va *adj* invasive *(procedure, surgery)*; **mínimamente** — minimally invasive; **no** — noninvasive

invasor -ra *adj* invasive *(disease, etc.)*; **tumor** — invasive tumor

investigación *f* research; **en** — *(medicamento, etc.)* investigational

invierno *m* winter

invisible *adj* invisible

in vitro, in vitro

involuntario -ria *adj* involuntary

inyección *f* injection, shot *(fam)*; **¿Me van a poner una inyección?..** Are you going to give me an injection?

inyectable *adj* injectable

inyectar *vt* to inject, to give (someone) an injection; *vr* to inject oneself, to give oneself an injection

ion *m* ion

iontoforesis *f* iontophoresis

ipecacuana f ipecac; **jarabe** m **de —** syrup of ipecac

ir vi to go; **— al baño** (euph) to have a bowel movement, to go to the bathroom (euph); **— al médico** to go to the doctor; **— y venir** to come and go; **El dolor va y viene..** The pain comes and goes.

ira f anger, rage

irbesartán m irbesartan

iris m (pl **iris**) iris

iritis f iritis

irradiación f irradiation

irradiar vt (un tumor) to irradiate; vi (calor) to radiate; vr (dolor) to radiate

irregular adj irregular

irresecable adj unresectable

irreversible adj irreversible

irrigación f irrigation

irrigar vt to irrigate

irritabilidad f irritability

irritable adj irritable

irritación f irritation

irritante adj irritating; **agente** m **—** irritant; m irritant

irritar vt to irritate; vr to become irritated

irrompible adj unbreakable

islote m islet; **islotes pancreáticos** pancreatic islets

isoleucina f isoleucine

isométrico -ca adj isometric

isoniazida, isoniacida f isoniazid (INH)

isosorbida f isosorbide

isótopo m isotope

isotretinoína f isotretinoin

isquemia f ischemia; **— cerebral transitoria** (esp. Mex) transient ischemic attack (TIA)

isquémico -ca adj ischemic

isradipina f (esp. SA) isradipine

isradipino m isradipine

itraconazol m itraconazole

ITS abbr infección de transmisión sexual. See **infección**.

ITU abbr infección del tracto urinario. See **infección**.

IV See **intravenoso**.

ivermectina f ivermectin

izquierdo -da adj left; f left, left-hand side

J

jabón m soap

jadear vi to pant

jadeo m panting

jalea f (medicinal) jelly

jamón m ham

jaqueca f migraine headache, migraine (fam)

jarabe m syrup; **— para la tos** cough syrup

jardinero -ra mf gardener

jardín preescolar, jardín infantil, jardín de niños (Mex) m nursery school, preschool

jarra f pitcher

jefe -fa mf head; **— de enfermeras** head nurse; **— de la familia** head of the family

jején m gnat (type that bite), no-see-um (fam)

jelepate m (CA) bedbug

jengibre *m* (*bot*) ginger
jeringa *f* syringe; — **de goma** bulb syringe
jeringuilla *f* (*esp. Carib*) syringe
jet lag *m* (*Ang*) jet lag
jimagua *mf* (*Cub*) twin
jogging *m* (*Ang*) jogging
joroba *f* humpback, hunchback, hump
jorobado -da *adj* humpbacked; *mf* hunchback
joven *adj* young; *m* young man, young person; *f* young woman
juanete *m* bunion
judías *fpl* (*Esp*) beans
judo *m* judo
jugo *m* juice; — **de fruta** fruit juice
juicio *m* sanity
juntar *vt* (*dos objetos*) to join
Juramento Hipocrático *m* Hippocratic Oath
juvenil *adj* juvenile
juventud *f* youth

K

karate *m* karate
kava *m&f* (*bot*) kava
kernicterus *m* kernicterus
ketamina *f* ketamine
ketoconazol *m* ketoconazole
ketoprofeno *m* ketoprofen
ketorolaco *m* ketorolac
kilo (*fam*) *See* **kilogram**.
kilocaloría *f* kilocalorie
kilogramo *m* kilogram, kilo (*fam*)
kwashiorkor *m* kwashiorkor

L

laberintitis *f* labyrinthitis
laberinto *m* (*anat*) labyrinth
labetolol *m* labetolol
labial *adj* labial
labio *m* lip; (*genital*) labium (*form*), lip (*fam*); — **inferior** lower lip; —

leporino cleft lip; — **superior** upper lip

laboral *adj* work-related, occupational

laboratorio *m* laboratory; — **de cateterismo** catheterization laboratory, cath lab (*fam*)

laca *f* (*para el cabello, en aerosol*) hair spray

laceración *f* laceration

lacerar *vt* to lacerate

lacrimal *See* **lagrimal**.

lacrimógeno *m* tear gas

lactancia *f* lactation, breastfeeding; (*primer período de la vida*) infancy, period of breastfeeding; — **materna** (*form*) breastfeeding

lactante *mf* (*form*) infant, nursing infant

lactar *vi* to lactate

lactasa *f* lactase

lácteo -a *adj* pertaining to milk; **producto** — milk product

láctico -ca *adj* lactic

lactobacilo *m* lactobacillus

lactosa *f* lactose; **intolerancia a la** — lactose intolerance

lactulosa *f* lactulose

ladilla *f* crab louse, pubic louse, crab (*fam*)

lado *m* side; **por el lado de mi madre**..on my mother's side; **dormir de** — to sleep on one's side

lagaña *f* (*Amer*) eye secretions, sleep (*fam*)

lagartija *f* push-up

lágrima *f* tear

lagrimal *adj* lacrimal

laguna mental *f* blackout, lapse of memory

lamentar *vi* to be sorry; **Lo lamento**..I'm sorry (about that).

lamento *m* (*duelo*) grief

lamer *vt* to lick

laminaria *f* laminaria

laminectomía *f* laminectomy

lamivudina *f* lamivudine

lamotrigina *f* lamotrigine

lámpara *f* lamp; — **de calor** heat lamp; — **de hendidura** slitlamp; — **de noche** nightlight; — **de rayos ultravioleta** sunlamp; — **de Wood** Wood's lamp

lamparita de noche *f* nightlight

lampazo *m* (*bot*) burdock

lana *f* wool; — **de oveja** lamb's wool

lanceta *f* lancet

lanolina *f* lanolin

lansoprazol *m* lansoprazole

lanugo *m* lanugo

laparoscópico -ca *adj* laparoscopic

laparoscopia, laparoscopía (*Amer, esp. spoken*) *f* laparoscopy

laparoscopio *m* laparoscope

laparotomía *f* laparotomy; — **exploradora** exploratory laparotomy

largo -ga *adj* long; **a** — **plazo** long-term; **hacer más** — to lengthen; *m* length

laringe *f* larynx

laringectomía *f* laryngectomy

laríngeo -a *adj* laryngeal

laringitis *f* laryngitis

laringoplastia *f* laryngoplasty

laringoscopia, laringoscopía (*Amer, esp. spoken*) *f* laryngoscopy

laringoscopio *m* laryngoscope

larva migrans, larva migratoria *f* larva migrans; — — **cutánea** cutaneous larva migrans; — — **visceral** visceral larva migrans

láser *m* laser

lastimadura *f* minor injury

lastimar *vt* to hurt, injure; *vr* to get hurt, to hurt oneself; **¿Se lastimó?**.. Did you hurt yourself?...**¿Se lastimó la cabeza?**..Did you hurt your head?

lata *f* can

latanoprost *m* latanoprost

latente *adj* latent

lateral *adj* (*anat*) lateral

látex *m* latex

latido *m* beat; — **del corazón** heartbeat

latigazo cervical *m* whiplash

latir *vi* (*el corazón*) to beat

lavado *m* lavage; (*intestinal*) enema; — **broncoalveolar** bronchoalveolar lavage; — **gástrico** gastric lavage; — **peritoneal** peritoneal lavage; — **vaginal** douche

lavar *vt* to wash; *vr* — **el pelo (la cara, las manos, etc.)** to wash one's hair (one's face, one's hands, etc.)

lavativa *f* enema

laxante *adj & m* laxative; — **emoliente** stool softener
laxo -xa *adj* lax
lazo *m* (*obst*) loop; — **afectivo** bond, emotional bond
lb *See* **libra.**
L-carnitina *f* L-carnitine
leche *f* milk; — **baja en grasas** low-fat milk; — **bronca** (*Mex*) raw milk; — **condensada** condensed milk; — **cruda** raw milk; — **de cabra** goat's milk; — **descremada** *or* **desnatada** non-fat *o* skim milk; — **de soja** soy milk; — **de vaca** cow's milk; — **en polvo** powdered milk; — **entera** whole milk; — **evaporada** evaporated milk; — **materna** breast milk; — **pasteurizada** pasteurized milk; — **sin lactosa** lactose-free milk; — **sin procesar** raw milk;
leche de magnesia *f* milk of magnesia
lecho *m* bed, sickbed; — **de muerte** deathbed; — **ungueal** nail bed; — **vascular** vascular bed
lechoso -sa *adj* milky
lecitina *f* lecithin
lectura *f* (*de un instrumento*) reading
leer *vt, vi* to read; — **los labios** to lipread
legaña *f* (*Esp*) eye secretions, sleep (*fam*)
lego -ga *adj* (*opinión, etc.*) lay
legra *f* curette
legrado *m* curettage; — **por succión** suction curettage
legumbre *f* legume
leiomioma *m* leiomyoma; — **uterino** uterine leiomyoma, fibroid (*fam*)
leiomiosarcoma *m* leiomyosarcoma
leishmaniasis, leishmaniosis *f* leishmaniasis; — **cutánea** cutaneous leishmaniasis; — **mucocutánea** mucocutaneous leishmaniasis; — **visceral** visceral leishmaniasis
lejía *f* lye
lengua *f* tongue; — **saburral** coated tongue; **sacar la** — to stick out one's tongue; **Saque la lengua..** Stick out your tongue.
lenguaje *m* language, speech; — **corporal** body language

lengüeta *f* barb
lente *m&f* lens; — **bifocal** bifocal lens; — **de contacto (duro** *or* **rígido, blando)** (hard, soft) contact lens; — **progresivo** progressive lens; — **trifocal** trifocal lens; *mpl* glasses, eyeglasses; — **bifocales** bifocal glasses *o* eyeglasses, bifocals (*fam*); — **de lectura** reading glasses; — **oscuros** sunglasses; — **protectores** (*esp. Mex*) safety glasses *o* goggles; — **trifocales** trifocal glasses *o* eyeglasses, trifocals (*fam*)
lentigo *m* lentigo
lento -ta *adj* slow
lepra *f* leprosy, Hansen's disease; — **dimorfa** borderline leprosy; — **lepromatosa** lepromatous leprosy; — **tuberculoide** tuberculoid leprosy
lepromatoso -sa *adj* lepromatous
leptospirosis *f* leptospirosis
lesbiana *adj* lesbian; *f* lesbian, gay woman
lesión *f* lesion, injury; — **de la médula espinal** spinal cord injury; — **deportiva** sports injury; — **por sobrecarga** overuse syndrome
lesionar *vt* to injure; *vr* to get *o* become injured, to hurt oneself
letal *adj* lethal
letárgico -ca *adj* lethargic
letargo *m* lethargy
letra *f* handwriting
letrina *f* latrine
leucemia *f* leukemia; — **linfoblástica** *or* **linfocítica aguda** acute lymphoblastic *o* lymphocytic leukemia; — **linfocítica** *or* **linfática crónica** chronic lymphocytic leukemia; — **mieloide crónica** chronic myelogenous *o* myeloid leukemia; — **mieloide** *or* **mielógena aguda** acute myeloid *o* myelogenous leukemia
leucina *f* leucine
leucocito *m* leukocyte
leucoencefalopatía *f* leukoencephalopathy; — **multifocal progresiva** progressive multifocal leukoencephalopathy
leucoplaquia *f* leukoplakia
leuprorelina *f* leuprolide
levadura *f* (*frec. pl*) yeast; **infección**

f **por levaduras** yeast infection; — **de cerveza** brewer's yeast

levamisol *m* levamisol

levantamiento *m* — **de pesas** weight lifting

levantar *vt* to raise, to lift; **Levante la pierna..**Raise your leg; — **pesas** to lift weights, to work out; *vr* to get up, to stand (up)

leve *adj* (*herida*) slight, (*caso de enfermedad*) light, mild, (*fiebre, infección*) low-grade

levofloxacina *f* (*esp. Amer*) levofloxacin

levofloxacino *m* levofloxacin

levonorgestrel *m* levonorgestrel

levotiroxina *f* levothyroxine

liberación *f* release; **de — controlada** controlled-release, timed-release; **de — lenta** slow-release; **de — prolongada** extended-release, slow-release; **de — sostenida** sustained-release; — **del túnel carpiano** carpal tunnel release

liberador -ra *adj* releasing, eluting; — **de cobre,** — **de hormona, etc.** copper-releasing, hormone-releasing, etc.; — **de fármacos** (*stent*) drug-eluting

liberar *vt* to release, (*virus, etc.*) to shed

libido *f* libido

libra (lb) *f* pound (lb)

libre *adj* free

libreta *f* log; — **de autocontrol** (*del diabético*) glucose log

lidiar *vi* — **con** to cope with

lidocaína *f* lidocaine

liendre *f* nit

ligado -da *adj* linked; — **al cromosoma X** X-linked; — **al sexo** sex-linked

ligadura *f* ligation; — **de trompas** or **tubárica** tubal ligation

ligamento *m* ligament

ligar *vt* to attach

ligero -ra *adj* light, slight; gentle

lima *f* file (*for nails, etc.*); (*fruta*) lime (*fruit*); — **de uñas** nail file

limar *vt* to file

limitar *vt* to limit

límite *adj* (*psych*) borderline; *m* limit; **dentro de límites normales** within normal limits; — **inferior normal** lower limit of normal; — **superior normal** upper limit of normal

limítrofe *adj* (*psych*) borderline

limón *m* lemon

limpiar *vt* to clean; *vr* (*después de defecar*) to wipe (oneself)

limpieza *f* cleaning; (*aseo*) cleanliness

limpio -pia *adj* clean

lindano *m* lindane

línea *f* line, streak; (*de una persona*) figure; — **de la(s) encía(s)** gum line; — **media (del cuerpo)** midline

linezolid *m* linezolid

linfa *f* lymph

linfadenitis *f* lymphadenitis

linfangitis *f* lymphangitis

linfático -ca *adj* lymphatic

linfedema *m* lymphedema

linfocito *m* lymphocyte; — **B,** — **CD4, etc.** B lymphocyte, CD4 lymphocyte, etc.

linfogranuloma venéreo *m* lymphogranuloma venereum (LGV)

linfoide *adj* lymphoid

linfoma *m* lymphoma; — **de células B** B cell lymphoma; — **de células T** T cell lymphoma; — **del tejido linfoide asociado a mucosas** or — **MALT** mucosa-associated lymphoid tissue (MALT) lymphoma; — **no Hodgkin** or **no hodgkiniano** non-Hodgkin's lymphoma

linimento *m* liniment

linoleico -ca *adj* linoleic

liofilizado -da *adj* lyophilized, freeze-dried

lipasa *f* lipase

lípido *m* lipid

lipodistrofia *f* lipodystrophy

lipoma *m* lipoma

lipoproteína *f* lipoprotein; — **de alta densidad** high density lipoprotein (HDL); — **de baja densidad** low density lipoprotein (LDL); — **de muy baja densidad** very low density lipoprotein (VLDL)

liposarcoma *m* liposarcoma

liposucción *f* liposuction

liquen plano *m* lichen planus

líquido -da *adj* liquid, runny; *m* li-

quid, fluid; — **amniótico** amniotic
fluid; — **cefalorraquídeo** (LCR)
cerebrospinal fluid (CSF); — **pleu-**
ral pleural fluid; — **seminal** seminal fluid; — **sinovial** synovial fluid
lisiado -da *adj* injured, disabled,
crippled (*ant*); *mf* injured person,
disabled person, cripple (*ant*)
lisiar *vt* to injure, to disable, to cripple (*ant*)
lisina *f* lysine
lisinopril *m* lisinopril
lisis *f* lysis; — **de adherencias** lysis
of adhesions
liso -sa *adj* smooth
lista de espera *f* waiting list
listeriosis *f* listeriosis
litio *m* lithium
litotricia, litotripsia (*esp. Mex*) *f*
lithotripsy; — **extracorpórea por**
ondas de choque extracorporeal
shock wave lithotripsy
litro *m* liter
liviano -na *adj* light (*in weight*)
llaga *f* ulcer, sore
llama *f* flame
llamada *f* call; (*por biper*) page; —
de atención wakeup call
llamar *vt, vi* to call; (*por biper*) to
page
llenar *vt* to fill
lleno -na *adj* full
llevar *vt* (*ropa, etc.*) to wear
llorando -da *adj* tearful
llorar *vi* to cry
lluvia radiactiva *f* fallout
lobar *adj* lobar
lobectomía *f* lobectomy
lobelia *f* (*bot*) lobelia
lobotomía *f* lobotomy
lobular *adj* lobar
lóbulo *m* lobe; (*de la oreja*) earlobe
local *adj* local
localización *f* localization
localizado -da *adj* localized
loción *f* lotion
loco -ca *adj* crazy, insane; **volver (a**

alguien) — to drive (someone)
crazy; **volverse** — to go crazy; *mf*
crazy person
locura *f* insanity, craziness
logopeda *mf* (*form*) speech pathologist, speech therapist
lombriz *f* (*pl* **-brices**) worm, intestinal worm; — **solitaria** tapeworm
longevidad *f* longevity
longitud *f* length; — **de onda** wavelength
loperamida *f* loperamide
lopinavir *m* lopinavir
loquios *mpl* lochia
loracepam *m* lorazepam
loratadina *f* loratadine
lorazepam *m* lorazepam
lordosis *f* lordosis
losartán *m* losartan
lote *m* (*pharm*) lot
lovastatina *f* lovastatin
LSD *See* **dietilamida del ácido lisér-**
gico.
lubricación *f* lubrication
lubricante *adj & m* lubricant
lubricar *vt* to lubricate
luces *pl of* **luz**
lucha *f* battle; — **contra el SIDA**
battle against AIDS
lugar del trabajo *m* workplace
lumbar *adj* lumbar
lumpectomía *f* (*Ang*) lumpectomy
lunar *m* mole
lupa *f* magnifying glass, hand lens
lúpulo *m* (*bot*) hops
lupus *m* lupus; — **(eritematoso) dis-**
coide discoid lupus; — **eritema-**
toso sistémico *or* **diseminado** systemic lupus erythematosus (SLE)
luteínico -ca *adj* luteal
lúteo -a *adj* luteal
luto *m* grief (*due to death*)
luxación *f* (*form*) dislocation
luxar *vt* to dislocate; *vr* to become
dislocated
luz *f* (*pl* **luces**) light; — **del sol**
sunlight

M

macerar *vt* to macerate
macho *adj* male
machucadura *f* mash, small crush injury
machucar *vt* to mash, crush
machucón *m* mash, small crush injury
macrobiótico -ca *adj* macrobiotic
madrastra *f* stepmother
madre *f* mother; — **biológica** biological mother; — **subrogada, — de alquiler** (*fam*) surrogate mother
madrugada *f* early morning (*before dawn*)
madurar *vi* to mature; (*un absceso*) to come to a head
madurez *f* maturity
maduro -ra *adj* mature; (*fruta*) ripe
maestro -tra *mf* teacher
magnesio *m* magnesium
magro -gra *adj* (*carne*) lean
magullado -da *adj* bruised, sore
magulladura *f* bruise
magullar *vt* to bruise; *vr* to bruise, to get bruised
maicena *f* cornstarch
maíz *m* corn
mal *adj See* **malo**; *adv* bad, sick; **sentirse —** to feel bad, to feel sick; **Me siento mal por haberla maltratado**..I feel bad for having mistreated her...**Me siento mal del estómago**.. I feel sick to my stomach; *m* illness, sickness, ailment, disease; — **del pinto** (*esp. Mex*) pinta, tropical skin infection; — **de montaña** mountain sickness; — **de ojo** evil eye, pediatric folk illness believed to occur when a person with magical powers eyes an infant with ill intent (*in some areas this applies to adults as well*); — **de orín** (*fam*) urinary tract infection; — **de Pott** Pott's disease
malabsorción *f* malabsorption
malaria *f* malaria
malatión *m* malathion

maléolo *m* malleolus
malestar *m* malaise, vague illness
maletín del médico *m* doctor's bag
malformación *f* malformation; — **arteriovenosa** arteriovenous malformation
malignidad *f* malignancy
maligno -na *adj* malignant
malla *f* mesh
malo -la *adj* bad
maloclusión *f* malocclusion
malos tratos *See* **maltrato**.
maltratado -da *adj* abused, battered; **refugio para mujeres maltratadas** battered women's shelter
maltratar *vt* to mistreat, to abuse
maltrato *m* mistreatment, abuse; — **a las personas mayores** elderly abuse; — **físico** physical abuse; — **infantil** child abuse; — **psicológico** psychological abuse
malvavisco *m* (*bot*) marshmallow
mama *f* (female) breast
mamá *f* (*pl* **mamás**) mom
mamadera *f* (*Amer, biberón*) baby bottle
mamar *vi* to nurse, to suck (*at mother's breast*); **dar de —** to breastfeed
mamario -ria *adj* mammary
mami *f* (*pl* **mamis**) mommy
mamila *f* (*de un biberón*) nipple (*of a baby bottle*)
mamita *f* mommy
mamografía *f* (*técnica imagenológica*) mammography; (*estudio imagenológico*) mammogram; — **digital** digital mammography; digital mammogram
mamoplastia *f* mammoplasty; — **de aumento** breast augmentation
mancha *f* spot, stain; — **en vino de Oporto** port-wine stain
manco -ca *adj* one-handed, one-armed
mandíbula *f* jaw, lower jaw, jawbone
mandil *m* apron; — **de plomo** lead

apron
mandrágora *f* (*bot*) ginseng
manejar *vt, vi* to manage; (*un vehículo*) to drive
manejo *m* management; — **del dolor** pain management
manga *f* sleeve; **camisa de — larga** long sleeve *o* long-sleeved shirt
manganeso *m* manganese
manguera *f* hose, tube
manguito *m* cuff; — **del tensiómetro** *or* **esfigmomanómetro** blood pressure cuff; — **rotador** rotator cuff
maní *m* peanut
manía *f* mania
maníaco -ca *adj* manic
maníaco-depresivo -va *adj* manic-depressive
manicomio *m* (*ant*) psychiatric hospital, insane asylum (*ant*)
manicura *f* manicure
manifestación *f* manifestation
maniobra *f* maneuver; — **de Heimlich** Heimlich maneuver
maniobrar *vt, vi* to maneuver
manipulación *f* manipulation
manipulador -ra *adj* manipulative; *mf* — **de alimentos** food handler
manipular *vt* to manipulate
mano *f* hand; — **péndula** wrist drop
manometría *f* manometry
manta *f* blanket, light blanket; — **térmica** *or* **eléctrica** electric blanket
manteca *f* cooking grease (*of animal origin*); — **de cerdo** lard
mantener *vt* to maintain
mantenimiento *m* maintenance; — **con metadona** methadone maintenance
mantequilla *f* butter; — **de maní** *or* **cacahuate** peanut butter
manual *adj* manual, handheld
manubrio *m* manubrium
manzana *f* apple; — **de Adán** (*esp. Mex*) Adam's apple
manzanilla *f* (*bot*) chamomile
mañana *adv* tomorrow; **pasado —** the day after tomorrow; *f* morning
mapache *m* raccoon
maquillaje *m* makeup, cosmetic(s)
maquillarse *vr* to put on makeup
máquina de afeitar *f* shaver, electric

shaver
maquinilla de afeitar *f* (*Esp*) shaver, electric shaver
marca *f* mark; — **de nacimiento** birthmark
marcador *m* marker
marcapasos *m* (*pl* **-sos**) pacemaker
marcha *f* gait
mareado -da *adj* dizzy, lightheaded, faint
mareo *m* dizziness, lightheadedness, (*en avión*) airsickness, (*en barco*) seasickness, (*en vehículo*) carsickness, (*producido por el movimiento en general*) motion sickness; **dar- (le) (a uno) —** to make (one) dizzy; **tener —** to feel dizzy, to feel lightheaded
margarina *f* margarine
margen *m* margin, border, edge
marido *m* husband
marihuana, mariguana (*Mex*) *f* marijuana, pot (*fam*), grass (*fam*)
marisco *m* (*frec. pl*) shellfish
marital *adj* marital
marrón *adj* brown
martillo *m* hammer
más *adj* (*comp and super of* **mucho**) more; **más pastillas**..more pills; *adv* more, most; **una opción más conservadora**..a more conservative option...**la opción más conservadora de las tres**..the most conservative option of the three; *n* más; — **de** more than (*a number*); **más de 12**..more than 12; — **que** more than; **más que ayer**..more than yesterday; [*Nota: Muchos adjetivos en inglés toman una forma comparativa en una sola palabra:* redder (más rojo), bigger (más grande), *etc. Lo mismo se aplica a las formas superlativas* (reddest, biggest, *etc.*)]
masa *f* mass, lump; — **muscular** muscle mass; — **ósea** bone mass
masaje *m* massage; — **cardíaco** cardiac massage; — **cardíaco externo** chest compressions; **dar un —** *or* **dar —** (*esp. Mex*) to give a massage
masajear *vt* to massage
masajista *m* massage therapist, body

worker

máscara f mask, face mask, (*para filtrar el aire*) respirator; — **de oxígeno** oxygen mask

mascarilla f mask, face mask, (*para filtrar el aire*) respirator; — **de oxígeno** oxygen mask; — **quirúrgica** surgical mask

mascota f pet

masculinidad f masculinity, manhood

masculino -na *adj* masculine, male

masivo -va *adj* massive

masoquismo m masochism

masoquista mf masochist

mastectomía f mastectomy; — **radical modificada** modified radical mastectomy

masticable *adj* chewable

masticar vt, vi to chew

mastitis f mastitis

mastocitosis f mastocytosis

mastoidectomía f mastoidectomy

mastoideo -a *adj* mastoid

mastoiditis f mastoiditis

masturbación f masturbation

masturbar vt, vr to masturbate

matar vt to kill

matasanos mf (*pl* **-nos**) quack

materia f matter

material m material, equipment

maternal *adj* maternal, motherly

maternidad f maternity

materno -na *adj* maternal; **tío** — maternal uncle

matricaria f (*bot*) feverfew

matrimonial *adj* marital; **problemas matrimoniales** marital problems

matriz f (*pl* **-trices**) matrix; (*útero*) uterus; — **ungueal** nail matrix

maxilar *adj* maxillary; m jaw, jawbone; — **inferior** lower jaw; — **superior** maxilla, upper jaw

maxilofacial *adj* maxillofacial

maximizar vt to maximize

máximo -ma *adj* maximum, maximal; m maximum

mayor (*comp of* **grande**) *adj* bigger, larger; older; (*anat, surg*) major

mear vt, vi (*vulg*) to urinate, to pee (*fam*), to piss (*vulg*)

meato m meatus

mebendazol m mebendazole

mecánico -ca *adj* mechanical; mf mechanic

mecanismo m mechanism; — **de defensa** or **defensivo** defense mechanism

mecha f wick

meclozina f meclizine; [*Nota: la* i *no es un error de imprenta.*]

meconio m meconium

medial *adj* (*anat*) medial

Media Luna Roja f Red Crescent

mediano -na *adj* medium; (*nervio*) median; f (*stat*) median; — **de peso** median weight, median of the weights

medias fpl hose, stockings; — **de compresión** or **compresivas** compression stockings; — **elásticas** support hose

mediastínico -ca *adj* mediastinal

mediastino m mediastinum

mediastinoscopia, mediastinoscopía (*Amer, esp. spoken*) f mediastinoscopy

medicado -da *adj* (*champú, etc.*) medicated

medicamento m medication, medicine, drug

medicar vt to medicate

medicina f medicine; (*medicamento*) medicine, medication; — **alternativa** alternative medicine; — **basada en la evidencia** evidence-based medicine; — **de familia** family medicine, family practice; — **de las adicciones** or **de la adicción** addiction medicine; — **del trabajo** occupational medicine; — **deportiva** sports medicine; — **familiar** family medicine, family practice; — **física** physical medicine; — **interna** internal medicine; — **laboral** occupational medicine; — **nuclear** nuclear medicine; — **popular** folk medicine; — **preventiva** preventive medicine; — **socializada** socialized medicine; — **tradicional** folk medicine; — **veterinaria** veterinary medicine

medicinal *adj* medicinal; (*champú, etc.*) medicated

médico -ca *adj* medical; m doctor, physician; — **de atención prima-**

ria primary care physician *o* doctor; — **de cabecera** family physician *o* doctor, personal physician, primary care physician *o* doctor; — **de familia** family practice physician *o* doctor; family physician *o* doctor; — **de guardia** physician *o* doctor on call, on-call physician *o* doctor; — **de la familia** family physician *o* doctor; — **familiar** (*Mex*) family practice physician *o* doctor; — **forense** coroner; — **general** *or* **generalista** general practitioner; — **personal** personal physician; — **primario** (*Esp*) primary care physician *o* doctor; — **privado** private physician *o* doctor; — **residente** resident; — **tratante** attending physician, treating physician

medicolegal *adj* medicolegal

medida *f* measure, measurement; **medidas heroicas** heroic measures

medidor *m* meter, measuring device, monitor; — **de glucosa** glucose meter *o* monitor

medio -dia *adj* half, half a, a half; (*stat*) mean, average; middle, mid-; **dedo** — middle finger; — **ciclo** mid-cycle; — **dormido** half asleep; — **hermana** half sister; — **hermano** half brother; — **pastilla** half a pill, a half pill; **peso** — mean *or* average weight; *m* middle; medium; — **ambiente** environment; — **de contraste** contrast medium, contrast, (*fam*); *f* mean, average

mediodía *m* noon

medir *vt* to measure

meditación *f* meditation

meditar *vi* to meditate

medroxiprogesterona *f* medroxyprogesterone

médula *f* medulla; marrow; — **espinal** spinal cord; — **ósea** bone marrow

medular *adj* medullary

medusa *f* jellyfish

mefloquina *f* mefloquin

megacolon *m* megacolon

megadosis *f* (*pl* -sis) megadose

megestrol *m* megestrol

meglumina *f* meglumine

mejilla *f* cheek

mejor (*comp of* **bueno** *and* **bien**) *adj* & *adv* better

mejorar *vt* to improve, to make better; *vr* to improve, get better

mejoría *f* improvement

melancolía *f* melancholy

melanina *f* melanin

melanoma *m* melanoma

melarsoprol *m* melarsoprol

melasma *m* melasma

melatonina *f* melatonin

melfalán *m* melphalan

mellizo -za *adj* & *mf* twin, fraternal twin

membrana *f* membrane, web; — **esofágica** esophageal web; — **mucosa** mucous membrane; — **timpánica** tympanic membrane; — **vitelina** yolk sac

memoria *f* memory, recall; — **a corto plazo** short-term memory; — **a largo plazo** long-term memory

menarquia, menarca (*Amer*) *f* menarche

meninge *f* meninx; [*Nota: en inglés se usa casi siempre el plural*: meninges.]

meningioma *m* meningioma

meningitis *f* meningitis

meningocele *m* meningocele

meningocócico -ca *adj* meningococcal

meningococo *m* meningococcus

meniscal *adj* meniscal

meniscectomía *f* meniscectomy

menisco *m* meniscus; **rotura de** — torn meniscus

menopausia *f* menopause

menopáusico -ca *adj* menopausal

menor (*comp of* **pequeño**) *adj* smaller; younger; least; (*anat, surg*) minor; **el menor tamaño**..the smaller size...**la hermana menor**..the younger sister...**el menor riesgo posible**..the least possible risk; *mf* (*de edad*) minor; — **emancipado** emacipated minor

menos *adj* (*comp de* **poco**) less; — **náusea**..less nausea; — **de** less than; **menos de 70**..less than 70; **menos lesiones de las que tenía antes**..less lesions than you had

menstruación f menstruation, (menstrual) period

before; *adv* less, least; **menos eficaz que el otro**..less effective than the other...**el menos eficaz de todos**..the least effective of all; — **que** less than; **menos que antes**.. less than before

menstrual *adj* menstrual

menstruar *vi* to menstruate

menta f (*bot*) mint; — **verde** spearmint

mental *adj* mental

mente f mind

mentiroso -sa *mf* **compulsivo** pathological liar

mentol *m* menthol

mentón *m* chin

mentoniano -na *adj* mental, pertaining to the chin

menudo *adj* **a** — often, frequently

mepacrina f quinacrine

meperidina f meperidine

mercaptopurina f mercaptopurine

mercurio *m* mercury

merienda f snack

mes *m* month

mesa f table, exam table; — **basculante** tilt table; — **de cirugía** operating table; — **de exploración** (*form*) examination table, exam table; — **de operaciones** operating table

mesalazina f mesalamine; [*Nota: la m no es un error de imprenta.*]

mescalina, mezcalina f mescaline

mesencéfalo *m* midbrain

mesentérico -ca *adj* mesenteric

mesenterio *m* mesentery

mesotelioma *m* mesothelioma

mesoterapia f mesotherapy

meta f goal

metabólico -ca *adj* metabolic

metabolismo *m* metabolism; — **basal** basal metabolism

metacarpiano -na *adj* & *m* metacarpal

metacualona f methaqualone

metadona f methadone

metal *m* metal; — **pesado** heavy metal

metálico -ca *adj* metallic

metamizol *m* methimazole

metanfetamina f methamphetamine

metano *m* methane

metanol *m* methanol, methyl alcohol

metaproterenol *m* metaproterenol

metastásico -ca *adj* metastatic

metástasis f (*pl* -sis) metastasis

metastatizar *vi* to metastasize

metatarsiano -na *adj* & *m* metatarsal

metaxalona f metaxalone

meter *vt* (*insertar*) to insert; *vr* — **el dedo en la nariz** (*para sacarse los mocos*) to pick one's nose

metformina f metformin

meticilina f methicillin

metilcelulosa f methylcellulose

metildopa f methyldopa

metilendioxianfetamina (MDA) f methylene dioxyamphetamine (MDA)

metilendioximetanfetamina, metilenodioximetanfetamina (MDMA) f methylene dioxymethamphetamine (MDMA), ecstacy (*fam*)

metilfenidato *m* methylphenidate

metimazol *m* methimazole

metionina f methionine

metisergida f methysergide

metocarbamol *m* methocarbamol

metoclopramida f metoclopramide

método *m* method, technique; — **del ritmo** *or* **del calendario** rhythm method; — **Lamaze** Lamaze method *o* technique

metolazona f metolazone

metoprolol *m* metoprolol

metotrexato, metotrexate *m* methotrexate

metralla f shrapnel

metro *m* meter; — **cuadrado** square meter

metronidazol *m* metronidazole

mezcal *m* mescal

mezcla f mixture

mezclar *vt* to mix

mezquino *m* (*Mex, CA*) wart

mialgia f myalgia

miastenia gravis, miastenia grave f myasthenia gravis

miconazol *m* miconazole

micosis fungoides f mycosis fungoides

micótico -ca *adj* mycotic, fungal

microalbuminuria f microalbuminu-

ria
microbiano -na *adj* microbial
microbio *m* microbe, microorganism, germ (*fam*)
microbiología *f* microbiology
microcirugía *f* microsurgery
microflora *f* flora
microgramo *m* microgram
micrometástasis *f* (*pl* **-sis**) micrometastasis
micronutriente *m* micronutrient
microondas *f* microwave [*Nota: en inglés la forma singular es más común.*]
microorganismo *m* microorganism, organism, germ (*fam*)
microscopia, microscopía *f* microscopy
microscópico -ca *adj* microscopic
microscopio *m* microscope; — **de luz** light microscope; — **electrónico** electron microscope
microvascular *adj* microvascular
midodrina *f* midodrine
miedo *m* fear; **tener** — to be afraid
miel (de abeja) *f* honey
mielina *f* myelin
mielografía *f* (*técnica imagenológica*) myelography; (*estudio imagenológico*) myelogram
mieloma múltiple *m* multiple myeloma
mielomeningocele *m* myelomeningocele
mieloproliferativo -va *adj* myeloproliferative
miembro *m* member, limb; (*fam, pene*) penis, member (*fam*)
migraña *f* migraine headache, migraine
milagro *m* miracle
milenrama *f* (*bot*) yarrow
milia *f* milia
miliar *adj* miliary
miliaria *f* miliaria, heat rash (*fam*), prickly heat (*fam*)
miligramo *m* milligram
mililitro *m* milliliter
milímetro *m* millimeter
milisegundo *m* millisecond
mimar *vt* to pamper, coddle, spoil
mime *m* (*PR, SD*) biting gnat
mineral *adj* & *m* mineral

minero -ra *mf* miner
minimizar *vt* to minimize
mínimo -ma *adj* minimum, minimal; *m* minimum
minociclina *f* minocycline
minoxidil *m* minoxidil
minusvalía *f* disability (*esp. partial*)
minusválido -da *adj* disabled (*esp. partially*)
minuto *m* minute
miocárdico -ca *adj* myocardial
miocardio *m* myocardium
miocardiopatía *f* cardiomyopathy; — **dilatada** dilated cardiomyopathy; — **hipertrófica** hypertrophic cardiomyopathy; — **restrictiva** restrictive cardiomyopathy
miocarditis *f* myocarditis
mioglobina *f* myoglobin
mioma *m* leiomyoma, myoma; — **uterino** uterine leiomyoma *o* myoma, fibroid (*fam*)
miopatía *f* myopathy
miope *adj* myopic, nearsighted (*fam*)
miopía *f* myopia, nearsightedness (*fam*)
miositis *f* myositis
mirada *f* gaze
mirar *vi* to look; **Mire hacia abajo..** Look downward.
miringitis *f* myringitis
miringoplastia *f* myringoplasty
mirtazapina *f* mirtazapine
miseria *f* misery
mitad *f* half; middle; **Tome la mitad de una pastilla..** Take half a pill.
mitral *adj* mitral
mixedema *m* myxedema
mixoma *m* myxoma
mixto -ta *adj* mixed (*in medical nomenclature*)
moco *m* mucus
modelo a seguir *m* role model
moderación *f* moderation
moderado -da *adj* moderate;
modificación *f* modification; — **de (la) conducta** behavior modification
modificado -da *adj* modified
modificador *m* modifier; — **de la respuesta biológica** biological response modifier
modificar *vt* to modify

modulador *m* modulator; — **selectivo de los receptores estrogénicos** *or* **de estrógenos** selective estrogen receptor modulator

mofeta *f* (*esp. Esp*) skunk

moho *m* mold, mildew

moisés *m* (*pl* -**sés**) cradle, bassinet

mojado -da *adj* wet, damp

mojar *vt* to wet; — **la cama** to wet the bed; *vr* to get wet

mola *f* (*obst*) mole; — **hidatiforme** hydatidiform mole

molar *adj* (*obst*) molar; *m* (*dent*) molar; **tercer** — third molar

molde *m* (*dent, etc.*) mold

moldear *vt* to mold

molécula *f* molecule

molecular *adj* molecular

moler *vt* to grind, crush

molestar *vt* to bother, to upset, to tease; (*sexualmente*) to fondle, to molest; **Me molesta el brazo**..My arm is bothering me...**¿Ha sido molestada?**..Has she been molested? *vr* to get *o* become upset

molestia *f* discomfort, (*frec. pl*) trouble; **Tengo molestias en el pie**..I have trouble with my foot.

molesto -ta *adj* annoying, irritating; (*trastornado*) upset

mollera *f* fontanelle *o* fontanel

molusco contagioso *m* molluscum contagiosum

mometasona *f* mometasone

monitor *m* monitor; — **cardíaco** cardiac monitor; — **fetal** fetal heart monitor

monitorear *vt* (*Amer*) to monitor

monitoreo *m* (*Amer*) monitoring

monitorización *f* (*Esp*) monitoring

monitorizar *vt* (*Esp*) to monitor

monoclonal *adj* monoclonal

monogamia *f* monogamy

monógamo -ma *adj* monogamous

monoinsaturado -da *adj* monounsaturated

mononucleosis *f* mononucleosis

monóxido de carbono *m* carbon monoxide

monstruo *m* monster; — **de Gila** Gila monster

montaña *f* mountain

montañismo *m* mountaineering

montelukast *m* montelukast

montura *f* (*Esp, para lentes*) frames (*for eyeglasses*)

morado -da *adj* purple; *m* bruise

moradura *f* bruise

mórbido -da *adj* morbid

morbilidad *f* morbidity

mordedura *f* bite (*wound*)

morder *vt, vi* to bite

mordida *f* (*dent*) bite

moreno -na *adj* dark, (*azúcar, pan*) brown

morete *m* bruise

moretón *m* bruise; **hacerse** *or* **salirle moretones** to bruise, get bruises, to get bruised

morfea *f* morphea

morfina *f* morphine

morfología *f* morphology

morgue *f* morgue

morir *vi, vr* (*pp* **muerto**) to die, expire; — **de hambre** to starve

mormado -da *adj* (*Mex, fam*) congested, having nasal congestion

mortal *adj* fatal, deadly

mortalidad *f* mortality, death rate; — **infantil** infant mortality

mortinato -ta *adj* (*form*) stillborn

mosca *f* fly; — **doméstica** housefly; — **volante** (*ophth*) floater

mosquito *m* mosquito

mostrar *vt* to show

mota *f* (*Mex, CA; fam*) marijuana, pot (*fam*), grass (*fam*)

motilidad *f* motility; — **espermática** sperm motility

motivación *f* motivation

motivar *vt* to motivate

motocicleta, moto (*fam*) *f* motorcycle

motoneta *f* scooter

motor -ra *adj* (*neuro*) motor

mover *vi, vr* to move, to wiggle; **No se mueva**..Don't move...**Mueva los dedos del pie**..Wiggle your toes.

móvil *adj* mobile

movilidad *f* mobility, motility; — **de los espermatozoides** sperm motility

movilización *f* mobilization; — **pasiva** passive mobilization

movilizar *vt* to mobilize

movimiento *m* movement, motion; **movimientos oculares rápidos**

rapid eye movements (REM);
rango de — range of motion
moxibustión *f* moxibustion
muchacho -cha *m* boy, child; *f* girl
mucho -cha *adj* (*comp and super*
más) much, a lot of (*fam*), (*plural*)
many, a lot of (*fam*); **mucho dolor**..
much pain..a lot of pain...**muchas**
picaduras..many bites..a lot of
bites; *adv* much, a lot; **mucho peor**
..much worse..a lot worse
mucinoso -sa *adj* mucinous
mucocele *m* mucocele
mucocutáneo -a *adj* mucocutaneous
mucolítico -ca *adj & m* mucolytic
mucormicosis *f* mucormycosis
mucosa *f* mucosa
mucosidad *f* mucus
mucoso -sa *adj* mucous
mudez *f* mutism
mudo -da *adj & mf* mute
muela *f* molar, back tooth (*fam*),
tooth; **— del juicio** *or* **cordal**
wisdom tooth
muerte *f* death; **— cerebral** brain
death; **— digna** death with dignity;
— natural natural death; **— pia-**
dosa mercy killing; **— súbita** sudden death
muerto -ta (*pp of* **morir**) *adj* dead,
deceased; *mf* dead person, corpse
muestra *f* sample, specimen
mujer *f* woman, (*fam, esposa*) wife
muleta *f* crutch
multidisciplinar *adj* (*Esp*) multidisciplinary
multidisciplinario -ria *adj* (*Amer*)
multidisciplinary

multifactorial *adj* multifactorial
multifocal *adj* multifocal
multinodular *adj* multinodular
múltiple *adj* multiple
multiplicar *vt, vr* to multiply
multivitamínico -ca *adj & m* multivitamin
muñeca *f* wrist
muñón *m* (*anat*) stump
mupirocina *f* mupirocin
murciélago *m* (*zool*) bat
muscular *adj* muscular (*pertaining to*
muscle)
músculo *m* muscle; **— bíceps** biceps
muscle, biceps; **— cuádriceps**
quadriceps muscle, quadriceps; **—**
deltoides deltoid muscle, deltoid;
— gastrocnemio or **gemelo** gastrocnemius muscle, gastrocnemius;
— glúteo gluteus muscle, gluteus;
— liso smooth muscle; **— pectoral**
pectoral muscle, pectoral; **— psoas**
psoas muscle, psoas; **— sóleo**
soleus muscle, soleus; **— trapecio**
trapezius muscle, trapezius; **—**
tríceps triceps muscle, triceps
musculoesquelético -ca *adj* musculoskeletal
musculoso -sa *adj* muscular (*person*)
músico -ca *mf* musician
muslo *m* thigh
mutación *f* mutation
mutante *adj & m* mutant
mutilación *f* mutilation
mutilar *vt* to mutilate
mutismo *m* mutism; **— selectivo** *or*
electivo elective mutism

N

nabumetona *f* nabumetone
nacer *vi* to be born
nacido -da (*pp of* nacer) *adj* born; —
  muerto stillborn; recién — newborn; *m* (*forúnculo*) boil
nacimiento *m* birth; (ciego, sordo,
  etc.) de — (blind, deaf, etc.) from
  birth
nadar *vi* to swim; ir a — to go swimming
nadolol *m* nadolol
nailon *m* nylon
nalga *f* (*frec. pl*) buttock
naloxona *f* naloxone
napalm *m* napalm
naproxeno, naproxén *m* naproxen
naranja *adj* orange; *f* (*fruta*) orange
naratriptán *m* naratriptan
narcisismo *m* narcissism
narcisista *adj* narcissistic; *mf* narcissist
narcolepsia *f* narcolepsy
narcótico -ca *adj & m* narcotic
nariz *f* (*pl* narices) nose
nasal *adj* nasal; voz — nasal voice
nasofaringe *f* nasopharynx
nasogástrico -ca *adj* nasogastric
nata *f* cream
natación *f* swimming
natalidad *f* birth rate
natural *adj* natural
naturaleza *f* nature
naturismo *m* naturopathy
naturista *adj* naturopathic; *mf* naturopath
naturópata *mf* naturopath
naturopatía *f* naturopathy
naturopático -ca *adj* naturopathic
náusea *f* (*frec. pl*) nausea; náuseas
  matutinas (*form*) *or* del embarazo
  morning sickness; náuseas y vómitos nausea and vomiting; producir
  náuseas to nauseate, make nauseated; sentir náuseas to feel nauseated; tener náuseas to be nauseated
nauseabundo -da *adj* nauseating
navaja (de afeitar) *f* razor blade

nebulizador *m* nebulizer, inhaler
nebulización *f* nebulization,
  breathing treatment
necesidad *f* need; necesidades especiales special needs
necesitar *vt* to need
necrobiosis lipoídica (diabeticorum) *f* necrobiosis lipoidica diabeticorum
necrofilia *f* necrophilia
necrofobia *f* necrophobia
necrólisis *f* necrolysis; — epidérmica tóxica toxic epidermal necrolysis
necropsia *f* autopsy
necrosante *adj* necrotizing
necrosis *f* necrosis
necrótico -ca *adj* necrotic
necrotizante *adj* necrotizing
nedocromilo *m* nedocromil
nefrectomía *f* nephrectomy
nefritis *f* nephritis
nefrogénico -ca *adj* nephrogenic
nefrolitiasis *f* nephrolithiasis
nefrología *f* nephrology
nefrólogo -ga *mf* nephrologist
nefroma *m* nephroma
nefropatía *f* nephropathy; — diabética diabetic nephropathy
nefrosis *f* nephrosis
nefrostomía *f* nephrostomy
nefrótico -ca *adj* nephrotic
negación *f* denial
negativo -va *adj & m* negative; falso
  — false negative; verdadero —
  true negative
negligencia *f* negligence, carelessness, neglect; — médica malpractice
negligente *adj* negligent, careless
negruzco -ca *adj* blackish
nelfinavir *m* nelfinavir
nene -na *mf* (*fam*) baby, infant
neoadyuvante *adj* neoadjuvant
neomicina *f* neomycin
neonatal *adj* neonatal
neonato *m* neonate, newborn

neonatología f neonatology
neonatólogo -ga mf neonatologist
neoplasia f (proceso) neoplasia; (tumor) neoplasm
neoplásico -ca adj neoplastic
neostigmina f neostigmine
nervio m nerve; — **auditivo** or **acústico** acoustic nerve; — **ciático** sciatic nerve; — **crural** femoral nerve; — **cubital** ulnar nerve; — **espinal** spinal nerve; — **facial** facial nerve; — **femoral** femoral nerve; — **frénico** phrenic nerve; — **mediano** median nerve; — **óptico** optic nerve; — **radial** radial nerve; — **raquídeo** spinal nerve; — **trigémino** trigeminal nerve; — **vago** vagus nerve
nervios mpl (fam, nerviosismo) nervousness, nerves (fam); **Tengo nervios**..I'm nervous.
nerviosismo m nervousness
nervioso -sa adj nervous, anxious; **estar** — to be nervous
neumococo m pneumococcus
neumoconiosis f pneumoconiosis
neumología f pulmonology
neumólogo -ga mf pulmonologist
neumonectomía f pneumonectomy
neumonía f pneumonia; — **adquirida en la comunidad** community-acquired pneumonia; — **por aspiración** aspiration pneumonia
neumonitis f pneumonitis; — **por hipersensibilidad** hypersensitivity pneumonitis
neumonología (SA) f pulmonology
neumonólogo -ga mf (SA) pulmonologist
neumotórax m pneumothorax
neural adj neural
neuralgia f neuralgia; — **del trigémino** trigeminal neuralgia; — **postherpética** postherpetic neuralgia
neurinoma m neurinoma; — **del acústico** acoustic neuroma
neuritis f neuritis
neuro-oftalmología f neuro-ophthalmology
neuroblastoma m neuroblastoma
neurocirugía f neurosurgery
neurocirujano -na mf neurosurgeon
neurofibroma m neurofibroma

neurofibromatosis f neurofibromatosis
neurofisiología f neurophysiology
neurogénico -ca, neurógeno -na adj neurogenic
neuroléptico -ca adj & m neuroleptic
neurología f neurology
neurológico -ca adj neurological, neurologic
neurólogo -ga mf neurologist
neuroma m neuroma; — **acústico** (esp. Mex) acoustic neuroma; — **de Morton** Morton's neuroma
neuromuscular adj neuromuscular
neurona f neuron
neuropatía f neuropathy; — **diabética** diabetic neuropathy; — **periférica** peripheral neuropathy; — **sensitiva, — sensorial** (esp. Mex) sensory neuropathy
neurosífilis f neurosyphilis
neurosis f (pl -sis) anxiety disorder, neurosis (ant); — **de guerra** shell shock
neurótico -ca adj chronically anxious, neurotic (ant); mf person who is chronically anxious, neurotic (ant)
neutralizar vt to neutralize
neutro -tra adj (chem) neutral
neutrófilo m neutrophil
neutropenia f neutropenia
nevirapina f nevirapine
nevo m nevus; — **displásico** dysplastic nevus
niacina f niacin
nicardipina f (esp. SA) nicardipine
nicardipino m nicardipine
niclosamida f niclosamide
nicotina f nicotine
nieto -ta m grandson, grandchild; f granddaughter
nifedipina f (esp. SA) nifedipine
nifedipino m nifedipine
nifurtimox m nifurtimox
nigua f chigoe, chigger
nilón m nylon
nimodipina f (esp. SA) nimodipine
nimodipino m nimodipine
niñero -ra mf baby-sitter
niñez f childhood
niño -ña m boy, child; f girl; (del ojo) pupil (of the eye)

níquel *m* nickel

nistagmus (*form*), **nistagmo** *m* nystagmus

nistatina *f* nystatin

nitrato *m* nitrate; — **de plata** silver nitrate

nitrito *m* nitrite

nitrofurantoína *f* nitrofurantoin

nitrógeno *m* nitrogen; — **líquido** liquid nitrogen

nitroglicerina *f* nitroglycerin

nivel *m* level; **de tercer** — tertiary; — **de conciencia** level of consciousness; — **terapéutico** therapeutic level

nizatidina *f* nizatidine

nocardiosis *f* nocardiosis

noche *f* night, nighttime, late evening; **por la** — at night, in the night

nocivo -va *adj* harmful; — **para la salud** bad for one's health

nocturno -na *adj* nocturnal; **polución** — nocturnal emission; **terrores nocturnos** night terrors

nodo (*card*) *See* **nódulo.**

nodriza *f* wet nurse

nodular *adj* nodular, lumpy (*fam*)

nódulo *m* nodule, lump (*fam*), bump (*fam*); (*card*) node; — **auriculoventricular** atrioventricular node; — **sinusal** sinoatrial node

nombre *m* name, first name

noradrenalina *f* norepinephrine

norepinefrina *f* norepinephrine

norfloxacina *f* (*esp. Amer*) norfloxacin

norfloxacino *m* norfloxacin

norgestimato *m* norgestimate

norma *f* norm, standard; (*pauta*) guideline

normal *adj* normal

normalizar *vt* to normalize

normalmente *adv* normally, usually

nortriptilina *f* nortriptyline

nosocomio *m* (*Amer*) hospital, clinic

nostalgia *f* homesickness; **sentir** — (*del hogar*) to be homesick

nostálgico -ca *adj* homesick

notar *vt* to notice

notificar *vt* to notify

novio -via *m* fiancé, boyfriend; *f* fiancée, girlfriend

NR *abbr* **no reanimar.** *See* **reanimar.**

nublado -da *adj* (*la visión*) cloudy

nubosidad *f* (*en el ojo*) cloudy spot, opacity (*in the eye*)

nuca *f* (*fam*) back of the neck

nuclear *adj* nuclear

nudillo *m* knuckle, joint of a finger

nudo *m* knot

nuera *f* daughter-in-law

nuez *f* (*pl* **nueces**) nut; — **de Adán** Adam's apple

número *m* number, (*Mex, recuento*) count; — **de glóbulos rojos** red blood cell count

nutricio -cia *adj* nutritional

nutrición *f* nutrition; — **enteral** enteral nutrition; — **parenteral total** (NPT) total parenteral nutrition (TPN)

nutricional *adj* nutritional

nutricionista *mf* nutritionist

nutriente *m* nutrient

nutrimento *m* nutrient

nutrir *vt* to nourish, to feed; to nurture

nutritivo -va *adj* nutritional, nutritious, nourishing

O

obedecer *vt* to obey, to mind
obesidad *f* obesity; — **central** central obesity; — **mórbida** morbid obesity
obeso -sa *adj* obese
obrar *vi* (*Mex, CA; defecar*) to have a bowel movement
obrero -ra *mf* worker
obscuro -ra *adj* dark, dim
observación *f* observation
obsesión *f* obsession
obsesivo-compulsivo -va *adj* obsessive-compulsive
obstetra *mf* obstetrician
obstetricia *f* obstetrics
obstétrico -ca *adj* obstetric, obstetrical
obstrucción *f* obstruction, blockage; — **de la vía aérea superior** upper airway obstruction; — **intestinal parcial** partial small bowel obstruction
obstructivo -va *adj* obstructive
obstruído -da *adj* obstructed, blocked
obstruir *vt* to obstruct, block; *vr* to become obstructed *o* blocked
occipital *adj* occipital
ocio *m* leisure
oclusión *f* occlusion
oclusivo -va *adj* occlusive
ocronosis *f* ochronosis
octogenario -ria *mf* octogenarian
ocular *adj* ocular
oculista *mf* ophthalmologist, eye doctor (*fam*)
ocupación *f* occupation
ocupacional *adj* occupational
odiar *vt* to hate
odio *m* hate
odontología *f* dentistry
odontólogo -ga *mf* (*form*) dentist
oficina *f* office
ofloxacina *f* (*esp. Amer*) ofloxacin
ofloxacino *m* ofloxacin
oftálmico -ca *adj* ophthalmic
oftalmología *f* ophthalmology
oftalmólogo -ga *mf* ophthalmologist

oftalmoscopio *m* ophthalmoscope
oído *m* ear (*organ of hearing*); (*audición*) hearing, sense of hearing; — **externo** external *o* outer ear; — **interno** inner ear; — **medio** middle ear; **oídos, nariz, y garganta** ear, nose, and throat (ENT)
oír *vt, vi* to hear
ojeras *fpl* dark circles under one's eyes
ojeroso -sa *adj* having dark circles under one's eyes
ojo *m* eye; — **morado** black eye; — **perezoso** (*esp. Mex*) lazy eye; — **rojo** conjunctivitis (*form*), pinkeye; — **vago** lazy eye
ola de calor *f* heat wave
olanzapina *f* olanzapine
olécranon *m* olecranon
oler *vt, vi* to smell; — **a** to smell like; — **mal** to smell bad
olfativo -va *adj* olfactory
olfatorio -ria *adj* olfactory
oligoelemento *m* trace element
olmo americano *m* (*bot*) slippery elm
olor *m* odor, smell; — **corporal** body odor; — **de pies** foot odor
olsalazina *f* olsalazine
olvidadizo -za *adj* forgetful, absent-minded
olvidar *vt* to forget
ombligo *m* umbilicus (*form*), navel, bellybutton (*fam*)
ombudsman *mf* ombudsman
omento *m* omentum
omeprazol *m* omeprazole
omóplato, omoplato *m* scapula, shoulder blade (*fam*)
OMS *abbr* **Organización Mundial de la Salud.** *See* **organización.**
oncocercosis *f* onchocerciasis
oncología *f* oncology
oncólogo -ga *mf* oncologist; — **radioterapeuta** radiation oncologist
onda *f* wave; — **cerebral** brain wave; — **de choque** shock wave
ONR *abbr* **orden de no reanimar.** *See* **reanimar.**

onza (onz.) f ounce (oz.)
ooforectomía f oophorectomy
opacidad f opacity
opaco -ca adj opaque
opción f option; **opciones de tratamiento** treatment options
operable adj operable
operación f operation; — **cesárea** cesarean section
operar vt, vi to operate; **Tenemos que operarle (de) la mano..**We need to operate on your hand... **operar maquinaria..**to operate machinery; vr to have an operation
operatorio -ria adj operative
opiáceo -a adj & m opiate
opinión f opinion; **segunda —** second opinion
opio m opium
opioide adj & m opioid
oportunidad f chance
oportunista adj opportunistic
opresivo -va adj (dolor) crushing
óptico -ca adj optical, optic; mf optician; f optics
optimismo m optimism
optimista adj optimistic
óptimo -ma adj optimum
optometrista mf optometrist
oral adj oral
órbita f (anat) orbit, eye socket (fam)
orbitario -ria adj orbital
orciprenalina f metaproterenol
orden f (del médico) order
ordenador m computer
ordenar vt to order
oreja f ear; **orejas de soplillo** (Esp) ears that stick out
orejeras fpl earmuffs
orf m orf
orfanato m orphanage
orfanatorio m (esp. Mex, CA) orphanage
orfelinato m orphanage
orgánico -ca adj organic; **alimentos orgánicos** organic food(s)
organismo m body, organism; **efecto sobre el organismo..**effect on your body; — **modificado genéticamente (OMG)** genetically modified organism (GMO)
organización f organization; **Organización Mundial de la Salud**

(OMS) World Health Organization (WHO)
órgano m organ; — **hueco** hollow organ; — **vital** vital organ
organoclorado m organochlorate
organofosforado m organophosphate
orgasmo m orgasm, climax
orientación f orientation; (guía) guidance; — **sexual** sexual orientation
orificio m orifice, hole; — **de entrada** entrance wound; — **de salida** exit wound
origen m source
orín m (fam, frec. pl) urine
orina f urine
orinadera f (Amer, fam) bout of frequent urination
orinal m urinal
orinar vt, vi to urinate; vr to urinate on oneself; — **en la cama** to wet the bed
orlistat m orlistat
oro m gold
orofaringe f oropharynx
orquiectomía, orquidectomía f orchiectomy
orquitis f orchitis
ortesis f (pl -sis) orthosis, orthotic device
ortiga f (bot) nettle
ortodoncia f orthodontia; (tratamiento) orthodontics
ortodóncico -ca adj orthodontic
ortodoncista mf orthodontist
ortopedia f orthopedics
ortopédico -ca adj orthopedic
ortopedista mf orthopedist, orthopedic surgeon
oruga f caterpillar
orzuelo m sty o stye
oscilar vi to fluctuate, to vary
oscurecer vt (la piel, etc.) to darken (one's skin, etc.)
oscuro -ra adj dark
oseltamivir m oseltamivir
óseo -a adj osseous (form), pertaining to bone; **médula —** bone marrow
ósmosis f osmosis
osteítis f osteitis; — **fibrosa quística** osteitis fibrosa cystica
osteoartritis f osteoarthritis, degenerative joint disease

osteofito *m* osteophyte
osteogénesis imperfecta *f* osteogenesis imperfecta
osteoma *m* osteoma
osteomalacia *f* osteomalacia
osteomielitis *f* osteomyelitis
osteonecrosis *f* osteonecrosis
osteópata *mf* osteopath
osteopatía *f* osteopathy
osteoporosis *f* osteoporosis
osteosarcoma *m* osteosarcoma
ostomía *f* ostomy
ótico -ca *adj* otic
otitis *f* otitis; — **externa** otitis externa, swimmer's ear (*fam*); — **media** otitis media
otoesclerosis *f* otosclerosis
otoño *m* fall, autumn
otorrinolaringología *f* otolaryngology; ear, nose and throat (ENT)
otorrinolaringólogo -ga *mf* otolaryngologist; ear, nose and throat specialist
otosclerosis *f* otosclerosis
otoscopio *m* otoscope
ovárico -ca *adj* ovarian

ovariectomía *f* oophorectomy
ovario *m* ovary; — **poliquístico** polycystic ovary
ovulación *f* ovulation
ovular *vi* to ovulate
óvulo *m* ovum, egg (*fam*); (*supositorio vaginal*) vaginal suppository
oxalato *m* oxalate
oxibutinina *f* oxybutynin
oxicodona *f* oxycodone
oxidado -da *adj* rusty; **clavo** — rusty nail
oxidante *m* oxidant
óxido *m* oxide; — **de titanio** titanium oxide; — **de zinc** zinc oxide; — **nitroso** nitrous oxide
oxígeno *m* oxygen
oxigenoterapia *f* oxygen (*as therapy*); — **domiciliaria** home oxygen; — **hiperbárica** hyperbaric oxygen
oximetría *f* oximetry; — **de pulso** (*Amer*) pulse oximetry
oxitocina *f* oxytocin
oxiuro *m* pinworm
ozono *m* ozone

P

PABA *abbr* **ácido paraaminobenzoico**. *See* **ácido.**
pabellón *m* (*de un hospital*) pavillion, ward
pacha *f* (*CA, biberón*) baby bottle
paciente *adj* patient; *mf* patient; — **ambulatorio** outpatient; — **hospitalizado** inpatient
paclitaxel *m* paclitaxel
padecer *vt, vi* to suffer, to have (*a disease, symptom, etc.*); **Padezco**

dolores de espalda..I suffer from back pains..I have back pains.
padecimiento *m* (*esp. Mex*) affliction, ailment
padrastro *m* stepfather; (*en el dedo*) hangnail
padre *m* father, parent; (*sacerdote*) priest; **padres adoptivos** adoptive parents; **padres biológicos** biological parents
paidofilia *f* pedophilia

paidopsiquiatría *f (form)* child psychiatry
pájaro *m* bird
palabra *f* word
paladar *m* palate, roof of the mouth *(fam)*; — **blando** soft palate; — **duro** hard palate
palangana *f* basin
paleta *f (fam, escápula)* scapula, shoulder blade *(fam)*; *(depresor de lengua)* tongue depressor, tongue blade *(fam)*
paletilla *f (fam, escápula)* scapula, shoulder blade *(fam)*
paliación *f* palliation
paliativo -va *adj* palliative
palidez *f* pallor
pálido -da *adj* pale
palidotomía *f* pallidotomy
palillo de algodón *m (Esp)* cotton swab
palma *f (anat, bot)* palm
palmada, palmadita *f* pat; **dar palmadas** *or* **palmaditas** to pat
palmar *adj* palmar
palmilla *f (de un zapato)* insole
palpar *vt* to palpate
palpitación *f* palpitation
palpitar *vi* to palpitate
paludismo *m* malaria
pamplina *f (bot)* chickweed
pan *m* bread
panadero -ra *mf* baker
panadizo *m* felon, whitlow
panarteritis nodosa, panarteritis nudosa *f* polyarteritis nodosa
páncreas *m (pl -creas)* pancreas
pancreatectomía *f* pancreatectomy
pancreático -ca *adj* pancreatic
pancreatitis *f* pancreatitis
pandemia *f* pandemic
pandilla *f* gang
panhipopituitarismo *m* panhypopituitarism
pánico *m* panic; **ataque** *m* **de —** panic attack
pantaletas *fpl (Mex)* panties, (women's) underpants
pantalones *mpl* pants
panties *mpl (esp. Carib)* (women's) underpants, panties
pantimedias *fpl* pantyhose
pantoprazol *m* pantoprazole

pantorrilla *f (anat)* calf
panza *f (fam)* belly, paunch *(fam)*, tummy *(ped, fam)*
panzón -zona *adj* potbellied, having a potbelly; *m* potbelly
pañal *m* diaper; — **desechable** disposable diaper; — **de tela** cloth diaper
paño *m* towel, drape; *(derm)* melasma; — **quirúrgico** surgical drape
pañuelo *m* handkerchief, *(de papel)* tissue; — **desechable** *(esp. Mex)* tissue
papa *f (Amer)* potato
papá *m (pl papás)* dad
papada *f* double chin
papel *m* paper; *(función)* role; — **higiénico,** — **sanitario** *(Mex, CA, Carib)*, — **de baño** *(Mex)* toilet paper
paperas *fpl* mumps
papi *m* daddy
papila *f* papilla; — **gustativa** taste bud
papilar *adj* papillary
papilomavirus *m (pl -rus)* papillomavirus
papito *m* daddy
paquete *m (de cigarillos)* pack *(of cigarettes)*; **paquetes diarios** packs per day
par *m (neuro)* cranial nerve; *(igual)* peer; **grupo de pares** peer group; — **craneal** cranial nerve; **presión** *f* **de (los) pares** peer pressure
paracentesis *f* paracentesis
paracetamol *m* acetaminophen
paracoccidioidomicosis *f* paracoccidioidomycosis
parado -da *adj (de pie)* standing; **estar —** to stand, to be standing; *f (Esp)* arrest; — **cardíaca** cardiac arrest; — **respiratoria** respiratory arrest
paradójico -ca *adj* paradoxical
paraespinal *adj* paraspinal
parafimosis *f* paraphimosis
paragonimiasis *f* paragonimiasis
parainfluenza *f* parainfluenza
parálisis *f* paralysis, palsy; — **cerebral** cerebral palsy; — **de Bell** Bell's palsy; — **del sueño** sleep paralysis; — **facial** facial paralysis,

facial palsy
paralizador m (*Amer*) stun gun
paralizante adj paralyzing
paralizar vt to paralyze
paramédico -ca adj & mf paramedic
paranasal adj paranasal
paranoia f paranoia
paranoide, paranoico -ca adj paranoid
paraparesia f paraparesis; — **espástica tropical** tropical spastic paraparesis
paraplejia, paraplejía f paraplegia
parapléjico -ca adj & mf paraplegic
paraquat m paraquat
pararse vr to stand, stand up
parasimpático -ca adj parasympathetic
parasitario -ria adj parasitic
parásito m parasite
parasitología f parasitology
paratifoidea f paratyphoid
paratión m parathion
paratiroidectomía f parathyroidectomy
paratiroideo -a adj parathyroid
paratiroides f (*pl* **-des**) (*fam*) parathyroid gland
parche m patch; — **de nicotina** nicotine patch
parcial adj partial
parecerse vr to look like; **Te pareces a tu madre**..You look like your mother.
pared f (*anat*) wall; — **abdominal** abdominal wall
paregórico m paregoric
pareja f (*compañero*) partner; (*dos personas*) couple
parental adj parental
parenteral adj parenteral
paresia f paresis
pariente mf relative; — **consanguíneo** (*form*) blood relative
parietal adj parietal
parir vt (*Carib, fam*) to give birth
parkinsonismo m Parkinsonism
paro m arrest; — **cardíaco** cardiac arrest; — **respiratorio** respiratory arrest
paroniquia f paronychia
parótida f (*fam*) parotid gland
parotídeo -a adj parotid

parotiditis f parotitis, (*paperas*) mumps
paroxetina f paroxetine
paroxismal adj paroxysmal
paroxismo m paroxysm
paroxístico -ca adj paroxysmal
parpadear vi to blink
parpadeo m blinking, blink
párpado m eyelid
parte f part; **cuarta** — quarter, fourth; **la cuarta parte de una tableta**..a quarter of a tablet; **partes blandas** soft tissue(s); **partes íntimas** (*euph*) genitals, private parts (*euph*); **tercera** — third; **dos terceras partes**..two thirds
partero -ra m male midwife; f midwife
participación f participation, involvement
partícula f particle
partida f certificate; — **de nacimiento** birth certificate
partido -da adj cracked, split, (*labios, piel*) chapped
partidura f (*Cub, ortho*) fracture, break
partir vt, vr to crack, split, (*labios, piel*) to chap; (*Cub, ortho*) to break
parto m birth, childbirth; delivery; **dolor** m **del** — labor pain; **estar de** — (*esp. Esp*) or **estar en trabajo de** — to be in labor; — **de nalgas** breech birth; — **natural** natural childbirth; **ponerse de** — (*Esp*) to go into labor; **sala de partos** delivery room, Labor and Delivery; **trabajo de** — labor
parvovirus m (*pl* **-rus**) parvovirus
pasado -da adj — **de peso** overweight
pasaje m passage; **pasajes nasales** nasal passages
pasajero -ra adj (*dolor, etc.*) fleeting, transient
pasar vt (*fam, una enfermedad*) to give; (*fam, tragar*) to swallow; — **saliva** (*fam*) to swallow (*dry swallow*); — **visita** to round, to make rounds; vr to wear off; **El dolor se le va a pasar**..The pain will wear off.
pasatiempo m pastime, hobby

pase *m* — **de visita** rounds
pasiflora *f* (*bot*) passion flower
pasillo *m* hallway
pasionaria *f* (*bot*) passion flower
pasivo -va *adj* passive
pasivo-agresivo -va *adj* passive-aggressive
paso *m* step; pass; **dar un** — to step, take a step; **el próximo** — the next step
pasta *f* paste; — **dentífrica** (*form*), — **de dientes**, *or* — **dental** toothpaste
pasteurizado -da *adj* pasteurized
pastilla *f* pill; — **para dormir** sleeping pill; — **para el dolor** pain pill
patada *f* kick; **dar patadas** to kick
patas *fpl* — **de gallo** *or* **gallina** crow's feet
patata *f* (*Esp*) potato
patear *vt, vi* to kick
patela *f* patella, kneecap (*fam*)
paternidad *f* paternity, fatherhood
paterno -na *adj* paternal
pato (*Amer*) *m* (*orinal*) urinal; (*bacinilla*) bedpan
patología *f* pathology
patológico -ca *adj* pathological, pathologic
patólogo -ga *mf* pathologist
patrón -trona *mf* employer; *m* pattern; — **oro** gold standard
pauta *f* guideline
PCP *See* **fenciclidina**.
peca *f* freckle
peces *pl of* **pez**
pecho *m* chest, breast; **dar el** — to breast-feed
pectoral *adj* pectoral
pedacito *m* small piece, chip
pedazo *m* piece
pediatra *mf* pediatrician
pediatría *f* pediatrics
pediátrico -ca *adj* pediatric
pediculosis *f* pediculosis
pedicura *f* pedicure
pedicure *m* pedicure
pedo *m* (*vulg*) gas (*expelled from rectum*), fart (*vulg*); **tirarse pedos** *or* **tirarse un** — to pass gas, to fart (*vulg*)
pedofilia *f* pedophilia
pegajoso -sa *adj* sticky

pegamento *m* (*como droga de abuso*) glue
pegar *vt* to strike, to hit
pegilado -da *adj* pegylated
peginterferón *m* peginterferon
peinar *vt* to comb; *vr* to comb one's hair
peine *m* comb
pelado -da *adj* (*la piel*) raw
pelagra *f* pellagra
pelarse *vr* (*la piel*) to peel
peligro *m* danger, hazard
peligroso -sa *adj* dangerous, hazardous
pelo *m* hair
pelota *f* ball; (*fam, nódulo*) bump, lump
peluca *f* wig
peludo -da *adj* hirsute (*form*), hairy
peluquero -ra *mf* barber, haircutter
pelviano -na *adj* pelvic
pélvico -ca *adj* pelvic
pelvis *f* (*pl* -vis) pelvis
pena *f* grief; (*vergüenza*) embarrassment
penciclovir *m* penciclovir
pendiente *adj* pending
pene *m* penis
peneano -na *adj* penile
penetración *f* penetration
penetrante *adj* penetrating
penetrar *vt* to penetrate
pénfigo *m* pemphigus
penfigoide *m* pemphigoid
penicilamina *f* penicillamine
penicilina *f* penicillin
pensamiento *m* thought
pensar *vi* to think
pentaclorofenol *m* pentachlorophenol
pentamidina *f* pentamidine
pentoxifilina *f* pentoxifylline
peor (*comp of* **malo** *and* **mal**) *adj* & *adv* worse
pepe *m* (*El Salv, Guat*) pacifier
pepsina *f* pepsin
péptico -ca *adj* peptic
pequeño -ña *adj* small, little
pera de goma *f* bulb syringe
percepción *f* perception; — **de la profundidad** depth perception
perclorato *m* perchlorate
percutáneo -a *adj* percutaneous

perder *vt* to lose; — **el conocimiento** *or* **la conciencia** to lose consciousness, to pass out, black out; — **la razón** to lose one's mind, to go crazy; — **la voz** to lose one's voice; — **peso** to lose weight

pérdida *f* loss; — **de audición** hearing loss; — **de peso** weight loss

perfeccionismo *m* perfectionism

perfeccionista *adj & mf* perfectionist

perfil *m* profile

perforación *f* perforation

perforado -da *adj* perforated

perforar *vt* to perforate, to pierce

perfume *m* perfume

perfusión *f* perfusion

perianal *adj* perianal

periarteritis nodosa, periarteritis nudosa *f* polyarteritis nodosa

pericárdico -ca *adj* pericardial

pericardio *m* pericardium

pericarditis *f* pericarditis; — **constrictiva** constrictive pericarditis

periferia *f* periphery

periférico -ca *adj* peripheral

perifonear *vt* (*form*) to page (*overhead*)

perímetro *m* circumference, girth

perinatal *adj* perinatal

perineal *adj* perineal

periódico -ca *adj* periodic

periodoncia *f* periodontics

periodoncista *mf* periodontist

periodontal *adj* periodontal

período, periodo *m* period; **su último período**..your last period; — **de incubación** incubation period

perioral *adj* perioral

periorbitario -ria *adj* periorbital

perirrenal *adj* perinephric

peristalsis *f* (*Ang*) peristalsis

peristaltismo *m* peristalsis

peritoneal *adj* peritoneal

peritoneo *m* peritoneum

peritonitis *f* peritonitis

periungueal *adj* periungual

perjudicar *vt* to damage, harm, to impair

permanente *adj* permanent

permetrina *f* permethrin

permiso *m* permission, consent

peroné *m* (*pl* **-nés**) fibula

peroneal (*Ang*) peroneal

peroneo -a *adj* peroneal

peróxido *m* peroxide; — **de benzoílo** benzoyl peroxide; —**de carbamida** carbamide peroxide; — **de hidrógeno** hydrogen peroxide

perrilla *f* (*Mex, fam*) sty *o* stye

perro *m* dog; — **guía** *or* **lazarillo** guide dog

persistente *adj* persistent

persistir *vi* to persist

persona *f* person; — **con SIDA** person with AIDS; *fpl* persons, people

personal *adj* personal

personalidad *f* personality; — **antisocial** antisocial personality; — **borderline** borderline personality; — **ciclotímica** cyclothymic personality; — **esquizoide** schizoid personality; — **histriónica** histrionic personality; — **límite** *or* **limítrofe** borderline personality; — **narcisista** narcissistic personality; — **obsesivo-compulsiva** obsessive-compulsive personality; — **paranoide** paranoid personality; — **pasivo-agresiva** passive-aggressive personality; — **tipo A** type A personality

pesa *f* (*deporte*) weight; **levantar pesas** to weight lift, weight lifting

pesadez *f* heaviness

pesadilla *f* nightmare

pesado -da *adj* heavy

pesar *vt, vi* to weigh; ¿**Cuánto pesa Ud.?**..How much do you weigh?

pesario *m* pessary

pescado *m* fish (*after being caught, as food*)

pescador -ra *m* fisherman; *f* fisherwoman

pesimismo *m* pessimism

pesimista *adj* pessimistic

peso *m* weight; — **al nacer** birth weight; — **ideal** ideal weight; — **magro** lean body weight

pestaña *f* eyelash

peste *f* plague; — **bubónica** bubonic plague

pesticida *m* pesticide

petidina *f* meperidine

petrolato *m* petroleum jelly

petróleo *m* petroleum

peyote *m* peyote

pez *m* (*pl* **peces**) fish; — **piedra** stonefish

pezón *m* nipple (*of a female*)

pezonera *f* nipple shield

pH *m* pH

pian *m* yaws

picada *f* (*de insecto*) sting (*of an insect*)

picadura *f* (*de insecto*) bite, sting; (*Mex, pinchazo*) puncture, stick, prick

picante *adj* hot, spicy; **salsa** — hot sauce

picar *vt* (*insecto*) to bite, to sting; (*Mex, punzar*) to puncture, to stick, prick; *vi* to itch; **¿Le pica el brazo?**..Does your arm itch? *vr* (*Mex, punzarse*) to puncture oneself, to stick *o* prick oneself

picaridina *f* picaridin

picazón *f* itch, itching, itchiness; **sentir** *or* **tener** — to itch

pico *m* peak

picor (*Esp*) *m* itch, itching, itchiness; (*de garganta*) tickle, irritation

pie *m* foot; **de** — standing; **estar de** — to stand, to be standing; — **caído** foot drop; — **de atleta** athlete's foot; — **diabético** diabetic foot; — **péndulo** foot drop; — **plano** flatfoot; — **zambo** *or* **zopo** clubfoot; **ponerse de** — to stand up

piedra *f* stone; **de** *or* **en la vesícula** gallstone; — **en el riñón** kidney stone; — **pómez** pumice stone

piel *f* skin; — **de gallina** goosebumps; — **de cordero** *or* **oveja** sheepskin

pielografía *f* urography, pyelography

pielonefritis *f* pyelonephritis

piercing *m* piercing

pierna *f* leg

pigmentación *f* pigmentation

pigmentado -da *adj* pigmented

pigmento *m* pigment

pilar *adj* pilar

píldora *f* pill; **la** — (*fam, anticonceptiva*) birth control pill, the pill (*fam*); — **anticonceptiva** birth control pill; — **del amor** (*fam*) methylenedioxyamphetamine (MDA); — **postcoital** (*form*), — **del día siguiente**, *or* — **del día después**

morning after pill

pilonidal *adj* pilonidal

pilórico -ca *adj* pyloric

píloro *m* pylorus

piloroplastia *f* pyloroplasty

pimienta *f* pepper

pinchar *vt* to puncture, to stick, prick; *vr* to puncture oneself, to stick *o* prick oneself

pinchazo *m* puncture, stick, prick; — **en el dedo** finger-stick

pindolol *m* pindolol

pineal *adj* pineal

pinguécula *f* pinguecula

pinta *f* pinta

pintarse *vr* — **las uñas** to put on nail polish, to paint one's nails; — **los labios** to put on lipstick

pintura *f* paint

pinza *f* clamp; *fpl* tweezers

pinzamiento *m* impingement

pinzar *vt* to clamp

piña *f* pineapple

pioderma gangrenoso *m* pyoderma gangrenosum

piogénico -ca *adj* pyogenic

piógeno -na *adj* pyogenic

pioglitazona *f* pioglitazone

piojo *m* louse; — **de la cabeza** head louse; — **del cuerpo** body louse; — **del pubis** *or* **púbico** crab louse, pubic louse

piorrea *f* pyorrhea

pipa *f* (*para fumar*) pipe (*for smoking*)

pipí (*esp. ped, fam*) *m* (*orina*) urine, pee (*fam*); (*pene*) penis, pee pee (*ped, fam*); **hacer** — to urinate, to pee (*fam*)

piquete (*esp. Mex*) *m* puncture, stick, prick; (*de insecto*) bite, sting; — **en el dedo** finger-stick

pirantel *m* pyrantel

pirazinamida *f* pyrazinamide

piretrina *f* pyrethrin

piridoxina *f* pyridoxine, vitamin B$_6$

pirimetamina *f* pyrimethamine

piroxicam *m* piroxicam

pis (*fam or vulg*) *m* urine, pee (*esp. ped, fam*); **hacer** — to urinate, to pee (*esp. ped, fam*)

piso *m* floor; — **de la boca** floor of the mouth; — **pélvico** pelvic floor

pispelo m (*El Salv*) sty o stye

pistola f gun, handgun; — **paralizante** (*Esp*) stun gun

pitarle el pecho, (*esp. PR*) to wheeze

pitiriasis f pityriasis; — **alba** pityriasis alba; — **rosada** pityriasis rosea; — **versicolor** tenia versicolor

pituitario -ria adj pituitary

placa f (*card, dent*) plaque; (*surg*) plate; (*radiología*) film, x-ray

placebo m placebo

placenta f placenta; **desprendimiento prematuro de** — placental abruption; — **previa** placenta previa

placentario -ria adj placental

placer m pleasure

plaguicida m pesticide

plan m plan

planificación familiar f family planning, planned parenthood

plano -na adj flat, level; **pie** — flatfoot, fallen arch; m plane

planta f (*del pie*) sole (*of the foot*); (*bot*) plant

plantar adj plantar

plantilla f insole, arch suport

plaqueta f platelet

plasma m plasma; — **fresco congelado** fresh frozen plasma

plasmaféresis f plasmapheresis

plasmático -ca adj pertaining to plasma; **potasio** — plasma potassium

plástico -ca adj & m plastic

plata f silver

plátano m banana

platelminto m flatworm

platino m platinum

plazo m **a corto** — short-term; **a largo** — long-term

pleito (legal) m lawsuit

plenitud f (*form*) fullness

pletismografía f plethysmography

pleura f pleura

pleural adj pleural

pleuresía f pleurisy

pleurítico -ca adj pleuritic

pleuritis f pleuritis

plexo m plexus; — **solar** solar plexus

pliegue m fold, crease; — **cutáneo** skin fold; — **palmar** palmar crease; — **ungueal** nail fold

plomo m lead

pluma f pen; — **de insulina** insulin pen

población f population

pobreza f poverty

poco -ca adj little, not much, few, not many; **poco dolor**..little pain..not much pain...**unas pocas veces**..a few times..not many times; m little; — **a** — little by little

poder m power; — **notarial** power of attorney

podofilina f podophyllin

podología f podiatry

podólogo -ga mf podiatrist

podrido -da (*pp of* **pudrir**) adj rotten

polen m pollen

poliarteritis nodosa, poliarteritis nudosa f polyarteritis nodosa

policitemia f polycythemia; — **vera** polycythemia vera

policlonal adj polyclonal

polietilenglicol m polyethylene glycol (PEG)

polietileno m polyethylene

poliinsaturado -da adj polyunsaturated

polimialgia reumática f polymyalgia rheumatica

polimiositis f polymyositis

polimixina B f polymyxin B

poliomielitis, polio (*fam*) f poliomyelitis, polio (*fam*)

polipectomía f polypectomy

pólipo m polyp; — **adenomatoso** adenomatous polyp; — **juvenil** juvenile polyp; — **nasal** nasal polyp

poliposis f polyposis; — **adenomatosa familiar** familial adenomatous polyposis

polipropileno m polypropylene

poliquístico -ca adj polycystic

poliquistosis renal f polycystic kidney disease

polisomnografía f polysomnography

polivitamínico m (*Esp*) multivitamin

póliza (de seguro) f (insurance) policy

pollo m chicken

polución nocturna f nocturnal emission

polvo m dust, powder; **en** — powdered; — **de ángel** (*fam*) phencyclidine (PCP), angel dust (*fam*); — **de casa** house dust; **polvos de talco** (*Esp*) talcum powder

pomada *f* cream, salve, ointment

pomelo *m* (*esp. Esp*) grapefruit

pomo *m* (*Mex, CA*) pill bottle

pómulo *m* cheekbone

poner *vt* (*pp* **puesto**) to place; *vr* (*vestirse*) to put on; (*volverse*) to turn; **Póngase esta bata**..Put on this gown...**¿Se le ponen blancos los dedos cuando hace frío?**..Do your fingers turn white when it gets cold? — **de pie** to stand up

ponzoña *f* poison, venom

pool *m* (*Ang*) pool; — **genético** gene pool

poplíteo -a *adj* popliteal

popó *m* (*fam*) stool, bowel movement, poo poo (*ped, fam*); **hacer** — to have a bowel movement, to go poo poo (*ped, fam*)

por *prep* per; — **ciento** percent; — **día** per day; — **minuto** per minute

porcelana *f* porcelain

porcentaje *m* percentage

porcino -na *adj* porcine

porción *f* portion, serving; **porciones por envase** servings per container

porfiria *f* porphyria; — **cutánea tarda** porphyria cutanea tarda

poro *m* pore

porro *m* (*fam*) marijuana cigarette, joint (*fam*)

porta *adj* (*vena*) portal

portador -ra *mf* (*de un virus o una bacteria*) carrier; **ser** — to carry, to have (*often chronically*); **Él es portador de SARM**..He is an MRSA carrier..He carries MRSA; **Ella es portadora de un catéter epidural**..She has a (chronic) epidural catheter.

portal *adj* portal

portátil *adj* portable

posibilidad *f* possibility, chance

posible *adj* possible

posición *f* position; **poner en** — to position; — **fetal** fetal position; — **misionera** missionary position

positivo -va *adj & m* positive; **falso** — false positive; **verdadero** — true positive

posmenopáusico *adj* postmenopausal

posnasal *adj* postnasal

posnatal *adj* postnatal

posos de café *mpl* coffee grounds

posparto *adj & adv* postpartum; **la tercera semana posparto**..the third week postpartum

posponer *vt* (*pp* **-puesto**) to postpone

posprandial *adj* postprandial

pospuesto *pp of* **posponer**

postemilla *f* (*Mex, CA; dent; fam*) abscess

posterior *adj* posterior

postexposición *adj* postexposure

postictal *adj* postictal

postizo -za *adj* prosthetic (*form*), artificial, false; **dientes postizos** false teeth

postmenopáusico -ca *adj* postmenopausal

post mortem *adj & adv* postmortem

postnasal *adj* postnasal

postnatal *adj* postnatal

postoperatorio -ria *adj* postoperative

postparto *See* **posparto**.

postraumático -ca *adj* posttraumatic

postre *m* dessert

postura *f* posture

postural *adj* postural

potable *adj* potable

potasio *m* potassium

potencia *f* potency

potencial *adj & m* potential; — **evocado** evoked potential

potente *adj* potent, powerful, strong

povidona yodada *f* povidone-iodine

PPD *m&f* PPD

práctica *f* practice; — **clínica** clinical practice

practicante *mf* practitioner (*of a sport, technique, etc.*); (*de la medicina*) medical student, physician in training

practicar *vt* (*la medicina, etc.*) to practice (*medicine, etc.*)

pramipexol *m* pramipexole

pramlintida *f* pramlintide

pravastatina *f* pravastatin

praziquantel, prazicuantel (*OMS*) *m* praziquantel

prazosina *f* prazosin

prebiótico *m* prebiotic

precanceroso -sa *adj* precancerous

precaución *f* precaution; **por pre-caución**..as a precaution; **precauciones de contacto** contact precautions; **precauciones de transmisión aérea** airborne precautions; **precauciones de transmisión por gotas** droplet precautions; **precauciones estándar** standard precautions; **precauciones universales** (*ant*) universal precautions (*ant*)

precio *m* (*de un servicio médico*) charge

precisión *f* precision

preciso -sa *adj* precise

precordial *adj* precordial

precoz *adj* precocious, premature, early; **pubertad** *f* — precocious puberty

precursor *m* precursor

predecir *vt* (*pp* -dicho) to predict

prediabetes *f* borderline diabetes, early diabetes

predicho *pp of* predecir

predisponente *adj* predisposing

predisponer *vt* (*pp* -puesto) to predispose

predisposición *f* predisposition

predispuesto -ta (*pp of* predisponer) *adj* predisposed, prone

prednisolona *f* prednisolone

prednisona *f* prednisone

preeclampsia *f* preeclampsia

preembrión *m* fertilized ovum prior to implantation

preexistente *adj* pre-existing

prehipertensión *f* borderline hypertension, early hypertension

preliminar *adj* preliminary

prellenado -da *adj* prefilled; **jeringa** *or* **jeringuilla** *f* — prefilled syringe

premaligno -na *adj* premalignant

prematuro -ra *adj* premature; *mf* (*fam*) premature newborn, preemie (*fam*)

premedicación *f* premedication

premenopáusico -ca *adj* premenopausal

premenstrual *adj* premenstrual

premolar *adj & m* premolar

prenatal *adj* prenatal

prensión *f* grip; **fuerza de** — grip strength

preñada *adj* (*fam*) pregnant

preñez *f* (*fam*) pregnancy

preocupación *f* worry (*frec. pl*)

preocuparse *vr* to worry; **¿Está preocupada?**..Are you worried?...**No se preocupe**..Don't worry.

preoperatorio -ria *adj* preoperative

preparación *f* preparation; — **quirúrgica** surgical prep, prep (*fam*)

preparado *m* (*pharm*) preparation

preparar *vt* to prepare

prepúber *adj* prepubertal; *mf* prepubertal child

prepuberal *adj* prepubertal

prepucio *m* foreskin

presbiacusia *f* presbycusis

presbicia *f* presbyopia

presbiopía *f* presbyopia

prescribir *vt* (*pp* -scrito) to prescribe

prescripción *f* prescription

prescrito *pp of* prescribir

presencia *f* presence

presentación *f* presentation; — **pelviana**, — **pélvica** (*esp. Mex*), *or* — **de nalgas** (*fam*) breech presentation

preservar *vt* to spare

preservativo *m* condom, rubber (*fam*)

presión *f* pressure; (*fam, de la sangre*) blood pressure; — **alta** hypertension (*form*), high blood pressure; — **arterial** (*form*) blood pressure; — **diastólica** diastolic pressure; — **positiva (de la vía aérea) a dos niveles** bi-level positive airway pressure (BiPAP); — **positiva continua (en la vía aérea)** continuous positive airway pressure (CPAP); — **sanguínea** (*form*) blood pressure; — **sistólica** systolic pressure

presionar *vt* to press, to apply pressure; **Presione el botón**..Press the button.

pretérmino *adj* preterm

prevalencia *f* prevalence

prevención *f* prevention

prevenible *adj* preventable; **enfermedad** — preventable disease

prevenir *vt* prevent

preventivo -va *adj* preventive

previo -via *adj* previous

priapismo *m* priapism

primaquina *f* primaquine

primario -ria *adj* primary
primavera *f* spring, springtime
primero -ra *adj* first; **primeros auxilios** first aid
primitivo -va *adj* primitive
primo -ma *mf* cousin
principio *m* principle; — **activo** active ingredient; — **del placer** pleasure principle
prión *m* prion
prisión *f* prison
privacidad *f* privacy
privación *f* deprivation; — **de sueño** sleep deprivation
privado -da *adj* private; **médico** — private doctor
probabilidad *f* probability
probablemente *adv* probably
probar *vt* to try (*as a test*)
probenecid *m* probenecid
probiótico *m* probiotic
problema *m* problem
probucol *m* probucol
procaína *f* procaine
procainamida *f* procainamide
proceder *m* (*Esp*) procedure
procedimiento *m* procedure
procesado -da *adj* (*alimentos, etc.*) processed
proceso *m* process
proctitis *f* proctitis
pródromo *m* prodrome
producir *vt* to produce
producto *m* product; — **de limpieza** cleanser; — **lácteo** *or* **de la leche** milk *o* dairy product; — **químico** chemical
pro-elección *adj* pro-choice
profesional *adj* & *mf* professional; — **de la salud,** — **sanitario** (*Esp*) health professional
profesor -ra *mf* (*en una escuela*) teacher
profiláctico -ca *adj* prophylactic; *m* condom
profilaxis *f* prophylaxis; — **postexposición** postexposure prophylaxis
profundidad *f* depth
profundo -da *adj* deep
progeria *f* progeria
progesterona *f* progesterone
programa *m* program
programado -da *adj* (*cita, etc.*)

scheduled; (*surg*) scheduled, elective
progresar *vi* to progress
progresión *f* progression
progresivo -va *adj* progressive
progreso *m* progress
proguanil *m* proguanil
prolactina *f* prolactin
prolactinoma *m* prolactinoma
prolapso *m* prolapse; — **de la válvula mitral** mitral-valve prolapse; — **de recto (de útero, de vejiga, etc.)** prolapsed rectum (uterus, bladder, etc.); — **valvular mitral** mitral-valve prolapse
proliferación *f* proliferation
proliferativo -va *adj* proliferative
prolina *f* proline
prolongación *f* prolongation
prolongar *vt* to prolong
promedio *adj* (*esp. Amer, inv*) average; **la estatura promedio**..the average height; *m* average, mean (*form*); **como** — on average; **debajo del** — below average; **encima del** — above average
prometazina *f* promethazine
prometido -da *m* fiancé; *f* fiancée
prominencia *f* prominence
pronosticar *vt* to predict
pronóstico -ca *adj* prognostic; *m* prognosis
pronto *adv* soon
propagación *f* spread
propagar *vt, vr* to spread
propensión *f* predisposition, susceptibility
propenso -sa *adj* prone, predisposed, susceptible; **propenso a infecciones**..prone to infections
propilenglicol *m* propylene glycol
propiltiouracilo *m* propylthiouracil
propiocepción *f* proprioception
propioceptivo -va *adj* proprioceptive
proporción *f* proportion
proporcionar *vt* to provide
propoxifeno *m* propoxyphene
propranolol *m* propranolol
proptosis *f* proptosis
prospecto (de envase) *m* package insert
prostaglandina *f* prostaglandin
próstata *f* (*fam*) prostate gland, pros-

tate (*fam*)
prostatectomía *f* prostatectomy
prostático -ca *adj* prostatic
prostatitis *f* prostatitis
prostituto -ta *mf* prostitute
proteasa *f* protease
protección *f* protection
protector -ra *adj* protective; *m* guard, shield; — **bucal** mouth guard; — **solar** sunscreen
proteger *vt* to protect; — **de** to protect against; *vr* to protect oneself
proteico -ca *adj* pertaining to protein; **restricción** — protein restriction
proteína *f (frec. pl)* protein; **rico en proteínas.**.rich in protein
proteinosis alveolar *f* alveolar proteinosis
protésico -ca *adj* prosthetic
prótesis *f (pl -sis)* prosthesis; — **dental** denture, false teeth (*fam*); — **mamaria** breast implant; — **total de cadera** total hip replacement; — **total de rodilla** total knee replacement
protocolo *m* protocol
protozoario -ria *adj & m* protozoan
protozoo *m* protozoan
protruir *vi* to protrude
protuberancia *f* protuberance; *(puente)* pons
proveedor -ra *mf* provider; — **de salud** health care provider
proveer *vt* to provide
pro-vida *adj* pro-life
provisional *adj* provisional, temporary
provocación *f* challenge; — **con alergenos** allergen challenge
provocar *vt* to bring on, trigger, induce, provoke; **¿Hay algo en particular que le provoque los dolores?**..Is there anything in particular that brings on the pains?
próximo -ma *adj* next
proyección *f (psych, etc.)* projection
proyectil *m* projectile
prueba *f* test, trial, assay, try; proof, evidence; **a** — **de agua, a** — **de niños, etc.** waterproof, childproof, etc.; **dosis** *f* **de** — test dose; — **cruzada** crossmatch; — **cutánea**

skin test; — **de audición** hearing test; — **de embarazo** pregnancy test; — **de esfuerzo** exercise stress test; — **de función pulmonar** *or* **respiratoria** pulmonary function test; — **del aliento** breath test; — **de la mesa basculante** tilt table test; — **de la tuberculina** (*form*) *or* — **de la tuberculosis** TB test, PPD; — **del parche** patch test; — **del VIH** HIV test; — **de Papanicolaou** Papanicolaou smear (*form*), Pap smear; — **de sangre** blood test; — **de tolerancia (oral) a la glucosa** (oral) glucose tolerance test
prurito *m* pruritis
pseudoaneurisma *m* pseudoaneurysm
pseudoefedrina *f* pseudoephedrine
pseudogota *f* pseudogout
pseudohipoparatiroidismo *m* pseudohypoparathyroidism
pseudoquiste *m* pseudocyst; — **pancreático** pancreatic pseudocyst
pseudotumor *m* pseudotumor; — **cerebral** pseudotumor cerebri
psicoactivo -va *adj* psychoactive
psicoanálisis *m* psychoanalysis, analysis (*fam*)
psicoanalista *mf* psychoanalyst, analyst (*fam*)
psicoanalizar *vt* to psychoanalyze
psicógeno -na *adj* psychogenic
psicología *f* psychology
psicológico -ca *adj* psychological
psicólogo -ga *mf* psychologist
psicomotor -ra *adj* psychomotor
psicópata *mf* psychopath
psicosis *f (pl -sis)* psychosis
psicosocial *adj* psychosocial
psicosomático -ca *adj* psychosomatic
psicoterapeuta *mf* psychotherapist, therapist (*fam*)
psicoterapia *f* psychotherapy
psicótico -ca *adj & mf* psychotic
psicotrópico -ca *adj & m* psychotropic
psilio *m* psyllium
psilocibina *f* psilocybin
psique, psiquis *f* psyche
psiquiatra *mf* psychiatrist
psiquiatría *f* psychiatry

psiquiátrico -ca *adj* psychiatric
psitacosis *f* psittacosis
psoas *m* (*pl* **psoas**) psoas
psoraleno *m* psoralen; — **más radiación ultravioleta A (PUVA)** psoralen plus ultraviolet A (PUVA)
psoriasis *f* psoriasis
pterigión *m* pterygium
PTI *abbr* **púrpura trombocitopénica idiopática.** *See* **purpura.**
ptosis *f* ptosis
PTT *abbr* **púrpura trombocitopénica trombótica.** *See* **purpura.**
puberal *adj* pubertal
pubertad *f* puberty
pubiano -na *adj* pubic
púbico -ca *adj* pubic
pubis *m* (*form*) pubic area
público -ca *adj* public
pudendo -da *adj* pudendal
pudrir *vt, vr* (*pp* **podrido**) to rot
puente *m* (*anat*) pons; (*dent, etc.*) bridge; — **nasal** nasal bridge, bridge of the nose
puerco *m* **carne** *f* **de** — pork
puerperal *adj* puerperal
puerperio *m* puerperium
puesto *pp* *of* **poner**
puff *m* (*Ang, de un inhalador*) puff (*on an inhaler*)
pujar *vi* to bear down, to strain (*at stool*); (*obst*) to push; ¿**Tiene que pujar para defecar?**..Do you have to strain to have a bowel movement?...(*obst*) ¡**Respire profundo y puje!**..Take a deep breath and push!
pujo *m* tenesmus (*form*), frequent often painful urge to defecate without the ability to do so
pulga *f* flea
pulgada *f* inch
pulgar *m* thumb
pulir *vt* (*dent, etc.*) to polish
pulmón *m* lung
pulmonar *adj* pulmonary, pulmonic
pulmonía (*fam*) *See* **neumonía.**
pulpectomía *f* root canal therapy, root canal (*fam*)
pulpejo *m* (*del dedo*) pad (*of finger*)
pulsación *f* pulsation; (*de un inhalador*) puff
pulsera *f* bracelet; — **de alerta médica** medic alert bracelet; — **de identificación** ID bracelet
pulsioximetría *f* (*Esp*) pulse oximetry
pulso *m* pulse; — **carotídeo (radial, etc.)** carotid (radial, etc.) pulse; **tomarle el** — to take someone's pulse
puna *f* mountain sickness
punción *f* (*form*) puncture, tap; — **aspiración con aguja fina** fine needle aspiration biopsy; — **digital** (*form*) finger-stick; — **lumbar** lumbar puncture, spinal tap
puncionar *vt* (*form*) to puncture, tap
punta *f* tip; — **del dedo** fingertip
puntaje de Apgar *m* Apgar score
puntiagudo -da *adj* sharp, pointed
punto *m* point; (*de sutura*) stitch; — **de corte** cutoff point; — **de presión** pressure point; — **gatillo** trigger point
punzada *f* shooting pain, twinge, pang
punzante *adj* (*dolor*) sharp, jabbing, piercing, shooting; **herida** — puncture wound; **objeto** — sharp object
punzar *vt* to puncture, to stick, prick
punzocortante *adj* (*esp. Mex*) sharp
puñalada *f* stab wound
puño *m* fist; **cerrar el** — to make a fist
pupa *f* (*Esp*) blister
pupila *f* (*del ojo*) pupil
pupú *m* *See* **popó.**
puré *m* (*pl* **purés**) purée
purga *f* laxative, purge (*ant*), purgative (*ant*)
purgación *f* (*fam, gonorrea*) gonorrhea, the clap (*fam, ant*)
purgante *adj* & *m* laxative, purgative (*ant*)
purificación *f* purification
purificado -da *adj* purified
purificador *m* purifier
purificar *vt* to purify
purina *f* purine
puro -ra *adj* pure; *m* cigar
púrpura *f* purpura; — **de Schönlein-Henoch** Henoch-Schönlein purpura; — **trombocitopénica idiopática (PTI)** idiopathic thrombocytopenic purpura (ITP); — **trombocitopénica trombótica (PTT)**

thrombotic thrombocytopenic purpura (TTP)
pus *m* pus
pústula *f* pustule

PUVA *abbr* **psoraleno más radiación ultravioleta A**. *See* **psoraleno**.

Q

quebradizo -za *adj* fragile
quebrado -da *adj* broken, split
quebradura *f* (*ortho*) break, split
quebrar *vt, vr* to break, fracture, split; **¿Cuándo se quebró la pierna?**..When did you break your leg?
quedar *vi* (*also* — **bien**) to fit; *vr* — **dormido** to fall asleep, to go to sleep; — **en cama** to stay in bed
queilitis *f* cheilitis
queja *f* complaint
quejarse *vr* to complain
quelación *f* chelation
quelante *adj* chelating; *m* chelating agent; — **del hierro** iron-chelating agent
queloide *m* keloid
quemador de grasa *m* fat burner
quemadura *f* burn; — **de primer (segundo, tercer) grado** first (second, third) degree burn; — **solar** sunburn
quemante *adj* burning
quemar *vt* to burn; *vr* to burn oneself, to get burned; (*con el sol*) to sunburn, to get sunburned *o* sunburnt; **¿Se quemó?**..Did you burn yourself?...**¿Se quemó el pie?**..Did you burn your foot?
quemazón *f* burning, burn
queratectomía *f* keratectomy; — **fotorrefractiva** photorefractive keratectomy (PRK)

queratina *f* keratin
queratitis *f* keratitis
queratomileusis *f* keratomileusis; — **in situ asistida con láser** laser-assisted in situ keratomileusis (LASIK)
queratosis *f* (*pl* -sis) keratosis; — **actínica** actinic keratosis; — **seborreica** seborrheic keratosis
queratotomía *f* keratotomy; — **radial** radial keratotomy
querer *vt, vi* (*amar*) to love
queso *m* cheese
quetiapina *f* quetiapine
quijada *f* jawbone, jaw
quilate *m* carat; **oro de 24 quilates** 24 carat gold
químico -ca *adj* chemical; *f* chemistry
quimioprofilaxis *f* chemoprophylaxis
quimioterapia *f* chemotherapy; — **a altas dosis** high-dose chemotherapy; — **de inducción** induction chemotherapy; — **neoadyuvante** neoadjuvant chemotherapy
quinacrina *f* quinacrine
quinapril *m* quinapril
quinidina *f* quinidine
quinina *f* quinine
quinta enfermedad *f* fifth disease
quintillizo -za *mf* quintuplet
quirófano *m* operating room (OR)
quiropráctico -ca *mf* chiropractor; *f*

chiropractic
quiropraxia *f* chiropractic
quirúrgico -ca *adj* surgical
quiste *m* cyst; — **de Baker** Baker's cyst; — **del conducto tirogloso** thyroglossal duct cyst; — **de ovario** ovarian cyst; — **dermoide** dermoid cyst; — **epidermoide** epidermal inclusion cyst (*form*), sebaceous cyst; — **hidatídico** hydatid cyst; — **ovárico** ovarian cyst; —

pilonidal pilonidal cyst; — **sebáceo** epidermal inclusion cyst (*form*), sebaceous cyst
quistectomía *f* cystectomy, removal of a cyst
quístico -ca *adj* cystic
quitar *vt* to remove; *vr* (*ropa, etc.*) to take off; (*dolor, hábito, etc.*) to go away; **Quítese la camisa**..Take off your shirt...**No se me quita el dolor**..The pain won't go away.

R

rabadilla *f* (*Amer, fam*) coccyx, tailbone (*fam*)
rabdomiólisis, rabdomiolisis *f* rhabdomyolysis
rabdomioma *m* rhabdomyoma
rabdomiosarcoma *m* rhabdomyosarcoma
rabeprazol *m* rabeprazole
rabia *f* (*enfermedad*) rabies; (*ira*) rage
rabieta *f* tantrum
rabioso -sa *adj* (*con el mal de rabia*) rabid
ración *f* ration, serving; **raciones por envase** servings per container
racionalización *f* (*psych*) rationalization
racionalizar *vi* (*psych*) to rationalize
radiación *f* radiation; **enfermedad por** — radiation sickness; — **ionizante** ionizing radiation
radiactividad *f* radioactivity
radiactivo -va *adj* radioactive
radial *adj* (*anat*) radial
radical *adj* radical

radiculopatía *f* radiculopathy; — **cervical** cervical radiculopathy
radio *m* radius; (*elemento*) radium
radioactividad *f* radioactivity
radioactivo -va *adj* radioactive
radiografía *f* (*técnica imagenológica*) radiography; (*estudio imagenológico*) x-ray, film; — **de tórax** chest x-ray
radioisótopo *m* radioisotope
radiología *f* radiology
radiólogo -ga *mf* radiologist
radionúclido *m* radionuclide
radioterapia *f* radiation therapy, radiotherapy
radioyodo *m* radioiodine
radón *m* radon
raíz *f* (*pl* **raíces**) root; — **del diente** tooth root *o* root of the tooth; — **del pelo** hair root; — **de regaliz** (*bot*) licorice root; — **nerviosa** nerve root
ralo -la *adj* (*cabello*) thin
raloxifeno *m* raloxifene
rama *f* branch

ramipril *m* ramipril
rango *m* range; **en rango normal**..in normal range; **— de movimiento** range of motion; **— de valores** range of values
ranitidina *f* ranitidine
ranurado -da *adj* (*tableta, etc.*) scored
rapé *m* (*tabaco*) snuff
rápido -da *adj* rapid
raquídeo -a *adj* spinal
raquitismo *m* rickets
raro -ra *adj* rare, unusual
rascarse *vr* to scratch (oneself); **Trate de no rascarse**..Try not to scratch (yourself).
rasgo *m* trait; **— drepanocítico** *or* **falciforme** sickle cell trait; *mpl* features
rasguñar *vt* to scratch
rasguño *m* scratch
rash *m* rash
raspa *f* fishbone
raspado *m* (*obst*) curettage
raspadura *f* (*fam*) abrasion, scrape (*fam*)
raspar *vt* to scrape, to skin (*fam*)
rasquiña *f* (*fam*) itching
rastreo *m* scan
rastrillo *m* (*Mex, navaja*) razor
rasuradora (eléctrica) *f* (*esp. Mex*) shaver, electric shaver
rasurar *vt, vr* to shave
rata *f* rat
raticida *m* rat poison, rodenticide
rato *m* short time, short while
ratón *m* mouse
raya *f* streak; (*zool*) stingray
rayo *m* ray; **los rayos del sol** *or* **solares** the sun's rays; **— X** x-ray
raza *f* race (*of people*)
razón *f* reason; (*math*) ratio; **perder la —** to lose one's mind, to go crazy; **— internacional normalizada (INR)** international normalized ratio (INR)
RCP *abbr* reanimación cardiopulmonar. *See* **reanimación.**
reabsorber *vt* to resorb; *vr* to get resorbed
reabsorbible *adj* (*sutura, etc.*) absorbable
reabsorción *f* resorption

reacción *f* reaction; **— adversa** adverse reaction; **— alérgica** allergic reaction; **— cruzada** cross reaction; **— en cadena** chain reaction; **— en cadena de la polimerasa** polymerase chain reaction (PCR); **— tardía** delayed reaction; **— transfusional** transfusion reaction
reaccionar *vi* to react
reactivación *f* reactivation
reactivar *vt* to reactivate
reactividad *f* reactivity; **— cruzada** cross-reactivity
reactivo -va *adj* reactive; *m* reagent
reagudización *f* exacerbation, flare
reagudizarse *vi* to get worse again, to flare
realidad *f* reality; **en —** actually
realimentación *f* refeeding
realmente *adv* actually
reanimación *f* resuscitation; **— cardiopulmonar (RCP)** cardiopulmonary resuscitation (CPR)
reanimar *vt* to resuscitate, to revive; **no —** **(NR)** Do Not Resuscitate (DNR); **orden** *f* **de no —** **(ONR)** DNR order; *vi,* to revive
reanudar *vt* to resume
rebote *m* rebound; **hipertensión** *f* **de —** rebound hypertension
recaer *vi* to relapse
recaída *f* relapse
recámara *f* bedroom
recepcionista *mf* receptionist
receptor *m* receptor; **positivo para receptores de estrógeno** estrogen-receptor-positive; *mf* (*de una transfusión, un trasplante, etc.*) recipient
recesivo -va *adj* recessive
receta *f* (*pharm*) prescription
recetar *vt* (*pharm*) to prescribe, to order
rechazar *vt* to reject
rechazo *m* rejection
rechinar *vi* (*los dientes*) to grind (*one's teeth*)
reciclaje *m* recycling
reciclamiento *m* recycling
reciclar *vt* to recycle
recidiva *f* (*form*) (*recurrencia*) recurrence; (*recaída*) relapse
recidivante *adj* (*form*) recurrent
recién nacido -da *mf* newborn

recientemente *adv* recently
recipiente *m* container
recobrar *vt, vr* to recover; — **el aliento** to catch one's breath; — **el conocimiento** to regain consciousness
recolocar *vt* to reattach
recombinante *adj* recombinant
recomendación *f* recommendation
recomendar *vt* to recommend
reconectar *vt* to reconnect, to reattach
reconocer *vt* to recognize; (*form, examinar*) to examine
reconocimiento *m* recognition; (*form, examen*) examination
reconstitución *f* reconstitution; — **inmunológica** *or* **inmune** immune reconstitution
reconstrucción *f* reconstruction
reconstructivo -va *adj* reconstructive
reconstruir *vt* to reconstruct
recordar *vt* to remember, recall
recostado -da *adj* recumbent, lying down
recostarse *vr* to lie down
recreación *f* recreation
recreacional *adj* recreational
recreo *m* recreation
recrudecer *vi, vr* to get worse again, to flare
rectal *adj* rectal
recto -ta *adj* straight; *m* rectum
rectocele *m* rectocele
recubrimiento *m* (*del estómago, etc.*) lining
recubrir *vt* (*el intestino, etc.*) to line
recuento *m* count; — **bacteriano** (*form*) *or* **de bacterias** bacterial *o* bacteria count; — **de eritrocitos** (*form*) red blood cell count; — **de espermatozoides** sperm count; — **de glóbulos blancos** white blood cell count; — **de glóbulos rojos** red blood cell count; — **de leucocitos** (*form*) white blood cell count; — **de pastillas** pill count; — **de plaquetas** platelet count; — **espermático** sperm count; — **leucocitario** (*form*) white blood cell count; — **plaquetario** (*form*) platelet count; — **sanguíneo completo** (*Esp*) complete blood count

recuerdo *m* recall
recuperación *f* recuperation, recovery; **sala de** — recovery room
recuperar *vt* to regain, recover; — **el aliento** to catch one's breath; — **peso** to regain weight; *vr* to recuperate, recover, to get better
recurrencia *f* recurrence
recurrente *adj* recurrent
recurso *m* resource, resort; **último** — last resort
red *f* net, network; **red de hospitales** ..network of hospitals; — **de seguridad** safety net
redondo -da *adj* round
reducción *f* reduction
reducible *adj* reducible
reducir *vt* (*ortho, etc.*) to reduce; *vr* to get smaller, shrink
reductible *adj* reducible
reemplazar *vt* to replace
reentrenamiento *m* retraining
reestenosis *f* (*pl* -**sis**) restenosis
reevaluar *vt* to reevaluate
referencia *f* reference
referido -da *adj* (*dolor*) referred
referir *vt* (*remitir*) to refer
reflejo *m* reflex; **martillo de reflejos** reflex hammer; — **condicionado** conditioned reflex; — **de eyección de la leche** (*obst, form*) letdown; — **de sobresalto** startle reflex; — **nauseoso** *or* **faríngeo** gag reflex; — **rotuliano** *or* **patelar** patellar reflex, knee jerk (*fam*)
reflexología *f* reflexology
reflujo *m* reflux; — **de ácido** acid reflux; — **gastroesofágico** esophageal reflux
reforzar *vt* to reinforce
refracción *f* refraction; **defecto de** — refractive error
refresco *m* soft drink
refrigeración *f* refrigeration
refrigerador *m* refrigerator
refrigerar *vt* to refrigerate
refrigerio *m* snack
refuerzo *m* reinforcement; **dosis** *f* **de** — booster dose
refugio *m* shelter; — **para mujeres,** — **para personas sin hogar, etc.** women's shelter, homeless shelter, etc.

regaliz *m* licorice
regazo *m* lap
regeneración *f* regeneration
regenerarse *vr* to regenerate
régimen *m* (*pl* **regímenes**) regimen; (*dieta*) diet; **seguir un —** to diet, to be on a diet
región *f* region, area
regional *adj* regional
registro *m* registry; (*de un ECG*) tracing; **— de tumores** tumor registry
regla *f* rule; (*período menstrual*) period; **bajarle la —** (*fam*) to have one's period, to start one's period
regresión *f* (*psych*) regression
regulable *adj* adjustable
regular *adj* regular
regurgitación *f* regurgitation, insufficiency; **— aórtica, — mitral, etc.** aortic regurgitation *o* insufficiency, mitral regurgitation *o* insufficiency, etc.
regurgitar *vt* to regurgitate
regusto *m* aftertaste
rehabilitación *f* rehabilitation
rehabilitar *vt* to rehabilitate; *vr* to become rehabilitated
rehidratación *f* rehydration
rehidratar *vt* to rehydrate
reinfección *f* reinfection
reinfectado -da *adj* reinfected
reír *vi, vr* to laugh
reiterativo -va *adj* repetitive
rejuvenecer *vt* to rejuvenate; *vr* to become rejuvenated
relación *f* relation, relationship; **Busco una relación seria**..I'm looking for a serious relationship; **relaciones sexuales** sexual intercourse, sex (*fam*); **¿Puedo tener relaciones sexuales?**..Can I have sexual intercourse?
relajación *f* relaxation; **técnicas de —** relaxation techniques
relajante *m* relaxant; **— muscular** muscle relaxant
relajar *vt, vr* to relax; **para relajar la tensión**..to relax the tension...**No puedo relajarme**..I can't relax.
relámpago *m* lightning
rellenar *vt* (*Amer, dent*) to fill (*a cavity*)

relleno *m* (*Amer, dent*) filling
reloj biológico *m* biological clock
remedio *m* remedy, cure; **— casero** home remedy; **— para** *or* **contra la tos** cough remedy
remisión *f* remission; (*a un especialista, etc.*) referral; **entrar en —** to go into remission; **— completa** complete remission; **— parcial** partial remission
remitir *vt* (*esp. Esp, a un paciente*) to refer
remodelación *f* remodeling; **— cardíaca** cardiac remodeling; **— ósea** bone remodeling
remodelamiento *m* remodeling; **— cardíaco** cardiac remodeling; **— óseo** bone remodeling
remojar *vt* to soak
remordimiento *m* remorse
remover *vt* to remove
removible *adj* removable
renal *adj* renal
rendimiento *m* performance
renguear *vi* (*esp. SA*) to limp
renovar *vt* to renew
renovascular *adj* renovascular
renquear *vi* (*esp. Esp*) to limp
rentabilidad *f* cost-effectiveness
rentable *adj* cost-effective
reparación *f* repair
reparar *vt* to repair, fix
repelente *m* repellent; **— de insectos** insect repellent
repente *m* **de —** suddenly
repetición *f* repetition
repetir *vt* to repeat
repetitivo -va *adj* repetitive
reponerse *vr* to recover
reportar *vt* (*declarar*) to report
reposabrazos *m* armrest
reposacabezas *m* headrest
reposapiés *m* footrest
reposar *vi* to rest
reposo *m* rest; **en —** at rest, resting; **frecuencia cardíaca en reposo**.. resting heart rate; **— en cama** bed rest
represión *f* (*psych*) repression
reprimir *vt* (*psych*) to repress
reproducción *f* reproduction; **— asistida** assisted reproduction
reproducir *vt, vr* to reproduce

reproductivo -va *adj* reproductive

reproductor -ra *adj* reproductive

reprogramar *vt* (*una cita*) to reschedule (*an appointment*)

resaca *f* hangover; **tener una —** to have a hangover, to be hungover

resbalar *vi, vr* to slip

rescatador -ra *mf* rescuer

rescatar *vt* to rescue

rescate *m* rescue; **— aéreo** air rescue; **tratamiento de —** salvage therapy

resecar *vt* to resect, to excise; *vr* to dry, dry out, get dry

resección *f* resection, excision; **— transuretral de la próstata** transurethral resection of the prostate (TURP)

reseco -ca *adj* dry, dried, dried out

resequedad *f* (*esp. Mex*) dryness

reserpina *f* reserpine

reserva *f* reserve, store

reservorio *m* reservoir

resfriado -da *adj* **estar —** to have a cold; *m* cold; **— común** common cold

resfriarse *vr* to catch a cold

residencia *f* home, institution; **— de ancianos** rest home

residente *mf* resident; **— de medicina familiar, — de cirugía, etc.** family practice resident, surgical resident, etc.

residual *adj* residual

residuo *m* residue, waste; **residuos peligrosos** hazardous waste

resina *f* resin

resincronización *f* resynchronization; **— cardíaca** cardiac resynchronization

resistencia *f* resistance; stamina; **— a la insulina** insulin resistance; **— cruzada** cross-resistance

resistente *adj* resistant; **— a la meticilina** methicillin-resistant

resistir *vt* to resist

resollar *vi* to breathe; (*jadear*) to breathe hard, to pant

resolución *f* resolution; **alta —** high resolution

resolverse *vr* (*pp* **resuelto**) to resolve, clear up

resonancia *f* resonance; **— magnética (nuclear) (RMN)** magnetic resonance imaging (MRI); **— magnética abierta** open MRI

respaldo *m* backup; **— quirúrgico** surgical backup

respetar *vt* to respect

respeto *m* respect; **— de uno mismo** self-respect

respiración *f* respiration, breath

respirador *m* respirator, ventilator

respirar *vt, vi* to breathe, breathe in; **Respire profundo.**.Breathe deeply ..Take a deep breath.

respiratorio -ria *adj* respiratory

responder *vi* to respond

respuesta *f* response; **— completa** complete response; **— inmune** immune response; **— parcial** partial response; **— sostenida** sustained response

restablecer *vt* to restore; *vr* (*de una enfermedad*) to recover

restablecimiento *m* recovery

restar *vt, vi* (*arith*) to subtract; **Reste 5 a 100.**.Subtract 5 from one 100.

restauración *f* (*dent, surg*) restoration

restaurar *vt* (*dent, surg*) to restore

restaurativo -va *adj* (*dent, surg*) restorative

resto *m* rest; **el resto de su convalecencia**..the rest of your convalescence

restricción *f* restriction

restringir *vt* to restrict

resucitación *f* resuscitation

resucitar *vt* to resuscitate

resuelto *pp of* **resolver**

resultado *m* result, outcome

resultar *vi* to turn out; **¿Y si resulta positivo?**..And if it turns out positive?

retardado -da *adj* delayed

retardante de fuego *m* flame *o* fire retardant

retardar *vt* to delay

retardo *m* retardation, delay; **— del crecimiento intrauterino** intrauterine growth retardation

retención *f* retention; **— urinaria** urinary retention

retenedor *m* (*orthodontia*) retainer

retener *vt* to retain; **— agua** to retain water

retenido -da *adj* (*dent, etc.*) impacted
reticulocito *m* reticulocyte
retina *f* retina
retiniano -na *adj* retinal
retinitis *f* retinitis; — **pigmentaria** *or* **pigmentosa** retinitis pigmentosa
retinoblastoma *m* retinoblastoma
retinoide *m* retinoid
retinol *m* retinol
retinopatía *f* retinopathy; — **diabética** diabetic retinopathy
retirada *f* removal; (*de un producto defectuoso*) recall
retirar *vt* (*catéter, suturas, etc.*) to remove; (*un producto defectuoso*) to recall
reto *m* challenge; **un reto diagnóstico y terapéutico**..a diagnostic and therapeutic challenge
retorcerse *vr* to writhe
retortijón, retorcijón *m* abdominal cramp
retrasado -da *adj* delayed, retarded; — **mental** developmentally delayed, mentally retarded (*ant*)
retrasar *vt* to delay; *vr* to lag
retraso *m* delay, lag; — **mental** developmental delay, mental retardation (*ant*)
retroalimentación *f* feedback
retrógrado -da *adj* retrograde
retroperitoneal *adj* retroperitoneal
retroviral *adj* retroviral
retrovírico -ca *adj* retroviral
retrovirus *m* (*pl* **-rus**) retrovirus
reuma *m* rheumatism
reumático -ca *adj* rheumatic
reumatismo *m* rheumatism; — **palindrómico** palindromic rheumatism
reumatoide *adj* rheumatoid
reumatología *f* rheumatology
reumatólogo -ga *mf* rheumatologist
reusable *adj* reusable
revacunación *f* revaccination; additional vaccination (*in a series*), booster vaccination
revalorar *vt* to reevaluate
revascularización *f* revascularization
reventar *vt, vr* to rupture, burst
reversible *adj* reversible
reversión *f* reversal
revestimiento *m* (*del estómago, etc.*) lining
revestir *vt* to line; **Células mucosas revisten el intestino**..Mucous cells line the intestine.
revisar *vt* to examine, to check
revisión *f* revision; (*examen*) examination; — **médica** medical examination, checkup (*fam*); — **por sistemas** review of systems
revitalizador -ra *adj* revitalizing
revitalizante *adj* revitalizing
revitalizar *vt* to revitalize
revivir *vi* to revive
ribavirina *f* ribavirin
riboflavina *f* riboflavin, vitamin B₂
ricina *f* ricin
rico -ca *adj* rich; — **en grasa** rich, greasy; — **en proteínas** rich in protein
riesgo *m* risk, hazard; **correr el — de** to run the risk of; **de alto —** high-risk; **de bajo —** low-risk; **factor** *m* **de —** risk factor; — **biológico** biohazard; — **calculado** calculated risk; **riesgos y beneficios** risks and benefits
riesgoso -sa *adj* hazardous
rifabutina *f* rifabutin
rifamicina *f* rifamycin
rifampicina *f* rifampin
rifaximina *f* rifaximin
rigidez *f* rigidity, stiffness
rígido -da *adj* rigid, stiff
rigor mortis *m* rigor mortis
rimantadina *f* rimantadine
rímel *m* mascara
rinitis *f* rhinitis; — **alérgica** allergic rhinitis
rinofima *m* rhinophyma
rinoplastia *f* rhinoplasty
rinovirus *m* (*pl* **-rus**) rhinovirus
riñón *m* kidney
riñonera *f* emesis basin
risa *f* laugh
risedronato *m* risedronate
risperidona *f* risperidone
ritidectomía *f* (*form*) face-lift
ritmo *m* rhythm; **método del —** rhythm method; — **biológico** biorhythm; — **circadiano** circadian rhythm
ritonavir *m* ritonavir
ritual *m* ritual

rivalidad *f* rivalry; — **entre hermanos** sibling rivalry
rizatriptán *m* rizatriptan
RMN *abbr* **resonancia magnética
nuclear.** *See* **resonancia.**
roble venenoso *m* poison oak
robótico -ca *adj* robotic
robusto -ta *adj* stocky
rodar *vi* — **por encima de** to run
over
rodilla *f* knee
rodillera *f* kneepad
roedor *m* rodent
rofecoxib *m* rofecoxib
rojizo -za *adj* reddish
rojo -ja *adj* red
rollos (de grasa) *mpl* flab
romero *m* (*bot*) rosemary
romo -ma *adj* dull, blunt
romper *vt, vr* (*pp* **roto**) (*ortho, etc.*)
to break
ron *m* rum
roncar *vi* to snore
roncha *f* (*frec. pl*) wheal, hive (*frec.
pl*)
ronchitas *fpl* (*fam*) spots (*on the
skin*), fine rash
ronco -ca *adj* hoarse; **tener la voz —**
to be hoarse
rondas (médicas) *fpl* rounds
ronquera *f* hoarseness
ronquidos *m* snoring
roña *f* (*Mex, fam*) scabies
ropa *f* clothes, clothing; — **de cama**
bedclothes, bedding; — **interior**
underwear
rosado -da *adj* pink
rosiglitazona *f* rosiglitazone
rostro *m* face
rosuvastatina *f* rosuvastatin
roto -ta (*pp of* **romper**) *adj* broken
rótula *f* patella, kneecap (*fam*)
rotura *f* rupture; (*esp. Esp, desgarro*)
tear; — **prematura de membranas**
premature rupture of membranes
rozadura *f* abrasion (*due to chafing*)
rozar *vt* to graze, to chafe, rub; *vi* to
chafe, rub
rozón *m* (*esp. Mex*) scratch, graze
rubefacción *f* (*physio, form*) flush,
flushing
rubéola *f* rubella, German measles
(*fam*)
rubio -bia *adj* blond; *m* blond; *f*
blonde
rubor *m* (*form*) redness, flush, flushing; (*debido a la menopausia*) hot
flush (*form*), hot flash
ruborizarse *vr* to flush, to blush
rugir *vi* (*el estómago*) to growl
ruido *m* noise; — **blanco** white
noise; **ruidos cardíacos** heart
sounds
ruptura *f* rupture; — **prematura de
membranas** premature rupture of
membranes
rural *adj* rural
rutina *f* routine; — **diaria** daily routine
rutinario -ria *adj* routine

S

sábana *f* sheet, bedsheet
sabañón *m* chilblain
saber *vi* to taste; — **a** to taste like; — **mal** to taste bad
sábila *f* aloe
sabor *m* flavor, taste; **con — a cereza, con — a plátano, etc.** cherry-flavored, banana-flavored, etc.
sacaleches *m* breast pump
sacar *vt* to remove, take out; — **aire** (*esp. Mex, CA; fam*) to breathe out; — **la lengua** to stick out one's tongue; — **sangre** to draw blood; *vr* — **los mocos** to pick one's nose
sacarina *f* saccharin
sacerdote *m* priest
saciedad *f* (*form*) satiety (*form*), fullness
saco *m* (*anat*) sac
sacro -cra *adj* sacral; *m* sacrum
sacroilíaco, sacroiliaco -ca (*esp. Mex*) *adj* sacroiliac
sacudida (muscular) *f* twitch
sacudir *vt* to shake; **sacudir a un bebé**..to shake a baby; *vr* — **la nariz** (*esp. Carib*) to blow one's nose
sádico -ca *adj* sadistic; *mf* sadist
sadismo *m* sadism
sadomasoquismo *m* sadomasochism
sadomasoquista *mf* sadomasochist
safeno -na *adj* saphenous
sal *f* salt; — **de Epsom** *or* **de la Higuera** Epsom salt; — **yodada** iodized salt; **sustituto de la —** salt substitute
sala *f* ward, room, suite; — **de emergencias** emergency room (ER); — **de endoscopia** endoscopy suite; — **de espera** waiting room; — **de maternidad** maternity ward; — **de neonatología** (*form*) newborn nursery; — **de observación** observation ward; — **de operaciones** operating room (OR); — **de partos** delivery room, Labor & Delivery; — **de reanimación** (*Esp*) recovery room; — **de recién nacidos** new-

born nursery; — **de recuperación** recovery room; — **de urgencias** emergency room (ER)
salado -da *adj* salted, salty
salbutamol *m* salbutamol
salicilato *m* salicylate
salida *f* exit
salino -na *adj* saline
salir *vi* to drain; **¿Le sale pus?**..Is it draining pus? **salir(le) (a uno)** to appear, develop; **Me salió una úlcera**..An ulcer appeared (developed)..I developed an ulcer; **salir(le) (a uno) granos** to break out (*one's skin*); **Le están saliendo granos**..He's breaking out..His skin is breaking out; **salir(le) (a uno) los dientes** to teethe, to come in (*one's teeth*); **¿Le están saliendo los dientes?**..Is he teething?..Are his teeth coming in? *vr* to appear, develop
saliva *f* saliva, spit
salivación *f* salivation
salival, salivar *adj* salivary
salmeterol *m* salmeterol
salmonelosis *f* salmonellosis
salpingitis *f* salpingitis
salpingooforectomía *f* salpingo-oophorectomy
salpullido *m* (*esp. Mex*) rash, heat rash, miliaria
salsalato *m* salsalate
saltar *vi* to hop; **Salte en un pie**..Hop on one foot; *vr* to skip; — **una comida** to skip a meal
salto *m* hop
salud *f* health; — **de la mujer** women's health; — **laboral** occupational health; — **mental** mental health; — **ocupacional** occupational health; — **pública** public health
saludable *adj* healthful, healthy
salvado *m* bran
salvamento *m* rescue
salvar *vt* to save, rescue, to salvage

salvia *f (bot)* sage
sanador -ra *mf* folk *o* traditional healer; faith healer
sanar *vt, vi* to heal
sanatorio *m* sanatorium
saneamiento (ambiental) *m* sanitation
sangrado *m* bleeding, bleed; — **menstrual** menstrual bleeding; — **nasal** nosebleed
sangrador *m* phlebotomist
sangrante *adj* bleeding; **úlcera** — bleeding ulcer
sangrar *vi* to bleed
sangre *f* blood; **poner** — *(fam)* to give a transfusion *(of blood)*, to transfuse *(blood)*; **¿Me van a poner sangre?**..Are you going to give me a transfusion?
sangría *f* (therapeutic) phlebotomy
sanguijuela *f* leech
sanguíneo -a *adj* pertaining to blood; **flujo** — blood flow
sanguinolento -ta *adj (form)* bloody; **esputo** — bloody sputum
sanidad *f* sanitation; *(esp. Esp, salud)* health
sanitario -ria *adj* sanitary; *(esp. Esp)* pertaining to health *(esp. public health)*
sano -na *adj* healthy
santos óleos *mpl* last rites, anointing of the sick
sapo *m (PR, SD)* thrush
saquinavir *m* saquinavir
sarampión *m* measles; — **alemán** *(fam)* rubella, German measles *(fam)*
sarcoidosis *f* sarcoidosis
sarcoma *m* sarcoma; — **de Ewing** Ewing's sarcoma; — **de Kaposi** Kaposi's sarcoma
sarín *m* sarin
SARM *abbr* **Staphylococcus aureus resistente a meticilina.** *See* **Staphylococcus aureus.**
sarna *f* scabies; — **noruega** Norwegian scabies
sarpullido *m* rash, heat rash, miliaria
sarro *m (dental)* calculus *(form)*, tartar
sasafrás *m (bot)* sassafras
saturado -da *adj* saturated

saturar *vt* to saturate
sauna *m&f* sauna
scanner *m (Ang)* scanner
SDRA *abbr* **síndrome de dificultad respiratoria del adulto.** *See* **síndrome.**
sebáceo -a *adj* sebaceous
sebo *m* sebum
seborrea *f* seborrhea
seborreico -ca *adj* seborrheic
seca *f (CA, Carib)* enlarged tender lymph node
secante *adj* drying
secar *vt* to dry; *vr* to dry, get dry, dry out
sección *f* section
seco -ca *adj* dry; **boca** — dry mouth
secreción *f* secretion, discharge
secretar *vt* to secrete
secretario -ria *mf* secretary
secreto médico *m* doctor-patient confidentiality
secretorio -ria *adj* secretory
secundario -ria *adj* secondary
secundinas *fpl* afterbirth
sed *f* thirst; **dar** — to make thirsty; **tener** — to be thirsty; **¿Tiene sed?** ..Are you thirsty?
seda *f* silk; — **dental** dental floss
sedación *f* sedation; — **consciente** conscious sedation
sedante *adj & m* sedative
sedar *vt* to sedate
sedentario -ria *adj* sedentary
sedimento *m* sediment, deposit
segmento *m* segment
segregar *vt (form)* to secrete
seguido *adv (esp. Mex)* often; **¿Qué tan seguido le dan las contracciones?**..How often are the contractions coming?
seguimiento *m* follow-up
segundo -da *adj* second; *m* second
seguridad *f* safety; — **en uno mismo** self-confidence
seguro -ra *adj* safe, sure; **para estar** — to be sure; **sexo** — safe sex; *m* insurance; *(Mex, imperdible)* safety pin; — **médico** medical insurance; — **privado** private insurance
selectivo -va *adj* selective
selegilina *f* selegiline
selenio *m* selenium

semana *f* week
semen *m* semen
seminal *adj* seminal
seminoma *m* seminoma
semivida *f* half-life
sen *m* (*bot*) senna
sena *f* (*bot*) senna
senderismo *m* hiking
senectud *f* old age
senil *adj* senile
seno *m* sinus; (*pecho*) breast; — **etmoidal** ethmoid sinus; — **frontal** frontal sinus; — **maxilar** maxillary sinus; — **pilonidal** pilonidal sinus
sensación *f* sensation, feeling
sensibilidad *f* sensitivity; feeling, (*tacto fino*) light touch sensation
sensibilizar *vt* to sensitize; *vr* to become sensitized
sensible *adj* sensitive; (*susceptible*) amenable; — **al tratamiento** amenable to treatment
sensitivo -va *adj* sensory (*nerves, etc.*)
sensorio -ria *adj* sensory (*perceptions, etc.*)
sentaderas *fpl* (*esp. Mex, fam*) buttocks, bottom (*fam*)
sentadilla *f* knee bend
sentado -da *adj* sitting; **quedarse —** to sit, to remain sitting; **Me quedé sentado más de una hora**..I sat for over an hour.
sentarse *vr* (*si está de pie*) to sit, sit down, (*si está acostado*) to sit up
sentido *m* sense; — **común** common sense; — **de la vista** sense of sight; — **del equilibrio** sense of balance; — **del gusto** sense of taste; — **del humor** sense of humor; — **del oído** sense of hearing; — **del olfato** sense of smell; — **del tacto** sense of touch
sentimiento *m* feeling, emotion
sentir *vt* to feel; (*lamentar*) to be sorry; **Va a sentir un poco de dolor**.. You're going to feel a little pain... **Lo siento**..I'm sorry; *vr* to feel; **¿Cómo se siente?**..How do you feel?...**¿Se siente cansada?**..Do you feel tired?
señal *f* sign, (*auditiva, visual, etc.*) cue; — **de alarma** warning sign

separado -da *adj* separate
separar *vt* to separate
sepsis *f* sepsis
septicemia *f* septicemia, blood poisoning (*fam*)
séptico -ca *adj* septic
septo *m* septum; — **interauricular** interatrial septum; — **interventricular** interventricular septum
septoplastia *f* septoplasty
sequedad *f* dryness; — **de boca** dry mouth
ser *m* — **amado** loved one; — **humano** human being
Serenoa repens, (*bot*) saw palmetto
seriado -da *adj* serial
sérico -ca *adj* pertaining to serum; **testosterona** — serum testosterone
serie *f* series; — **ósea** bone scan
serina *f* serine
serio -ria *adj* serious
seroconversión *f* seroconversion
serología *f* serology
serológico -ca *adj* serological, serologic
seronegativo -va *adj* seronegative
seropositivo -va *adj* seropositive
serotipo *m* serotype
serotonina *f* serotonin
serpiente *f* snake; — **de cascabel** rattlesnake
sertaconazol *m* sertaconazole
sertralina *f* sertraline
servicio *m* service; (*frec. pl, baño*) restroom; **servicios sociales** social services
seta *f* mushroom
seudoaneurisma *m* pseudoaneurysm
seudoefedrina *f* pseudoephedrine
seudogota *f* pseudogout
seudohipoparatiroidismo *m* pseudohypoparathyroidism
seudoquiste *m* pseudocyst — **pancreático** pancreatic pseudocyst
seudotumor *m* pseudotumor; — **cerebral** pseudotumor cerebri
severo -ra *adj* severe
sexo *m* sex, gender; — **oral** oral sex; — **seguro** safe sex
sexología *f* study of sexuality
sexual *adj* sexual
sexualidad *f* sexuality
shigelosis *f* shigellosis

shock *m* (*Ang*) shock; — **anafiláctico** anaphylactic shock; — **cardiogénico** cardiogenic shock; — **hipovolémico** hypovolemic shock; — **neurogénico** neurogenic shock; — **séptico** septic shock

sialoadenitis *f* sialoadenitis

sibilancia (*form*) *f* wheeze; *fpl* wheezes, wheezing

sibutramina *f* sibutramine

SIDA *abbr* **síndrome de inmunodeficiencia adquirida**. *See* **síndrome**.

siempre *adv* always; **casi** — almost always; **como** — as usual

sien *f* (*anat*) temple

siesta *f* afternoon nap, nap; **dormir una** —, **tomar una** — (*esp. Mex*) to take a nap, to nap

sietemesino -na *mf* (*fam*) baby born at 7 months, premature newborn, preemie (*fam*)

sietillo -lla *mf* (*fam, CA*) baby born at 7 months, premature newborn, preemie (*fam*)

sífilis *f* syphilis

sifilítico -ca *adj* syphilitic

sigmoide *adj* sigmoid

sigmoideo -a *adj* sigmoid

sigmoides *m* (*fam*) sigmoid colon

sigmoidoscopia, sigmoidoscopía (*Amer, esp. spoken*) *f* sigmoidoscopy; — **flexible** flexible sigmoidoscopy

sigmoidoscopio *m* sigmoidoscope

significado *m* significance

signo *m* (*de enfermedad*) sign; — **de alarma** warning sign; **signos vitales** vital signs

siguiente *adj* after, following, next

silbido (en el pecho) *m* wheeze; **tener silbidos (en el pecho)** to have wheezing, to wheeze; **Tengo silbidos (en el pecho)..**I have wheezing..I'm wheezing.

sildenafil *m* (*Amer*) sildenafil

sildenafilo *m* sildenafil

silicona *f* silicone; **implante** *m* **de** — silicone implant

silicosis *f* silicosis

silla *f* chair; — **de ruedas** wheelchair; — **de ruedas eléctrica** electric wheelchair; — **de ruedas ma-**

nual manual wheelchair; — **de ruedas motorizada** motorized wheelchair; — **de ruedas plegable** folding wheelchair

sillón dental *m* dental chair

simeticona *f* simethicone

simetría *f* symmetry

simétrico -ca *adj* symmetric, symmetrical

simpatectomía *f* sympathectomy

simpático -ca *adj* (*neuro*) sympathetic

simulado -da *adj* factitious

simvastatina *f* simvastatin

sin *prep* without, free; — **azúcar, — sal, etc.** sugar-free, salt-free, etc.; — **dolor** without pain, pain-free; — **fines de lucro** nonprofit, not-for-profit; — **olor** odorless; — **querer** by accident

sinapsis *f* (*pl* **-sis**) synapse

síncope *m* syncope (*form*), faint

sincronizar *vt* to synchronize

síndrome *m* syndrome; — **alcohólico fetal** fetal alcohol syndrome; — **antifosfolípido** antiphospholipid syndrome; — **carcinoide** carcinoid syndrome; — **compartimental** compartmental syndrome; — **de abstinencia** withdrawal; — **de Asherman** Asherman's syndrome; — **de cefalea postraumática** post-concussional syndrome; — **de choque tóxico** (*Mex*) toxic shock syndrome; — **de Cushing** Cushing's syndrome; — **de desgaste** wasting syndrome; — **de dificultad respiratoria del adulto** adult respiratory distress syndrome (ARDS); — **de dolor regional complejo** complex regional pain syndrome; — **de Down** Down's syndrome; — **de Ehlers-Danlos** Ehlers-Danlos syndrome; — **de fatiga crónica** chronic fatigue syndrome; — **de Felty** Felty's syndrome; — **de Gilbert** Gilbert's syndrome; — **de Gilles de la Tourette** Gilles de la Tourette syndrome; — **de Guillain-Barré** Guillain-Barré syndrome; — **de inmunodeficiencia adquirida (SIDA)** acquired immunodeficiency syndrome (AIDS); — **de intes-**

tino corto short bowel syndrome; — de intestino irritable irritable bowel syndrome; — de Klinefelter Klinefelter's syndrome; — de la muerte súbita infantil (*Amer*), — de la muerte súbita del lactante (*Esp*) sudden infant death syndrome (SIDS); — de la piel escaldada estafilocócica staphylococcal scalded skin syndrome; — del asa ciega blind loop syndrome; — del nido vacío empty nest syndrome; — del niño maltratado battered child syndrome; — del túnel carpiano carpal tunnel syndrome; — de Marfan Marfan's syndrome; — de Munchausen Munchausen syndrome; — de ovario poliquístico polycystic ovary syndrome; — de Peutz-Jeghers Peutz-Jeghers syndrome; — de Pickwick Pickwickian syndrome; — de piernas inquietas restless legs syndrome; — de Reiter Reiter's syndrome; — de Reye Reye's syndrome; — de Sheehan Sheehan's syndrome; — de shock tóxico toxic shock syndrome; — de Sjögren Sjögren's syndrome; — de sobrecarga overuse syndrome; — de Stevens-Johnson Stevens-Johnson syndrome; — de Turner Turner's syndrome; — de Wernicke-Korsakoff Wernicke-Korsakoff syndrome; — de Wolff-Parkinson-White Wolff-Parkinson-White syndrome; — hemolítico-urémico hemolytic-uremic syndrome; — hepatorrenal hepatorenal syndrome; — metabólico metabolic syndrome; — mielodisplásico myelodysplastic syndrome; — nefrótico nephrotic syndrome; — nefrótico de cambios mínimos minimal change disease; — neuroléptico maligno neuroleptic malignant syndrome; — postconmocional postconcussional syndrome; — post-polio post-polio syndrome; — premenstrual premenstrual syndrome (PMS); — respiratorio agudo severo (SRAS) severe acute respiratory syndrome (SARS)

sinergia *f* synergy
sínfisis *f* symphysis
sinoauricular *adj* sinoatrial
sinovial *adj* synovial
sinovitis *f* synovitis
sintético -ca *adj* synthetic
sintetizar *vt* to synthesize
síntoma *m* symptom
sintomático -ca *adj* symptomatic
sinus *m* sinus; — pilonidal pilonidal sinus
sinusal *adj* (*card*) sinoatrial
sinusitis *f* sinusitis
siringomielia *f* syringomyelia
sistema *m* system; — cardiovascular cardiovascular system; — endocrino endocrine system; — esquelético skeletal system; — inmunológico *or* inmune immune system; — métrico metric system; — musculoesquelético musculoskeletal system; — nervioso autónomo autonomic nervous system; — nervioso central (SNC) central nervous system (CNS); — nervioso parasimpático parasympathetic nervous system; — nervioso periférico peripheral nervous system; — nervioso simpático sympathetic nervous system
sistémico -ca *adj* systemic
sistólico -ca *adj* systolic
sitio *m* site; — quirúrgico surgical site
smog *m* (*Ang*) smog
SNC *abbr* sistema nervioso central. See sistema.
sobaco *m* (*fam*) axilla, armpit (*fam*)
sobador -ra (*Mex, CA*), sobandero -ra (*Amer*) *mf* folk healer who employs manipulations and massage to treat dislocations and other orthopedic conditions
sobar *vt* (*Amer*) to rub, to massage
sobre *adv* (*por encima de*) over; Su presión arterial es de 160 sobre 90..Your blood pressure is 160 over 90.
sobrecarga *f* overload; — de hierro iron overload
sobrecargar *vt* to overload
sobrecompensar *vi* to overcompensate

sobrecrecimiento *m* overgrowth
sobredosis *f (pl* **-sis)** overdose
sobreexcitar *vt* to overexcite; *vr* to become overexcited
sobremordida *f* overbite
sobrepeso *m* excess weight
sobreproducción *f* overproduction
sobrerreaccionar *vi* to overreact
sobresalir *vi* to protrude, to stick out
sobreuso *m* overuse; **lesión** *f* **por —** overuse injury
sobreutilización *f* overutilization
sobreviviente *mf* survivor; **— del cáncer** cancer survivor
sobrevivir *vt, vi* to survive
sobriedad *f* sobriety
sobrino -na *m* nephew; *f* niece
sobrio -ria *adj* sober
socio -cia *mf (profesional)* partner, associate
socioeconómico -ca *adj* socioeconomic
sociosanitario -ria *adj (esp. Esp)* pertaining to public health; **perspectiva —** public health perspective
socorrista *mf* rescuer
socorro *interj* Help! *m* help, assistance, *(después de un desastre)* aid, relief
sodio *m* sodium
sodomía *f* sodomy
sodomizar *vt* to sodomize
sofocación *f* suffocation
sofocar *vt* to suffocate
sofoco *m (debido a la menopausia)* hot flush *(form)*, hot flash
soja *f* soy
sol *m* sun; **tomar el —** to get sun
solar *adj* solar
soldado *m* soldier
soldar *vi (ortho)* to knit
sóleo *m* soleus
solicitud *f (para seguro médico, etc.)* application
sólido -da *adj & m* solid
solitario -ria *adj mf* loner
soltar *vt (pp* **suelto)** to loosen, free, *(fam, relajar)* to relax; **Suelte el cinturón.**.Loosen your belt...**Suelte la pierna.**.Relax your leg.
soltero -ra *adj* unmarried, single
soltura *f (Mex, fam)* diarrhea

soluble *adj* soluble
solución *f* solution; **— amortiguadora** buffer solution; **— salina normal** normal saline solution
solvente *m* solvent
somático -ca *adj* somatic
somatización *f* somatization
somatotropina *f* growth hormone
somatropina *f* somatropin
sombras *fpl* **— de** *or* **para ojos** eye shadow
sombrero *m* hat
someterse a *vi* to undergo
somnífero *m* sleeping pill
somnoliento -ta *adj* sleepy, drowsy
sonambulismo *m* sleepwalking
sonarse la nariz *vr* to blow one's nose
sonda *f* tube, (urinary) catheter; **— de alimentación** feeding tube; **— de gastrostomía** gastrostomy tube (G-tube); **— Foley** Foley catheter; **— nasogástrica** nasogastric tube; **— vesical** urinary catheter
sondaje *m* catheterization *(of the bladder)*
sondar *vt (form)* to catheterize *(the bladder)*
sonido *m* sound
sonografía *f (técnica imagenológica)* ultrasonography, ultrasound; *(estudio imagenológico)* sonogram
sonograma *m* sonogram
sonreír *vi, vr* to smile
sonrisa *f* smile
sonrojarse *vr (physio)* to flush, to blush
soñar *vt, vi* to dream; **— con** to dream of *o* about; **— despierto** to daydream
sopa *f* soup
soplar *vt, vi* to blow; *vr* **— la nariz** *(Carib)* to blow one's nose
soplo (cardíaco) *m* (heart) murmur
soportable *adj* tolerable, bearable
soportar *vt* to support, *(peso)* to bear *(weight)*
soporte *m* support; **— nutricional** nutritional support; **— vital** life support
sorber *vt* to sip
sorbitol *m* sorbitol
sorbo *m* sip; **— de jugo** sip of juice

sordera f deafness
sordo -da adj deaf; (dolor) dull; mf deaf person
sordomudez f deaf-mutism
sordomudo -da adj deaf and mute; mf deaf-mute
soroche m (SA) mountain sickness
sostén m brassiere, bra (fam)
sostener vt to support, to sustain
sotalol m sotalol
spa m spa, health resort
spray m (Ang) spray; — **de pimienta** pepper spray
SRAS abbr **síndrome respiratorio agudo severo**. See **síndrome**.
Staphylococcus aureus, Staphylococcus aureus; — — **resistente a meticilina (SARM)** methicillin-resistant Staphylococcus aureus (MRSA)
stent m (pl **stents**) stent
suave adj soft, (pelo, piel) smooth, (jabón) mild, (toque) light, gentle
suavizante adj (una loción, etc.) softening
suavizar vt (la piel, etc.) to soften
subacromial adj subacromial
subacuático -ca adj underwater
subagudo -da adj subacute
subalimentación f undernourishment
subalimentado -da adj undernourished
subaracnoideo -a adj subarachnoid
subclavio -via adj subclavian
subclínico -ca adj subclinical
subconciencia f subconscious
subconjunctival adj subconjunctival
subconsciencia f subconscious
subconsciente adj subconscious
subcutáneo -a adj subcutaneous
subdural adj subdural
subespecialidad f subspecialty
subespecialista mf subspecialist
subir vi to rise, go up; **Le subió el azúcar**..Your sugar rose (went up).
súbitamente adv suddenly
súbito -ta adj sudden
subletal adj sublethal
sublimación f (psych) sublimation
sublingual adj sublingual
subluxación f subluxation
submandibular adj submandibular
submarino -na adj underwater

submentoniano -na adj submental
subnormal adj subnormal
subtotal adj subtotal
subungueal adj subungual
succión f suction; — **del pulgar** (form) thumb sucking
suciedad f dirt
sucio -cia adj dirty
sucralfato m sucralfate
sudamina f heat rash
sudar vi to perspire (form), to sweat
sudor m perspiration (form), sweat
sudoración f sweating, sweats; — **nocturna** night sweats
sudoroso -sa adj sweaty
suegro -gra m father-in-law; f mother-in-law
suela f sole (of a shoe)
suelo m (Esp) floor; — **de la boca** floor of the mouth; — **pélvico** pelvic floor
suelto -ta (pp of **soltar**) adj loose, free
sueño m sleep; dream; **dar** — to make sleepy; — **húmedo** wet dream; — **ligero** light sleep; **tener** — to be sleepy
suero m serum; (solución) rehydration solution (usually IV); **¿Me van a poner suero?**..Are you going to give me fluids IV? — **de rehidratación oral,** — **oral** (fam) oral rehydration solution
sufentanilo m sufentanil
suficiente adj sufficient
sufrimiento m suffering
sufrir vi to suffer
suicida adj suicidal; **gesto** — suicide gesture
suicidarse vr to commit suicide
suicidio m suicide; **intento de** — suicide attempt; — **asistido** assisted suicide
sujetador m brassiere; mpl (physical) restraints
sujetar vt (a un paciente) to restrain (a patient)
sulfacetamida f sulfacetamide
sulfadiazina, sulfadiacina f sulfadiazine
sulfametoxazol m sulfamethoxazole
sulfas fpl sulfa drugs
sulfasalacina f sulfasalazine

sulfato *m* sulfate; — **cúprico** (*form*) *or* **de cobre** copper sulfate; — **de condroitina** chondroitin sulfate; — **de magnesio** magnesium sulfate, Epsom salt; — **ferroso** ferrous sulfate; — **magnésico** (*form*) magnesium sulfate, Epsom salt

sulfito *m* sulfite

sulfonamida *f* sulfonamide

sulindaco *m* sulindac

sumar *vt* (*arith*) to add; **¿Puede sumar 10 y 12?**..Can you add 10 and 12?

sumatriptán *m* sumatriptan

suministros médicos *mpl* medical supplies

superar *vt* to overcome; — **miedos** to overcome fears

superdotado -da *adj* gifted

superficial *adj* superficial

superficie *f* surface

superior *adj* (*anat*) superior, upper; **brazo** — upper arm; **espalda** — upper back; **maxilar** *m* — upper jaw; **parte** *f* — **del cuerpo** upper body; — **a** higher than, above; **superior a 90**..higher than 90.. above 90

supernumerario -ria *adj* supernumerary

supervivencia *f* survival

superviviente *mf* survivor; — **del cáncer** cancer survivor

superyó *m* superego

supino -na *adj* supine

suplementario -ria *adj* supplemental, supplementary

suplemento *m* supplement

supositorio *m* suppository; — **vaginal** vaginal suppository

suprarrenal *adj* adrenal; *f* (*fam*) adrenal gland

suprarrenalectomía *f* adrenalectomy

supresión *f* suppression

supresor -ra *adj* suppressive; *m* suppressant; — **del apetito** appetite suppressant

suprimir *vt* to suppress, (*apetito, deseo*) to curb

supuración *f* discharge

supurar *vi* to form pus, to drain pus

supurativo -va *adj* suppurative

suramina *f* suramin

surfactante *m* surfactant

surtido *m* supply

surtir *vt* (*un medicamento de acuerdo con una receta*) to fill (*a prescription*); — **de nuevo** (un medicamento de acuerdo con una receta hecha previamente) to refill (*a medication o prescription*); — **efecto** to take effect

susceptibilidad *f* susceptibility

susceptible *adj* susceptible

suspender *vt* (*un tratamiento, etc.*) to discontinue, to suspend

suspensión *f* suspension

suspensorio *m* athletic supporter, jockstrap (*fam*)

suspirar *vi* to sigh

suspiro *m* sigh

sustancia *f* substance, matter; — **blanca** white matter; — **gris** grey matter; — **química** chemical

sustitución *f* substitution, replacement; — **valvular aórtica**, — **valvular mitral, etc.** aortic valve replacement, mitral valve replacement, etc.

sustituir *vt* to replace, to substitute; **Ud. puede sustituir mantequilla por aceite de oliva**..You can replace butter with olive oil..You can substitute olive oil for butter; [*Nota: observe que al traducir* sustituir *a* to substitute *el orden de los dos objetos* mantequilla y aceite de oliva *se invierte, lo cual no ocurre al traducirlo* a to replace.]

sustituto *m* substitute; — **de la sal** salt substitute

susto *m* fright, scare; (*Amer*) folk illness manifest by anxiety and other symptoms and believed to be caused by a sudden fright

sutura *f* suture; — **reabsorbible** absorbable suture

suturar *vt* to suture, to stitch (*up*)

tab 265 TC

T

tabaco *m* tobacco; (*esp. Carib, puro*) cigar; — **de mascar** chewing tobacco

tábano *m* horsefly

tabáquico -ca *adj* pertaining to tobacco

tabaquismo *m* tobacco use

tabique *m* septum; — **desviado** deviated septum; — **interauricular** interatrial septum; — **interventricular** interventricular septum; — **nasal** nasal septum

tableta *f* tablet

tablilla *f* splint

tabú *adj & m* (*pl* **-búes**) taboo

TAC *m&f* CAT scan (*See also* **tomografía axial computarizada** *under* **tomografía.**)

tacón *m* heel (*of the sole of a shoe*); **de — alto** high-heeled; **de — bajo** low-heeled

tacrina *f* tacrine

tacrolimus, tacrolimús (*OMS*) *m* tacrolimus

tacto *m* touch, sense of touch; examination; — **fino** light touch sensation; — **rectal** rectal examination, rectal exam (*fam*)

tadalafilo *m* tadalafil

taladrar *vt* (*dent*) to drill

taladro *m* (*dent*) drill

tálamo *m* thalamus

talasemia *f* thalassemia

talco *m* talc, (*en polvo*) talcum powder

talidomida *m* thalidomide

talio *m* thallium

talla *f* (*altura*) height

taller *m* workshop; — **de entrenamiento en habilidades sociales para médicos** social skills training workshop for doctors

tallo *m* (*del pelo, pene, etc.*) shaft

talón *m* (*anat*) heel; — **de la mano** heel of the hand

tamaño *m* size; — **de porción** serving size

tambalear *vi, vr* to stagger

tamoxifeno *m* tamoxifen

tampón *m* tampon; (*amortiguador*) buffer, (*esp. Esp*) buffer solution

tamsulosina *f* tamsulosin

tanino *m* tannin

tanque *m* tank; — **de oxígeno** oxygen tank

tantalio *m* tantalum

tapa *f* (*de una botella*) cap (*of a bottle*); — **de seguridad** safety cap

tapado -da *adj* (*fam*) blocked, clogged, stopped up; (*la nariz*) stuffy, stuffed up

tapar *vt* to cover; (*dent, fam*) to fill (*a cavity*); *vi* (*la nariz*) to stop up

tapizar *vt* (*revestir*) to line

tapiz rodante *m* (*esp. Esp*) treadmill

tapón *m* plug; **tapones auditivos** (*form*) earplugs; — **de cerumen** cerumen impaction; **tapones para los oídos** earplugs

taponamiento *m* tamponade; (*de una herida o cavidad*) packing; — **cardíaco** cardiac tamponade; — **nasal** nasal packing

taquicardia *f* tachycardia

tarántula *f* tarantula

tarde *adj* late; *f* afternoon, early evening

tardío -a *adj* late, delayed

tarjeta *f* (*del seguro, etc.*) card

tarsal *adj* tarsal

tartamudear *vi* to stutter, stammer

tártaro *m* (*dent*) calculus (*form*), tartar

tasa *f* rate; — **de metabolismo basal** basal metabolic rate; — **de mortalidad** death rate; — **de mortalidad infantil** infant mortality rate; — **de natalidad** birth rate

tatuaje *m* tattoo

taurina *f* taurine

taza *f* cup, cupful

TB *See* **tuberculosis.**

TC *m&f* CT scan. *See also* **tomografía computada** *under* **tomografía.**

TDAH *abbr* **trastorno por déficit de atención con hiperactividad**. *See* **trastorno**.

té *m* tea

TEC *abbr* **terapia electrochoque** *or* **electroconvulsiva**. *See* **terapia**.

tecato -ta *mf* (*PR, fam*) heroin addict, junkie (*fam*)

tecnecio *m* technetium

técnico -ca *mf* technician; *f* technique; — **aséptica** sterile *o* aseptic technique; — **de relajación** relaxation technique; — **estéril** sterile *o* aseptic technique

tecnología *f* technology

tejido *m* tissue; — **cicatricial** scar tissue; — **conectivo** *or* **conjuntivo** connective tissue; — **de granulación** granulation tissue

tela *f* tape; — **adhesiva** adhesive tape

telangiectasia *f* telangiectasia; — **hemorrágica hereditaria** hereditary hemorrhagic telangiectasia

teléfono *m* telephone; — **celular** cellular telephone, cell phone (*fam*)

telemedicina *f* telemedicine

telemetría *f* telemetry

telepate *m* (*El Salv, Hond*) bedbug

telitromicina *f* telithromycin

temazepam *m* temazepam

temblar *vi* to tremble, shake; **¿Le tiemblan las manos?**..Do your hands shake?

temblor *m* tremor; (*de tierra*) earthquake; — **esencial** essential tremor; *mpl* (*fam*) tremor

tembloroso -sa *adj* tremulous, shaky (*fam*)

temor *m* fear

temperamento *m* temperament

temperatura *f* temperature; (*fam*) fever; — **ambiente** room temperature; — **axilar** axillary temperature; — **oral** oral temperature; — **rectal** rectal temperature; **tomarle la** — (**a alguien**) to take (someone's) temperature; **tomarse la** — to take one's (own) temperature

templado -da *adj* (*tibio*) lukewarm

temporada *f* season, time of year; — **gripal** *or* **de la gripe** flu season

temporal *adj* temporary; (*anat*) temporal

temporomandibular *adj* temporomandibular

temprano -na *adj & adv* early

tenazas *fpl* (*esp. Mex*) tweezers

tendencia *f* tendency, trend

tendinitis *f* tendinitis; — **calcificante** calcific tendinitis

tendón *m* tendon; — **de Aquiles** Achilles tendon; — **de la corva** hamstring

tendonitis *f* tendinitis

tener *vt* to have; **Tengo artritis**..I have arthritis.

tenesmo *m* tenesmus, frequent often painful urge to defecate without the ability to do so

tenia *f* taenia, tapeworm

tenis *m* tennis

tenofovir *m* tenofovir

tenosinovitis *f* tenosynovitis

tensar *vt* (*los músculos*) to tense (*one's muscles*)

tensiómetro *m* blood pressure monitor

tensión *f* tension, strain; — **arterial** (*form*) blood pressure; — **nerviosa** nervous tension

tenso -sa *adj* tense; **ponerse** — to tense up

teofilina *f* theophylline

teoría *f* theory

TEP *abbr* **tomografía por emisión de positrones**. *See* **tomografía**.

terapeuta *mf* therapist; — **del lenguaje** speech therapist; — **ocupacional** occupational therapist

terapéutico -ca *adj* therapeutic; *f* therapy

terapia *f* therapy; — **antirretroviral de gran actividad (TARGA)** highly active antiretroviral therapy (HAART); — **combinada** combination therapy; — **de consolidación** consolidation therapy; — **de grupo** group therapy; — **de inducción** induction therapy; — **del lenguaje** speech therapy; — **de mantenimiento** (*oncología, medicina de las adicciones, etc.*) maintenance therapy; — **de rescate** salvage therapy; — **de sustitución nicotínica** nicotine-replacement therapy; — **electroconvulsiva (TEC)**

electroconvulsive therapy (ECT); — **física** physical therapy; — **grupal** group therapy; — **hormonal sustitutiva** hormone-replacement therapy; — **intensiva** intensive therapy, (*SA, cuidados intensivos*) intensive care; — **ocupacional** occupational therapy; — **respiratoria** (*esp. Amer*) respiratory therapy; — **ultrasónica** ultrasound therapy

terapista *mf* therapist
teratogenicidad *f* teratogenicity
teratogénico -ca *adj* teratogenic
teratoma *m* teratoma
terazosina *f* terazosin
terbinafina *f* terbinafine
terbutalina *f* terbutaline
tercio *m* third; **dos tercios**..two thirds
terfenadina *f* terfenadine
termal *adj* thermal
terminal *adj* terminal; **en fase** — end-stage
término *m* term; **a** — at term
termómetro *m* thermometer; — **rectal** rectal thermometer
termoterapia *f* heat therapy
terremoto *m* earthquake
terrores nocturnos *mpl* night-terrors
terso -sa *adj* smooth
testamento vital *m* living will
testicular *adj* testicular
testículo *m* testicle; — **no descendido** undescended testicle
Testigo de Jehová *mpl* Jehovah's Witness
testosterona *f* testosterone
teta *f* (*vulg*) breast, nipple, tit (*vulg*)
tétanos *m* tetanus
tetero *m* (*Amer*) baby bottle
tetilla *f* nipple (*of a male*); (*Esp, del biberón*) nipple (*of a baby bottle*)
tetina *f* (*del biberón*) nipple (*of a baby bottle*)
tetraciclina *f* tetracycline
tetracloruro de carbono *m* carbon tetrachloride
tetrahidrocannabinol *m* tetrahydrocannabinol (THC)
tetralogía de Fallot *f* tetralogy of Fallot
tetraplejía *f* quadriplegia
tetrapléjico -ca *adj & n* quadriplegic

tez *f* complexion
TIA *See* **accidente** *or* **ataque isquémico transitorio** *under* **accidente** *or* **ataque**.
tía *f* aunt
tiabendazol *m* thiabendazole
tiagabina *f* tiagabine
tiamazol *m* methimazole
tiamina *f* thiamine
tiazida *f* thiazide
tibio -bia *adj* lukewarm, warm; *f* tibia, shinbone (*fam*); — **vara** tibia varus
tiburón *m* shark
tic *m* (*pl* **tics**) tic; — **doloroso** trigeminal neuralgia, tic douloureux
tiempo *m* time; weather; **¿Cuánto tiempo hace que no come?**..How long have you not eaten? **con el** — eventually, in time; **mucho** — a long time; **poco** — a short time; — **de ocio** leisure time; — **de protrombina (PT)** prothrombin time (PT); — **libre** free time; — **parcial de tromboplastina (TPT)** partial thromboplastin time (PTT); **todo el** — all the time
tienda *f* tent; store; — **de oxígeno** oxygen tent; — **de productos naturales** *or* — **naturista** health food store, natural food store
tieso -sa *adj* stiff
tifo *m* typhus
tifoideo -a *adj* typhoid; *f* typhoid fever
tifus *m* typhus
tijeras *fpl* scissors; **unas tijeras**..a pair of scissors; — **de uñas** nailscissors
tila *f* (*bot*) linden
timectomía *f* thymectomy
timidez *f* shyness
tímido -da *adj* timid, shy, bashful
timo *m* thymus
timolol *m* timolol
timoma *m* thymoma
timpánico -ca *adj* tympanic
tímpano *m* (*anat*) eardrum
timpanoplastia *f* tympanoplasty
tina *f* (*de baño*) bathtub; — **de hidromasaje** (*esp. Mex*) whirlpool
tinción *f* (*micro*) stain; — **de Gram** Gram's stain; — **de Papanicolaou**

Papanicolaou smear

tinea tinea; — **capitis** tinea capitis; — **corporis** tinea corporis; — **cruris** tinea cruris; — **pedis** tinea pedis, athlete's foot (*fam*)

tinidazol *m* tinidazole

tinnitus *m* tinnitus

tintura *f* tincture

tiña *f* tinea; — **crural** tinea cruris; — **de la cabeza** (*esp. Mex*) *or* — **del cuero cabelludo** tinea capitis; — **del cuerpo** tinea corporis, ringworm (*fam*); — **de los pies** tinea pedis, athlete's foot (*fam*); — **inguinal** tinea cruris

tío *m* uncle

tioridazina *f* thioridazine

tiotropio *m* tiotropium

típico -ca *adj* typical

tipo *m* type; — **de sangre A (B, O, etc.)** blood type A (B, O, etc.); — **de tejido** tissue type

tipranavir *m* tipranavir

tiraleche *m* (*esp. Mex*) breast pump

tiramina *f* tyramine

tira reactiva *f* (*para sangre*) test strip; (*para orina*) dipstick

tirita *f* (*esp. Esp*) small adhesive bandage

tiroglobulina *f* thyroglobulin

tiroidectomía *f* thyroidectomy

tiroideo -a *adj* thyroid

tiroides *m&f* (*pl* -**des**) (*fam*) thyroid gland, thyroid (*fam*)

tiroiditis *f* thyroiditis; — **de Hashimoto** Hashimoto's thyroiditis; — **subaguda** subacute thyroiditis

tirón (muscular) *m* muscle pull, pulled muscle, strain

tirosina *f* tyrosine

tirotóxico -ca *adj* thyrotoxic

tirotoxicosis *f* thyrotoxicosis

tirotropina, tirotrofina *f* thyrotropin, thyroid-stimulating hormone (TSH)

tiroxina *f* thyroxine

tisana *f* medicinal tea

titanio *m* titanium

titulación *f* titration

titulado -da *adj* (*certificado*) certified

titular *vt* to titrate

título *m* titer

toalla *f* towel; — **sanitaria** *or* **femenina** sanitary napkin

toallita *f* (*para lavarse*) washcloth; — **de alcohol** alcohol pad

tobillo *m* ankle

tocar *vt* to touch

tocoferol *m* tocopherol

tocolítico -ca *adj & m* tocolytic

tocología *f* obstetrics

tocólogo -ga *mf* obstetrician

tofo *m* tophus

tofu *m* tofu

tolazamida *f* tolazamide

tolbutamida *f* tolbutamide

tolerable *adj* tolerable, bearable

tolerancia *f* tolerance; **alta (baja)** — **al dolor** high (low) pain tolerance *o* tolerance of pain

tolerante *adj* tolerant

tolerar *vt* to tolerate, stand, bear

tolteradina *f* tolteradine

tolueno *m* toluene

toma *m* (*Amer, fam*) electrical outlet; *f* (*Esp*) dose; — **eléctrica** (*esp. Esp*) electrical outlet

tomacorriente *m* (*Amer*) electrical outlet

tomador -ra *mf* (*Amer*) drinker

tomaína *f* ptomaine

tomar *vt* (*una bebida*) to drink; (*medicamentos, etc.*) to take; **Tome una pastilla en la mañana y una en la tarde**..Take one pill in the morning and one in the evening; — **aire** (*fam, inspirar*) to breathe in

tomate *m* tomato

tomografía *f* (*técnica imagenológica*) tomography; (*estudio imagenológico*) tomogram, scan; — **axial computarizada (TAC)** computerized axial tomography (CAT); CAT scan; — **computada (TC)** computed tomography (CT); CT scan; — **computarizada helicoidal** spiral computed tomography; spiral CT scan; — **por emisión de positrones (PET** *or* **TEP)** positron emission tomography (PET); PET scan

tónico *m* tonic

tonificación *f* toning; **ejercicios de** — toning exercises

tonificar *vt* (*los músculos*) to tone (*one's muscles*)

tono m tone, pitch; **tonos cardíacos** heart sounds; **de — alto** high-pitched; **de — bajo** low-pitched; **— muscular** muscle tone

tonsilectomía f (Ang) tonsillectomy

tópico -ca adj topical

topiramato m topiramate

toque m touch

torácico -ca adj thoracic

toracocentesis f (pl -sis) thoracentesis

toracoscopia, toracoscopía (Amer, esp. spoken) f thoracoscopy

toracoscópico -ca adj thoracoscopic

toracotomía f thoracotomy

torasemida f torasemide

tórax m (form) thorax (form), chest

torcedura f sprain

torcerse vr to sprain, twist; **¿Cuándo se torció la muñeca?**..When did you sprain your wrist?

torcido -da adj crooked, twisted

tormenta tiroidea f thyroid storm

tornillo m screw

torniquete m tourniquet

toronja f grapefruit

torpe adj clumsy

torrente sanguíneo m bloodstream

torsión f torsion; **— testicular** testicular torsion

torso m torso

tortícolis f torticollis

tortura f torture

torturar vt to torture

torunda f (de algodón) cotton ball

torus m (pl **torus**) torus; **— palatino** torus palatinus

torzón m (Mex, fam) abdominal cramp

tos f cough; **jarabe** m **para la —** cough syrup; **pastilla para la —** cough drop; **— ferina** pertussis (form), whooping cough; **— perruna** barking cough; **— seca** dry cough

toser vi to cough; **Tosa fuerte**.. Cough hard.

tosferina (fam) **tos ferina**. See **tos**.

total adj & m total

toxemia f toxemia

toxémico -ca adj toxemic

toxicidad f toxicity

tóxico -ca adj toxic; **no —** nontoxic

toxicología f toxicology

toxicólogo -ga mf toxicologist

toxicomanía f drug addiction

toxicómano -na mf drug addict

toxina f toxin; **— botulínica** botulinum toxin

toxocariasis f toxocariasis

toxoide m toxoid; **— diftérico** diphtheria toxoid; **— tetánico** tetanus toxoid

toxoplasmosis f toxoplasmosis

trabajador -ra mf worker; **— social** social worker

trabajar vi to work

trabajo m work, job; **— corporal** bodywork; **— de parto** labor (See also **parto**.)

tracción f traction

tracoma m trachoma

tracto m tract; **— digestivo** digestive o gastrointestinal tract; **— genitourinario** genitourinary tract; **— respiratorio (superior, inferior)** (upper, lower) respiratory tract; **— urinario** urinary tract

traducir vt to translate

tragar vt, vi to swallow; **— saliva** to swallow (dry swallow)

trago m swallow; (Amer) drink (of an alcoholic beverage)

tramadol m tramadol

trancazo m (esp. Esp, fam) influenza, flu; (Mex, fam) dengue fever

trance m trance

tranquilizante adj sedative; m (sedante) sedative; (neuroléptico) neuroleptic

tranquilizar vt to sedate, to tranquilize (ant); vr to calm down, quiet down

tranquilo -la adj calm

transcurso m course

transcutáneo -a adj transcutaneous

transdérmico -ca adj transdermal

transexual adj & mf transsexual

transferencia f transfer; (psych, etc.) transference; **— embriónica** embryo transfer; **— intratubárica de gametos** gamete intrafallopian transfer (GIFT)

transferrina f transferrin

transformación f transformation

transfundir vt (form) to transfuse

transfusión *f* transfusion; **hacer una — ** to transfuse, to give a transfusion; **— de glóbulos rojos (plaquetas, etc.)** transfusion of red blood cells (platelets, etc.); **— de intercambio** exchange transfusion
transgenerismo *m* transgenderism
transgénero *adj* transgender; **mujer transgénero** transgender female
transición *f* transition
transicional *adj* transitional
transitorio -ria *adj* transient
translocación *f* translocation
transmisible *adj* communicable
transmisión *f* transmission; **de — aérea** (*form*) airborne; **de — alimentaria** (*form*) foodborne; **de — sanguínea** (*form*) bloodborne
transmitir *vt* to transmit
transpiración *f* perspiration
transpirar *vi* to perspire
transportar *vt* to transport
transporte *m* transport
transposición *f* transposition
transrectal *adj* transrectal
transuretral *adj* transurethral
transvaginal *adj* transvaginal
trapecio *m* (*anat*) trapezius; (*para una cama hospitalaria*) trapeze (*for a hospital bed*)
tráquea *f* trachea, windpipe (*fam*)
traqueítis *f* tracheitis
traqueobronquitis *f* tracheobronchitis
traqueostomía *f* tracheostomy
traqueotomía *f* tracheotomy
trasero *m* (*fam*) buttocks, bottom (*fam*)
trasladar *vt* (*a un paciente*) to transfer, to move
traspié *m* **dar un —** to stumble, trip
trasplantar *vt* to transplant
trasplante *m* transplant; **— cardíaco** *or* **de corazón** heart transplant; **— de hígado** liver transplant; **— de médula ósea** bone marrow transplant; **— de órganos** organ transplant; **— de pelo** hair transplant; **— de pulmón** lung transplant; **— de riñón** kidney transplant; **— hepático** liver transplant; **— pulmonar** lung transplant; **— renal** renal transplant, kidney transplant

trastornado -da *adj* crazy, (*molesto*) upset
trastornar *vt* to upset; *vr* to get *o* become upset
trastorno *m* disorder, disturbance, disability; **— bipolar** bipolar disorder; **— de ansiedad** *or* **angustia** anxiety disorder; **— de aprendizaje** learning disability; **— de comportamiento** behavioral disorder; **— de la excitación sexual en la mujer** female sexual arousal disorder; **— de la personalidad** personality disorder; **— del aprendizaje** learning disability; **— del lenguaje** speech *o* language disorder; **— del sueño** sleep disorder; **— de pánico** panic disorder; **— de somatización** somatoform disorder; **— dismórfico corporal** body dysmorphic disorder; **— límite de la personalidad** borderline personality disorder; **— obsesivo-compulsivo** obsessive-compulsive disorder; **— por atracón** binge-eating; **— por déficit de atención con hiperactividad (TDAH)** attention deficit-hyperactivity disorder (ADHD); **— por estrés postraumático** posttraumatic stress disorder; **— somatomorfo** *or* **somatoforme** somatoform disorder
tratable *adj* treatable
tratado -da *adj* treated; **no —** untreated
tratamiento *m* treatment; **— antirretroviral de gran actividad (TARGA)** highly active antiretroviral therapy (HAART); **— combinado** combination therapy; **— de conducto** root canal therapy, root canal (*fam*); **— de rescate** salvage therapy; **— directamente observado** directly observed therapy; **— hormonal sustitutivo** hormonal replacement therapy; **— quelante** chelation therapy
tratar *vt* (*una enfermedad*) to treat; (*un paciente*) to treat, to attend; **— de** to try
trauma *m* trauma (*esp. psychiatric*)
traumático -ca *adj* traumatic
traumatismo *m* trauma

traumatizar *vt* to traumatize
traumatología *f* trauma surgery; (*esp. Esp, cirugía ortopédica*) orthopedic surgery
traumatólogo -ga *mf* trauma surgeon; (*esp. Esp, cirujano ortopédico*) orthopedic surgeon
travesti *mf* transvestite
travestismo *m* transvestism
travieso -sa *adj* mischievous
trazado *m* (*ECG, etc.*) tracing
trazador *m* tracer
trazas *fpl* trace(s); **trazas de plomo..** trace(s) of lead
trazodona *f* trazodone
trematodo *m* fluke
trementina *f* turpentine
treonina *f* threonine
tretinoína *f* tretinoin
triage *m* triage
triamcinolona *f* triamcinolone
triamtereno *m* triamterene
triazolam *m* triazolam
tríceps *m* (*pl* -ceps) triceps
tricocéfalo *m* whipworm
tricomoniasis *f* trichomoniasis
tricúspide *adj* tricuspid
trifluoperazina *f* trifluoperazine
trifocal *adj* trifocal
trigémino -na *adj* trigeminal
triglicérido *m* triglyceride
trigo *m* wheat; **— integral** *or* **entero** whole wheat
trillizo -za *mf* triplet
trimestre *m* trimester
trimetoprim *m* trimethoprim
trimetoprima *f* trimethoprim
tripa *f* (*fam*) intestine, bowel, gut
tripanosomiasis *f* trypanosomiasis
tripsina *f* trypsin
triptófano *m* tryptophan
triquinosis *f* trichinosis
trismo *m* trismus
trisomía *f* trisomy; **— 21** trisomy 21
triste *adj* sad
tristeza *f* sadness
triturar *vt* (*form, una tableta*) to crush, to grind
trivalente *adj* trivalent
trocánter *m* trochanter
trocantéreo -a *adj* (*Esp*) trochanteric
trocantérico -ca *adj* (*Amer*) trochanteric

troglitazona *f* troglitazone
trombectomía *f* thrombectomy
trombo *m* thrombus
tromboangeítis obliterante *f* thromboangiitis obliterans
trombocitopenia *f* thrombocytopenia
trombocitosis *f* thrombocytosis; **— esencial** essential thrombocytosis
tromboembolia *f* thromboembolism
tromboflebitis *f* thrombophlebitis
trombolisis *f* thrombolysis
trombolítico -ca *adj & m* thrombolytic
trombosis *f* (*pl* -sis) thrombosis; **— cerebral** (thrombotic) stroke; **— venosa profunda** deep venous thrombosis (DVT)
trompa *f* tube; **— de Eustaquio** Eustachian tube; **— de Falopio** *or* **uterina** fallopian tube
tronco *m* (*anat*) trunk; **— del encéfalo** brainstem
tropezar *vi* to stumble, trip
tropical *adj* tropical
trotar *vi* (*forma de ejercicio*) to jog
tubárico -ca *adj* tubal
tuberculina *f* tuberculin
tuberculoide *adj* tuberculoid
tuberculosis (TB) *f* tuberculosis (TB)
tuberculoso -sa *adj* tuberculous
tubería *f* tubing
tubo *m* tube; **— de drenaje** drainage tube; **— de drenaje pleural** chest tube; **— de ensayo** test tube; **— digestivo** digestive tract; **— endotraqueal** endotracheal tube; **— torácico** chest tube
tubo-ovárico -ca *adj* tubo-ovarian
tubular *adj* tubular
túbulo *m* tubule
tuerto -ta *adj* lacking vision in one eye
tularemia *f* tularemia
tumor *m* tumor; **— benigno** benign tumor; **— cerebral** brain tumor; **— desmoide** desmoid tumor; **— de Wilms** Wilms' tumor; **— maligno** malignant tumor
tumoral *adj* pertaining to a tumor; **tamaño —** tumor size;
túnel *m* tunnel; **— carpiano** carpal tunnel
tupido -da *adj* (*esp. Carib*) **con la**

nariz — congested, having a stuffy *o* stuffed up nose
tusílago *m* (*bot*) coltsfoot

tutor -ra *mf* guardian, legal guardian, conservator

U

úlcera *f* ulcer, sore; — **de decúbito** decubitus ulcer, bedsore; — **de estrés** stress ulcer; — **duodenal** duodenal ulcer; — **gástrica** gastric ulcer; — **péptica** peptic ulcer; — **por presión** decubitus ulcer, pressure sore
ulceración *f* ulceration
ulcerado -da *adj* ulcerated
últimamente *adv* recently
último -ma *adj* last; **su última cirugía..**your last surgery
ultrafiltración *f* ultrafiltration
ultrasonido *m* ultrasound
ultrasonografía *f* ultrasonography, ultrasound
ultravioleta *adj* ultraviolet
umbral *m* threshold; — **de audición** auditory threshold; — **del dolor** pain threshold
ungueal *adj* ungual
ungüento *m* ointment, salve
unidad *f* unit, department; — **coronaria** coronary care unit; — **de cuidados intensivos (UCI)** intensive care unit (ICU); — **de sangre** unit of blood; — **de terapia intensiva** (*SA*) intensive care unit (ICU); — **de urgencias** emergency department, emergency room (ER); — **internacional** international unit
uniforme *adj* uniform; *m* uniform
unión *f* union, junction; — **auriculo-**

ventricular atrioventricular junction
unir *vt* to unite, join; *vr* to unite
universal *adj* universal
uno *m* **hacer del** — (*euph, orinar*) to urinate (*form*), to do number one (*euph*)
uña *f* nail; (*de la mano*) fingernail; (*del pie*) toenail; — **encarnada**, — **enterrada** (*Mex, CA, Carib*), — **encajada** ingrown nail
uñero *m* ingrown nail; (*panadizo*) whitlow, felon
uranio *m* uranium
urbano -na *adj* urban
urea *f* urea
uremia *f* uremia
urémico -ca *adj* uremic
uréter *m* ureter
ureteral *adj* ureteral
uretra *f* urethra
uretritis *f* urethritis; — **no gonocócica** non-gonococcal urethritis
urgencia *f* emergency; **cesárea de** — emergency C-section; **sala** *or* **unidad** *f* **de urgencias** emergency room (ER), emergency department
urgente *adj* urgent; **cesárea** — (*esp. Esp*) emergency C-section
urinario -ria *adj* urinary
urocinasa *f* urokinase
urocultivo *m* (*form*) urine culture
urodinámica *f* urodynamics

urogenital *adj* urogenital
urografía *f* (*técnica imagenológica*) urography, pyelography; (*estudio imagenológico*) pyelogram, urogram; — **intravenosa** intravenous pyelogram (IVP)
urograma *m* pyelogram, urogram
urokinasa *f* urokinase
urología *f* urology
urólogo -ga *mf* urologist
urosepsis *f* urosepsis
urticaria *f* urticaria, hives (*fam*)
usar *vt* to use
uso *m* use; **uso del brazo**..use of the arm; **para — repetido** reusable; —

compasivo (*pharm*) compassionate use; — **excesivo** excessive use
usual *adj* usual
usuario -ria *mf* user
uta *f* a mild form of American cutaneous leishmaniasis
uterino -na *adj* uterine
útero *m* uterus; **en el —** in utero
UTI *abbr* **unidad de terapia intensiva**. *See* **unidad**.
utilizar *vt* to use, utilize
úvea *f* uvea
uveítis *f* uveitis
úvula *f* uvula

V

vaciamiento *m* emptying; — **ganglionar** lymph node resection
vaciar *vt* to empty; **vaciar la vejiga** ..to empty one's bladder
vacío -a *adj* empty
vacuna *f* vaccine; vaccinia; — **antigripal** flu vaccine; — **antipoliomielítica oral** oral polio vaccine; — **atenuada** attenuated vaccine; — **BCG** BCG vaccine; — **conjugada** conjugated vaccine; — **contra Haemophilus influenzae tipo b** Haemophilus influenzae type b vaccine; — **contra la gripe** flu vaccine; — **contra la hepatitis B** hepatitis B vaccine; — **contra la rabia** rabies vaccine; — **contra la varicela** varicella vaccine; — **contra la viruela** smallpox vaccine; — **DTP** DPT vaccine; — **meningocócica** meningococcal vaccine; — **neumocócica** pneumococcal vac-

cine; — **Sabin** Sabin vaccine; — **Salk** Salk vaccine; — **triple viral, — triple vírica** (*Esp*) MMR vaccine; — **viva** live vaccine
vacunación *f* vaccination, immunization
vacunado -da *adj* vaccinated; **no —** unvaccinated; *mf* vaccinee
vacunal *adj* pertaining to vaccination; **cobertura —** vaccination coverage
vacunar *vt* to vaccinate, to immunize
vagal *adj* vagal
vagina *f* vagina
vaginal *adj* vaginal
vaginitis *f* vaginitis
vaginosis *f* vaginosis; — **bacteriana** bacterial vaginosis
vago *m* vagus
vagotomía *f* vagotomy; — **selectiva** selective vagotomy
vaina *f* sheath; — **nerviosa** nerve

sheath
valaciclovir *m* valacyclovir
valdecoxib *m* valdecoxib
valécula *See* **vallécula**.
valeriana *f* (*bot*) valerian
valgo -ga *adj* valgus; **genu** — genu valgus
valgus *adj* valgus; **hallux** — hallux valgus
validez *f* validity
válido -da *adj* valid
valiente *adj* brave; ¡**Sé valiente!**..Be brave!
valina *f* valine
vallécula *f* vallecula
valor *m* value, score; — **nutritivo** food value; — **T** T-score; — **Z** Z-score
valoración *f* evaluation, assessment, testing; — **de Apgar** (*Mex*) Apgar score; — **urodinámica** urodynamic testing
valorar *vt* to evaluate
valproato *m* valproate
valsartán *m* valsartan
válvula *f* valve; — **aórtica** aortic valve; — **mitral** mitral valve; — **pilórica** pyloric valve; — **pulmonar** pulmonic valve; — **tricúspide** tricuspid valve
valvuloplastia *f* valvuloplasty
vancomicina *f* vancomycin
vapor *m* vapor, steam; **cocer al** — to steam (*cook by steaming*)
vaporizador *m* vaporizer
vardenafil *m* vardenafil
vardenafilo *m* (*Esp*) vardenafil
variable *adj & f* variable
variación *f* variation
variante *adj & f* variant
variar *vi* to vary, to fluctuate
varice, várice *f* varix, varicose vein (*fam*); [*Nota: el término* varix *se usa casi siempre en el plural:* varices.]
varicela *f* varicella, chickenpox (*fam*)
varicocele *m* varicocele
varicoso -sa *adj* varicose; **vena** — varicose vein
variz *f* (*pl* **varices**) (*esp. Esp*) *See* **varice, várice**.
varo -ra *adj* varus
varón *m* male

varus *adj* varus
vascular *adj* vascular
vasculitis *f* vasculitis, angiitis; — **leucocitoclástica** leukocytoclastic vasculitis; — **necrotizante** *or* **necrosante** necrotizing vasculitis; — **por hipersensibilidad** hypersensitivity vasculitis
vasectomía *f* vasectomy
vaselina *f* petroleum jelly
vasija *f* basin, bedpan
vaso *m* vessel; glass; **un vaso de agua**..a glass of water; — **sanguíneo** blood vessel
vasoconstricción *f* vasoconstriction
vasoconstrictor *m* vasoconstrictor
vasodilatación *f* vasodilation
vasodilatador *m* vasodilator
vasoespasmo, vasospasmo *m* vasospasm
vasopresina *f* vasopressin, antidiuretic hormone (ADH)
vasovagal *adj* vasovagal
vecindad *f* neighborhood
vecino -na *mf* neighbor
vector *m* vector
veganismo *m* veganism
vegano -na *adj & mf* vegan
vegetación *f* vegetation
vegetal *adj & m* vegetable
vegetarianismo *m* vegetarianism
vegetariano -na *adj & mf* vegetarian
vegetativo -va *adj* vegetative; **estado — persistente** persistent vegetative state
vehículo *m* vehicle
vejez *f* old age
vejiga *f* bladder; blister; — **hiperactiva** hyperactive bladder, overactive bladder (*fam*); — **neurogénica**, — **neurógena** (*esp. Esp*) neurogenic bladder
vello *m* body hair
velocidad de sedimentación globular (VSG) *f* erythrocyte sedimentation rate (ESR)
velo del paladar *m* (*form*) soft palate
vena *f* vein; — **antecubital** antecubital vein; — **femoral** femoral vein; — **porta** portal vein; — **safena** saphenous vein; — **subclavia** subclavian vein; — **varicosa** varicose vein; — **yugular externa** ex-

ternal jugular vein; — **yugular interna** internal jugular vein

vena cava *f* vena cava; — — **inferior** inferior vena cava; — — **superior** superior vena cava

vencer *vt* to overcome; — **miedos** to overcome fears

vencido -da *adj* (*pharm*) outdated, out of date

vencimiento *m* (*pharm*) expiration; **fecha de** — expiration date

venda *f* bandage(s), dressing material; — **adhesiva** adhesive bandage; — **elástica** elastic bandage

vendaje *m* bandage, dressing; — **adhesivo** adhesive bandage; — **compresivo** compression *o* pressure bandage, pressure dressing; — **elástico** elastic bandage; — **funcional** taping; — **oclusivo** occlusive dressing; — **preventivo** taping; — **en ocho** figure-of-eight bandage

vendar *vt* to bandage, to dress (*a wound*)

veneno *m* poison, venom; — **para hormigas, — para ratas, etc.** ant poison, rat poison, etc.

venenoso -sa *adj* poisonous

venéreo -a *adj* sexually transmitted; **enfermedad** — sexually transmitted disease

venir *vi* to come; — **de familia** to run in one's family; *vr* (*fam, alcanzar el orgasmo*) to have an orgasm, to come (*fam*)

venlafaxina *f* venlafaxine

venoso -sa *adj* venous

venta *f* **de** — **libre** over-the-counter

ventaja *f* advantage

ventilación *f* ventilation; — **mecánica** mechanical ventilation

ventilador *m* electric fan; (*respirador*) ventilator

ventosear *vi* to pass gas

ventosidad *f* gas (*expelled from rectum*)

ventral *adj* ventral

ventricular *adj* ventricular

ventrículo *m* ventricle

vénula *f* venule

ver *vt, vi* (*pp* **visto**) to see; *vr* to look, to look like; **Se ve triste.**..You look

sad.

verano *m* summer

verapamilo, verapamil *m* verapamil

verdadero -ra *adj* true

verde *adj* green

verdoso -sa *adj* greenish

verdugón *m* wheal, welt

verdura *f* vegetable; *fpl* greens

vergüenza *f* shame, embarrassment

verruga *f* wart; — **genital** genital wart; — **plantar** plantar wart

vértebra *f* vertebra

vertebroplastia *f* vertebroplasty

vertical *adj* vertical

vértice *m* (*anat*) vertex

vértigo *m* vertigo

vesícula *f* vesicle, blister; (*fam*) gallbladder; — **biliar** gallbladder

vestibular *adj* vestibular

vestíbulo *m* vestibule

vestido *m* dress

vestir *vt* to dress; *vr* to dress (oneself), to get dressed

veterano -na *mf* veteran

veterinario -ria *adj* veterinary; *mf* veterinarian; *f* veterinary medicine

vez *f* (*pl* **veces**) time; **a veces** at times; **cada** — each time, every time; **de** — **en cuando** from time to time, occasionally; **dos veces al día** two times a day, twice daily; **la primera** — the first time; **la próxima** — the next time; **la última** — the last time; **muchas veces** many times, often; **raras veces** rarely; **una** — one time

VHB *abbr* **virus de la hepatitis B**. *See* **virus**.

VHC *abbr* **virus de la hepatitis C**. *See* **virus**.

VHS *abbr* **virus herpes simple**. *See* **virus**.

vía *f* tract, duct; route; **por** — **oral** (*form*) by mouth; — **aérea** (*frec. pl*) airway; — **biliar** (*frec. pl*) biliary tract; — **de administración** route of administration; — **lagrimal** lacrimal duct, tear duct (*fam*); **vías respiratorias (altas, bajas)** (upper, lower) respiratory tract

viable *adj* viable

viajes *mpl* travel; — **internacionales** foreign travel

vial *m* vial
víbora *f* viper
vibración *f* vibration
vibrador *m* vibrator
vicio *m* bad habit
víctima *f* victim
vida *f* life, lifetime; **de por** — for life, lifelong; — **media** half-life; — **sexual** sex life; — **social** social life
vidarabina *f* vidarabine
video (*Amer*), **vídeo** (*Esp*) *m* video
videotoracoscopia, videotoracoscopía (*Amer, esp. spoken*) *f* video-assisted thoracoscopy
vidrio *m* glass; **un pedazo de vidrio..** a piece of glass
viejo -ja *adj* old; *m* old man, old person; *f* old woman
viento *m* wind
vientre *m* belly, abdomen; (*útero*) womb
vigabatrina *f* vigabatrine
vigilancia *f* surveillance, monitoring
vigor *m* stamina
vigoroso -sa *adj* vigorous, strong; (*actividad*) strenuous
VIH *abbr* **virus de la inmunodeficiencia humana**. *See* **virus**.
vinagre *m* vinegar
vinblastina *f* vinblastine
vinchuca *f* (*esp. SA*) kissing bug
vincristina *f* vincristine
vínculo *m* (*obst, psych, etc.*) bond
vino *m* wine; — **blanco** white wine; — **tinto** red wine
violación (sexual) *f* rape
violar *vt* to rape
violencia *f* violence; — **doméstica** *or* **conyugal** domestic violence
violento -ta *adj* violent
violeta de genciana *f* Gentian violet
viral *adj* viral
viremia *f* viremia
virgen *mf* virgin
virginidad *f* virginity
vírico -ca *adj* viral
virilidad *f* virility, manhood
virilización *f* virilization
virología *f* virology
virológico -ca *adj* virologic, virological
virtual *adj* virtual; **endoscopia** — virtual endoscopy

viruela *f* smallpox
virulencia *f* virulence
virulento -ta *adj* virulent
virus *m* (*pl* **virus**) virus; — **atenuado** attenuated virus; — **de Epstein-Barr** Epstein-Barr virus (EBV); — **de la gripe** flu virus; — **de la hepatitis B (VHB), — de la hepatitis C (VHC), etc.** hepatitis B virus (HBV), hepatitis C virus (HCV), etc.; — **de la inmunodeficiencia humana (VIH)** human immunodeficiency virus (HIV); — **del Nilo Occidental** West Nile virus; — **del papiloma humano (VPH)** human papillomavirus (HPV); — **herpes simple (VHS)** herpes simplex virus (HSV); — **linfotrópico humano (de células T)** human T-lymphotrophic virus; — **Norwalk** Norwalk virus; — **sincitial respiratorio, — respiratorio sincitial** (*Esp*) respiratory syncytial virus; — **varicela-zoster** varicella-zoster virus; — **vivo** live virus
viruta *f* shaving (*of metal, etc.*)
víscera *f* organ; — **hueca** hollow organ
visceral *adj* visceral
viscosidad *f* viscosity
viscoso -sa *adj* viscous
visible *adj* visible
visión *f* vision, sight, eyesight; — **borrosa** blurred vision; — **cercana** near vision; — **doble** double vision; — **lejana** far vision; — **nocturna** night vision; — **periférica** peripheral vision; — **(en) túnel** tunnel vision
visita *f* visit; — **al médico** visit to the doctor, doctor's visit; — **domiciliaria** house call; — **no programada** unscheduled visit, drop-in (*fam*)
visitante *mf* visitor
visitar *vt* to visit
vista *f* vision, sight, eyesight; (*radiografía, etc.*) view; **a simple** — with the naked eye; — **cansada** (*fam*) presbyopia
visto *pp* of **ver**
visual *adj* visual
visualización *f* visualization
visualizar *vt* to visualize

vital *adj* vital
vitalidad *f* vitality
vitamina *f* vitamin; — **A, B₁₂, etc.** vitamin A, B₁₂, etc.; **vitaminas del complejo B** vitamin B complex; — **hidrosoluble** water-soluble vitamin; — **liposoluble** fat-soluble vitamin
vitamínico -ca *adj* pertaining to vitamins; **contenido —** vitamin content
vitíligo, vitiligo (*Amer*) *m* vitiligo
vítreo -a *adj* vitreous
viuda negra *f* black widow
viudo -da *adj* widowed; *m* widower; *f* widow
vivir *vi* to live; — **con** to live with; **vivir con un amigo**..to live with a friend...**vivir con (el) sida**..to live with AIDS
vivo -va *adj* alive, (*virus, vacuna*) live
vocal *adj* vocal
voltear *vt* (*a un encamado*) to turn; *vr* to turn over, roll over; **¿Me volteo?**..Should I turn over?
voltio *m* volt
volumen *m* volume; — **tidal** tidal volume
voluntad *f* will; **contra su —** against your will; **fuerza de —** will power; **la — de vivir** the will to live; **por**

su propia — of your own free will
voluntario -ria *adj* voluntary; *mf* volunteer
volver *vi* (*pp* **vuelto**) — **en sí** to regain consciousness; *vr* — **loco** to go crazy, to lose one's mind, to flip out (*fam*)
vólvulo *m* volvulus
vomitar *vt, vi* to vomit, to throw up (*fam*)
vomitivo -va *adj* & *m* emetic
vómito *m* (*frec. pl*) vomit; vomiting; **vómitos del embarazo** morning sickness; **vómito(s) en proyectil**, **vómitos en escopetazo** (*Esp*) projectile vomiting
voyeurismo *m* voyeurism
voz *f* (*pl* **voces**) voice, speech; **hablar** *or* **decir en — baja** to whisper; **perder la —** to lose one's voice; — **esofágica** esophageal speech
VPH *abbr* **virus del papiloma humano**. *See* **virus.**
VSG *abbr* **velocidad de sedimentación globular**. *See* **velocidad.**
vuelta *f* turn; **darse media —** to turn around; **darse —** to turn; (*voltearse*) to turn over, roll over; **dar vueltas** (*girar*) to spin
vuelto *pp of* **volver**
vulnerable *adj* vulnerable
vulva *f* vulva

W

warfarina *f* warfarin

X

xantoma *m* xanthoma

Y

ya visto, déjà vu
yema *f* yolk; (*del dedo*) pad (*of the finger*); — **de huevo** egg yolk
yerba *See* **hierba**.
yerbabuena *f* (*bot*) peppermint
yerbero -ra *mf* herbalist, person who sells herbs
yerna *f* (*esp. Carib*) daughter-in-law
yerno *m* son-in-law
yeso *m* (*ortho*) cast, plaster (*for a cast*)

yeyunal *adj* jejunal
yeyuno *m* jejunum
yo *m* (*psych*) ego
yodado -da *adj* iodized
yodo *m* iodine
yoga *m* yoga
yogur *m* yogurt
yohimbina *f* yohimbine
yuca *f* (*bot*) yucca
yugular *adj* jugular

Z

zafirlukast *m* zafirlukast
zalcitabina *f* zalcitabine
zaleplón *m* zaleplon

zanahoria *f* carrot
zanamivir *m* zanamivir
zancudo *m* (*Amer*) mosquito

zapato *m* shoe; **zapatos ortopédicos**
  orthopedic shoes
zarzaparrilla *f* (*bot*) sarsaparilla
zen *m* zen
zidovudina *f* zidovudine
zigoto *m* zygote
zinc *m* zinc; **óxido de** — zinc oxide
ziper *m* (*Ang*) zipper
ziprasidona *f* ziprasidone
zolmitriptán *m* zolmitriptan
zolpidem *m* zolpidem

zombi *m* zombie
zona *f* zone, area; *m* (*fam, zoster*)
  herpes zoster, shingles (*fam*); —
  afectada affected area
zorrillo *m* (*esp. Amer*) skunk
zorro -ra *mf* fox
zumba *f* (*El Salv, Guat; fam*) binge
zumbido *m* (*de oído, etc.*) ringing,
  buzzing, hum
zumo *m* juice
zurdo -da *adj* left-handed

DIALOGUES

DIÁLOGOS

HISTORY AND PHYSICAL/
HISTORIA CLÍNICA Y EXAMEN FÍSICO

PRESENT ILLNESS / ENFERMEDAD ACTUAL

Good morning. I'm Dr. Jones. / Buenos días. Soy la Dra. Jones.
Good afternoon. I'm Dr. Smith. / Buenas tardes. Soy el Dr. Smith.
Have a seat, ma'am. / Siéntese, señora.
How can I help you? / ¿En qué puedo servirle?
What brings you here today? / ¿Qué lo trae por aquí?
Do you have pain? / ¿Tiene Ud. dolor?
Where is the pain exactly? / ¿Dónde está el dolor exactamente?
Can you show me? / ¿Puede enseñarme?
Does the pain move to other areas? / ¿Se le mueve el dolor a otros lados?
Does the pain stay here? / ¿Se le queda aquí el dolor?
What is the pain like? / ¿Cómo es el dolor?
Sharp? / ¿Agudo?
Dull? / ¿Sordo?
Does it burn? / ¿Le arde?
Like quick jabs? / ¿Como punzadas (piquetes)?
Like pressure? / ¿Como una opresión?
Is it a severe pain? / ¿Es un dolor severo?
Moderate? / ¿Moderado?
Mild? / ¿Leve?
When did the pain begin? / ¿Cuándo le empezó el dolor?
When was the first time you ever had this pain? / ¿Cuándo fue la primera vez que sintió este dolor?
Did it go away for a while? / ¿Se le quitó por un tiempo?
By itself? / ¿Por sí solo?
When did it begin again? / ¿Cuándo le empezó de nuevo?
Does the pain come and go? / El dolor, ¿va y viene?
Is it a constant pain? / ¿Es un dolor constante?
When it comes, how long does it last? / ¿Cuando le viene, cuánto tiempo le dura?
How often do you get the pain? / ¿Cada cuánto tiempo le viene el dolor?

In the last week, how many times have you had the pain? / ¿En la última semana, cuántas veces ha tenido el dolor?

What were you doing when the pain came on? / ¿Qué estaba haciendo cuando empezó el dolor?

What time of day does the pain come on? / ¿A qué hora del día empieza el dolor?

Do you get it more often in the morning? / ¿Le viene más en la mañana?

In the afternoon? / ¿En la tarde?

Anytime? / ¿A cualquier hora?

Is it worse after you eat? / ¿Empeora después de comer?

Is it worse when you exert yourself? / ¿Empeora al hacer esfuerzos?

Is there anything which makes the pain worse? / ¿Hay algo que le agrave el dolor?

Is there anything which makes the pain better? / ¿Hay algo que le alivie el dolor?

Does it get better with exercise? / ¿Se alivia con el ejercicio?

It gets worse? / ¿Se pone peor?

Have you tried medications? / ¿Ha probado medicamentos?

Did it help? / ¿Le ayudó?

Are there relatives or friends who have the same problem? / ¿Hay familiares o amigos que tienen el mismo problema?

What do you think is causing the problem? / ¿Qué cree que está causando el problema?

Have you seen a doctor before for this problem? / ¿Ha consultado a un médico por este problema antes?

What did he say you had? / ¿Qué le dijo que tenía?

Did he do any studies? / ¿Le hizo estudios?

Did he draw blood? / ¿Le sacó sangre?

When was this? / ¿Cuándo fue esto?

What's the name of the doctor? / ¿Cómo se llama el médico?

Do you know his telephone number? / ¿Sabe su número de teléfono?

Why did you come to the hospital today instead of some other day? / ¿Porqué vino al hospital hoy en vez de cualquier otro día?

Do you have any other problems? / ¿Tiene algún otro problema?

How long have you been in the United States? / ¿Hace cuánto que está en los Estados Unidos?

When was the last time you left the country? / ¿Cuándo fue la última vez que salió del país?

Where did you go? / ¿A dónde fue?

By the way, how old are you? / ¿A propósito, cuántos años tiene Ud.?

PAST MEDICAL HISTORY / ANTECEDENTES MÉDICOS

How long have you had diabetes? / ¿Hace cuánto que tiene diabetes?
Who takes care of you for your diabetes? / ¿Quién lo trata por su diabetes?
Do you have a regular doctor? / ¿Tiene algún médico a quien consulta regularmente?
Where is he located? / ¿Dónde está ubicado?
Is he a private doctor? / ¿Es un médico privado?
When was the last time you saw a doctor? / ¿Cuándo fue la última vez que consultó a un médico?
Have you ever been hospitalized? / ¿Ha sido hospitalizado alguna vez?
Have you ever had surgery? / ¿Ha sido operado alguna vez?
Have you ever had any serious illness? / ¿Alguna vez ha tenido alguna enfermedad grave?
Have you ever had emotional problems? / ¿Ha tenido alguna vez problemas emocionales?

MEDICATIONS / MEDICAMENTOS

Are you taking any medications? / ¿Está tomando algún medicamento?
Have you taken any over-the-counter medications? / ¿Ha tomado algún medicamento que se vende sin receta médica?
Are you taking birth control pills? / ¿Está tomando píldoras anticonceptivas?
Do you have your medications with you? / ¿Trae sus medicamentos?
What color are the pills? / ¿De qué color son las pastillas?
Are they tablets or capsules? / ¿Son tabletas o cápsulas?
How many times a day do you take them? / ¿Cuántas veces al día las toma?
Who prescribed the pills for you? / ¿Quién le recetó las pastillas?
Do you take them every day or do you forget every now and then? / ¿Las toma todos los días o se le olvida de vez en cuando?
For example, in a week how many times do you forget to take the pills? / ¿Por ejemplo, durante una semana cuántas veces se le olvida tomar las pastillas?
When was the last time you took this pill? / ¿Cuándo fue la última vez que tomó esta pastilla?
How many of these did you take yesterday? / ¿Cuántas de estas tomó Ud. ayer?

Show me exactly which pills you took this morning. / Muéstreme exactamente cuales pastillas tomó esta mañana.
When did you run out of pills? / ¿Cuándo se le acabaron las pastillas?

ALLERGIES / ALERGIAS

Are you allergic to penicillin? / ¿Es Ud. alérgico a la penicilina?
Have you ever taken penicillin? / ¿Ha tomado penicilina alguna vez?
Are you allergic to any medication? / ¿Es Ud. alérgico a algún medicamento?
Have you ever had a bad reaction to a medicine? / ¿Ha tenido alguna vez una mala reacción después de tomar una medicina?
What happened? / ¿Qué le pasó?
Can you tolerate aspirin? / ¿Tolera bien la aspirina?

SOCIAL HISTORY / HISTORIA SOCIAL

What type of work do you do? / ¿Qué tipo de trabajo hace Ud.?
How long have you been out of work? / ¿Hace cuánto que no trabaja?
Why haven't you been able to work? / ¿Porqué no ha podido trabajar?
What kind of work did you use to do? / ¿Qué tipo de trabajo hacía Ud.?
Were there toxic chemicals or other hazards where you worked? / ¿Había sustancias químicas tóxicas u otros peligros donde trabajaba?
What do you do during the day? / ¿Qué hace Ud. durante el día?
Do you eat well? / ¿Come bien?
Do you sleep well? / ¿Duerme bien?
Do you have a place to live? / ¿Tiene donde vivir?
Who do you live with? / ¿Con quién vive Ud.?
Do you smoke? / ¿Fuma Ud.?
Did you use to smoke? / ¿Fumaba?
How many packs a day did you use to smoke? / ¿Cuántas cajetillas fumaba al día?
When did you quit smoking? / ¿Cuándo dejó de fumar?
Do you drink alcohol? / ¿Toma bebidas alcohólicas?
Wine? / ¿Vino?
Beer? / ¿Cerveza?
Did you use to drink? / ¿Tomaba?
How long has it been since you quit drinking? / ¿Hace cuánto que no toma?

When was the last time you had a drink? / ¿Cuándo fue la última vez que tomó un trago?

How much can you drink when you have a mind to? / ¿Cuánto puede tomar cuando tiene ganas?

Do your hands ever shake when you quit drinking? / ¿Le tiemblan las manos cuando deja de tomar?

Have you ever had the d.t.'s when you quit drinking? / ¿Ha delirado alguna vez cuando ha dejado de beber?

Have you ever had seizures when you quit drinking for a few days? / ¿Alguna vez ha tenido convulsiones cuando no ha bebido por unos días?

Have you tried to quit drinking? / ¿Ha tratado de dejar de tomar?

Have you ever used drugs? / ¿Ha usado drogas alguna vez?

Have you ever used I.V. drugs? / ¿Se ha inyectado drogas alguna vez?

How often do you use it? / ¿Cada cuánto la usa?

Do you share needles? / ¿Comparte agujas?

Have you had relations with other men? / ¿Ha tenido relaciones con otros hombres?

With prostitutes? / ¿Con prostitutas?

Did you use condoms? / ¿Usó preservativos (condones)?

Have you ever received a blood transfusion? / ¿Ha recibido alguna vez una transfusión de sangre?

Have you been tested for AIDS? / ¿Le han hecho la prueba del SIDA?

What was the result? / ¿Cuál fue el resultado?

FAMILY HISTORY / ANTECEDENTES FAMILIARES

Are there any diseases which run in the family? / ¿Hay enfermedades que vienen de familia?

Are there family members who have had colon cancer? / ¿Hay familiares que han tenido cáncer del colon?

Are your parents still living? / ¿Aún viven sus padres?

Does your mother have any medical problems? / ¿Tiene algún problema médico su madre?

What did your father die of? / ¿De qué murió su padre?

How old was he when he died? / ¿Qué edad tenía cuando murió?

REVIEW OF SYSTEMS / REVISIÓN POR SISTEMAS

General / General:

Has your weight changed recently? / ¿Ha cambiado de peso reciente-
mente?
How many kilograms have you gained? / ¿Cuántos kilos ha ganado?
How many pounds have you lost? / ¿Cuántas libras ha perdido?
Over what period of time? / ¿En cuánto tiempo?
Do you have as much energy as usual? / ¿Tiene la misma energía de
siempre?
How long have you felt tired? / ¿Hace cuánto que se siente cansado?
Have you had fever? / ¿Ha tenido fiebre?
Night sweats? / ¿Sudores durante la noche?

Skin / Piel:

Do you have problems with your skin? / ¿Tiene problemas con la piel?
/ **Rash?**
¿Erupción? (¿Sarpullido?)
Itching? / ¿Comezón? (¿Picazón?)
Sores? / ¿Úlceras? (¿Llagas?)
How often do you bathe? / ¿Cada cuánto se baña?
For how long? / ¿Por cuánto tiempo?
Do you use hot water? / ¿Usa Ud. agua caliente?

Head / Cabeza:

Do you have headaches? / ¿Tiene dolores de cabeza?
Have you hurt your head recently? / ¿Se ha lastimado la cabeza
recientemente?

Eyes / Ojos:

Can you see well? / ¿Puede ver bien?
Do you wear glasses? / ¿Usa lentes?
Does your vision get blurry at times? / ¿Ve borroso a veces?
Do you ever see double? / ¿Ve doble a veces?
Do you have cataracts? / ¿Tiene cataratas?
Glaucoma? / ¿Glaucoma?
Do you see halos around lights at night? / ¿Ve Ud. halos (círculos)
alrededor de las luces en la noche?
Have you ever had your vision tested? / ¿Le han revisado la vista
alguna vez?

When was the last time you saw an eye doctor? / ¿Cuándo fue la última vez que consultó a un médico de los ojos?

Ears / Oídos:

Do you hear well? / ¿Oye bien?
Do you hear equally well in both ears? / ¿Oye igual de bien con los dos oídos?
Has your hearing gotten worse recently? / ¿Oye menos últimamente?
 Do you have an earache? / ¿Tiene dolor de oído?
Have you had ear infections? / ¿Ha tenido infecciones del oído?
Is there liquid draining from your ear? / ¿Le sale líquido del oído?
Do you feel as though the room were spinning around you? / ¿Siente como si el cuarto le estuviera dando vueltas?

Nose / Nariz:

Do you get a lot of nosebleeds? / ¿Le sangra la nariz frecuentemente?
Are you allergic to pollen? / ¿Es Ud. alérgico al polen?
Do you have sinusitis? / ¿Tiene sinusitis?
Do you get a lot of colds? / ¿Le dan resfriados frecuentemente?
Can you smell all right? / ¿Puede distinguir bien los olores?

Oropharynx / Orofaringe:

Do any of your teeth hurt? / ¿Le duele algún diente?
Do you have false teeth? / ¿Tiene dientes postizos?
How often do you brush your teeth? / ¿Cada cuánto se cepilla los dientes?
Do your gums bleed easily? / ¿Le sangran con facilidad las encías?
When was the last time you saw a dentist? / ¿Cuándo fue la última vez que vio a un dentista?
Is your throat sore? / ¿Le duele la garganta?
Do you get canker sores frequently? / ¿Le salen pequeñas llagas en la boca frecuentemente?
Has your voice changed recently? / ¿Le ha cambiado la voz recientemente?

Neck / Cuello:

Is your neck sore? / ¿Le duele el cuello?
Do you have any lumps in your neck? / ¿Tiene bolitas en el cuello?

Breasts / Mamas (Senos):

Do you have any lumps in your breasts? / ¿Tiene algunos nódulos (bolitas) en los senos?

Have you ever had a mammogram? / ¿Le han hecho una mamografía alguna vez?

Do your nipples ever secrete milk? / ¿Le sale leche de los pezones a veces?

Lungs / Pulmones:

Do you have trouble breathing? / ¿Tiene dificultad para respirar?

Are you short of breath? / ¿Le falta el aire?

Can you climb stairs? / ¿Puede subir escaleras?

Do you have to stop to catch your breath? / ¿Tiene que parar para recuperar el aliento?

How may blocks can you walk without stopping? / ¿Cuántas cuadras puede caminar sin parar?

Do you use oxygen at home? / ¿Usa oxígeno en casa?

Do you have a cough? / ¿Tiene tos?

Are you bringing up phlegm? / ¿Le sale flema(s)?

Have you coughed up blood? / ¿Ha tosido sangre?

Do you have wheezing? / ¿Tiene sibilancias (silbidos) en el pecho?

Do you have asthma? / ¿Tiene asma?

Is there anything that brings on the asthma attacks? / ¿Hay algo que le provoque los ataques de asma?

Does it have anything to do with the time of year? / ¿Tiene algo que ver con las estaciones del año?

Do you have allergies? / ¿Tiene alergias?

Is there a lot of dust in your home? / ¿Hay mucho polvo en su casa?

Are there animals in your home? / ¿Hay animales en la casa?

Have you ever had a TB test? / ¿Le han hecho alguna vez la prueba para la tuberculosis?

What was the result? / ¿Cuál fue el resultado?

Have you ever had a chest x-ray? / ¿Le han tomado una radiografía (placa) de tórax alguna vez?

Heart / Corazón:

Do you have heart problems? / ¿Tiene problemas de corazón?

High blood pressure? / ¿Presión alta?

How do you know you have high blood pressure? / ¿Cómo sabe que tiene presión alta?

Do you ever have chest pain? / ¿Ha tenido dolor de pecho alguna vez?

Do you use pillows when you sleep? / ¿Usa Ud. almohadas cuando duerme?

What happens when you don't use pillows? / ¿Qué le pasa cuando no usa almohadas?

Have you ever woken up in the middle of the night with a smothering sensation? / ¿Alguna vez se ha despertado en la noche con una sensación de ahogo?

Have you ever been told you had a heart murmur? / ¿Le han dicho alguna vez que tiene un soplo cardíaco?

When you were a child, did you have a disease called rheumatic fever? / ¿Cuando era niño, le dio una enfermedad llamada fiebre reumática?

Gastrointestinal / Gastrointestinal:

Do you have trouble swallowing? / ¿Tiene dificultad para tragar (pasar) alimentos?

Does food stick in your throat? / ¿Se le atraganta (atora) la comida?

Do you have trouble swallowing liquids too? / ¿Tiene dificultad para tragar (pasar) líquidos también?

Do you have heartburn? / ¿Tiene acidez?

Nausea? / ¿Náusea(s)?

Vomiting? / ¿Vómito(s)?

Did you vomit blood? / ¿Vomitó sangre?

Do you have a stomachache? / ¿Tiene dolor de estómago?

Are there certain foods that bring on the pain? / ¿Hay ciertas comidas que le provoquen los dolores?

Do you have trouble going to the bathroom? / ¿Tiene problemas para ir al baño?

Are you constipated? / ¿Está Ud. estreñido?

Do you have diarrhea? / ¿Tiene Ud. diarrea?

Have you noticed blood in your stool? / ¿Ha notado sangre en sus heces fecales (popó, caca)?

Have you had stools that were black like asphalt? / ¿Ha tenido heces fecales negras (popó negro, caca negra) como el asfalto de la calle?

Do you have hemorrhoids? / ¿Tiene hemorroides (almorranas)?

Have you had your gallbladder taken out? / ¿Le han sacado la vesícula?

Have you had hepatitis? / ¿Ha tenido hepatitis?

Has your skin ever turned yellow? / ¿Se le ha puesto la piel amarilla alguna vez?

Genitourinary / Genitourinario:

Do you have problems urinating? / ¿Tiene problemas para orinar?

Are you urinating more often than usual? / ¿Orina más a menudo que de costumbre?

Do you have to get up in the middle of the night to urinate? / ¿Tiene que levantarse durante la noche para orinar?

Does it burn when you urinate? / ¿Le arde al orinar?

Have you ever had a urinary tract infection? / ¿Ha tenido alguna vez una infección de la orina?

Have you ever noticed blood in your urine? / ¿Ha notado sangre en la orina alguna vez?

Have you ever passed a stone? / ¿Ha eliminado un cálculo (una piedra) en la orina alguna vez?

Have you ever had a sexually transmitted disease? / ¿Ha tenido alguna vez una enfermedad de transmisión sexual?

Were you treated by a doctor? / ¿Recibió tratamiento de un médico?

Do you have any sexual problems? / ¿Tiene algún problema sexual?

(Men) / (Hombres)

Do you have to strain to get your urine out? / ¿Tiene que esforzarse para que salga la orina?

How is your stream? / ¿Cómo está el chorro?

Do you have problems with dribbling? / ¿Gotea después de haber terminado?

Do you have sores on your penis? / ¿Tiene llagas (heridas, úlceras) en el pene?

Do you have a discharge from your penis? / ¿Le sale alguna secreción por el pene?

(Women) / (Mujeres)

Do you ever lose your urine accidentally? / ¿Se le escapa la orina a veces sin querer?

When you laugh or cough? / ¿Cuándo se ríe o tose?

Do you still have periods? / ¿Todavía le viene la regla?

When was your last period? / ¿Cuándo fue su última regla?

Was it normal? / ¿Fue normal?

Do you have pain with your periods? / ¿Tiene dolor con la regla?

Do you bleed a lot during your periods? / ¿Sangra mucho durante la regla?

How many sanitary napkins do you use? / ¿Cuántas toallas sanitarias usa?

Do you use tampons? / ¿Usa tampones?

Are your periods regular? / ¿Sus reglas son regulares?

Have you had bleeding between periods? / ¿Ha sangrado entre las reglas?

How old were you when you had your first period? / ¿A qué edad le vino la primera regla?

When did you go through menopause? / ¿Cuándo le vino la menopausia?

Have you had bleeding since then? / ¿Ha sangrado desde entonces?

Do you get hot flashes? / ¿Le vienen sofocos (bochornos)?

How many children have you had? / ¿Cuántos hijos ha tenido?

Did you have problems with any of your pregnancies? / ¿Tuvo problemas con alguno de sus embarazos?

Have you had any abortions or miscarriages? / ¿Ha tenido algún aborto?

An abortion or a miscarriage? / ¿Provocado o espontáneo?

When was the last time you had sexual relations? / ¿Cuándo fue la última vez que tuvo relaciones sexuales?

Are you using any birth control? / ¿Usa algún método anticonceptivo?

The pill? / ¿La píldora?

The diaphragm? / ¿El diafragma?

An IUD? / ¿Un dispositivo intrauterino? (¿Un DIU?)

Condoms? / ¿Preservativos (condones)?

Could you be pregnant? / ¿Podría estar embarazada?

Do you have a vaginal discharge? / ¿Tiene secreción (flujo) vaginal?

As usual or different? / ¿Como siempre o diferente?

What is it like? / ¿Cómo es?

Do you have sores on your genitals? / ¿Tiene llagas (heridas, úlceras) en los genitales?

Do you have itching? / ¿Tiene comezón (picazón)?

Does it hurt when you have intercourse? / ¿Le duele cuando tiene relaciones?

Musculoskeletal / Musculoesquelético:

Do you have joint pains? / ¿Tiene dolores de las articulaciones (coyunturas)?

Do your joints swell up? / ¿Se le hinchan las articulaciones (coyunturas)?

Do you feel stiff in the morning? / ¿Se siente rígido (tieso) en la mañana?

Does your back hurt? / ¿Le duele la espalda?

Do you feel weak? / ¿Se siente débil?

Do you have trouble climbing stairs? / ¿Le dificulta subir escaleras?

Getting up from a chair? / ¿Levantarse de una silla?
Combing your hair? / ¿Peinarse?

Neurological / Neurológico:

Which hand do you write with? / ¿Con cuál mano escribe Ud.?
Have you had a stroke? / ¿Ha padecido un ataque cerebral (derrame, embolia)?
Has a single part of your body ever turned weak, like your arm or your leg? / ¿Se le ha puesto débil una sola parte del cuerpo alguna vez, como el brazo o la pierna?
Has your vision in one eye ever gone black? / ¿Se le ha puesto negra la vista en un solo ojo alguna vez?
Does any part of your body feel numb? / ¿Siente adormecida alguna parte del cuerpo?
Do you have tingling? / ¿Tiene hormigueo?
Do your hands shake? / ¿Le tiemblan las manos?
Do you have trouble remembering things? / ¿Tiene dificultad para recordar cosas?
Do you get dizzy at times? / ¿Tiene mareos a veces?
As if you were going to faint? / ¿Como si fuera a desmayarse?
Have you fainted? / ¿Se ha desmayado?
Have you ever had a seizure? / ¿Ha tenido alguna vez una convulsión?

Mental status / Estado mental:

What's your name? / ¿Cómo se llama Ud.?
Do you know where you are? / ¿Sabe donde está?
What type of building are we in? / ¿En qué tipo de edificio estamos?
What's the date? / ¿Cuál es la fecha?
What year is it? / ¿Qué año es?
Do you know who I am? / ¿Sabe quien soy yo?

Psychiatric / Psiquiátrico:

Would you say you are a nervous person? / ¿Diría que Ud. es una persona nerviosa?
Is something bothering you? / ¿Hay algo que le molesta?
Would you say you suffer from depression at times? / ¿Diría que padece de depresión a veces?
Have you ever seen a psychiatrist? / ¿Ha visto alguna vez a un psiquiatra?
Did it help? / ¿Le ayudó?
Have you ever thought of killing yourself? / ¿Ha pensado alguna vez en suicidarse?

Have you thought about how you would do it? / ¿Ha pensado en como lo haría?

Have you thought of hurting someone else? / ¿Ha pensado en hacerle daño a otra persona?

Do you think you can take care of yourself? / ¿Cree que puede valerse por sí mismo?

Are you going to be able to manage? / ¿Va a poder arreglárselas?

Endocrine / Endocrino:

Do you have thyroid problems? / ¿Tiene problemas de tiroides?
Did a doctor tell you? / ¿Se lo dijo un médico?
Do you feel hot frequently? / ¿Siente calor muy a menudo?
More than usual? / ¿Más que de costumbre?
Do you feel cold a lot when others don't? / ¿Siente frío muchas veces cuando los demás no lo sienten?
Are you thirsty a lot? / ¿Tiene mucha sed?
Have you always been thirsty or is this something new? / ¿Siempre ha tenido sed o es algo nuevo? /
Are you eating a lot? / ¿Está comiendo mucho?

PHYSICAL EXAMINATION / EXAMEN FÍSICO

General Examination / Examen General

Have a seat on the exam table. / Siéntese en la mesa (de exploración).
Take off your jacket. / Quítese la chaqueta (chamarra).
I need to take your blood pressure. / Necesito tomarle la presión.
Roll up your sleeve please. / Arremánguese la camisa, por favor.
Let your arm fall; I will hold it up. / Deje caer el brazo; yo se lo sostengo.
Your blood pressure is one hundred thirty over seventy. / Su presión es de 130 sobre 70.
Take off your clothes from the waist up please. / Desvístase de la cintura hacia arriba, por favor.
Take off all your clothes except your underwear. / Quítese toda la ropa menos la ropa interior.
Put on this gown with the opening at the back. / Póngase esta bata con la abertura hacia atrás.
Sit facing this wall please. / Siéntese mirando hacia esta pared, por favor.
Sit with your legs dangling. / Siéntese con las piernas colgando.

Let me take your pulse. / Déjeme tomarle el pulso.

Follow my finger with your eyes without moving your head. / Siga mi dedo con los ojos sin mover la cabeza.

Look at my nose. / Míreme la nariz.

Stare at that point on the wall. / Fije la vista en aquel punto en la pared.

Keep staring at it even if I get in the way of one eye. / Siga mirándolo aún cuando yo bloquee su visión en un ojo.

Try not to move your eyes. / Trate de no mover los ojos.

Now look directly at the light. / Ahora mire directamente a la luz.

Raise your eyebrows. / Levante las cejas.

Frown. / Frunza el ceño.

Wrinkle your nose. / Arrugue la nariz.

Smile. / Sonría.

Show me your teeth. / Enséñeme los dientes.

Clench your teeth. / Apriete los dientes.

Raise your shoulders against my hands. / Levante sus hombros contra mis manos.

Look up at the ceiling. / Mire al techo.

Open your mouth. / Abra la boca.

Stick your tongue out. / Saque la lengua.

Move it from side to side. / Muévala de lado a lado.

Say "Ah." / Diga "A."

Swallow. / Trague.

Breathe quietly through your nose while I listen your heart. / Respire suavemente por la nariz mientras le escucho el corazón.

Don't talk for a moment. / No hable por un momento.

Lean forward. / Inclínese hacia adelante.

Cross your arms. / Cruce los brazos.

Take deep breaths through your mouth while I listen to your lungs. / Respire profundo por la boca mientras le escucho los pulmones.

I need to examine your breasts. / Necesito examinarle las mamas (los senos).

Do you examine your own breasts regularly? / ¿Examina Ud. sus proprias mamas (senos) regularmente?

Place your hands on your hips and push inward. / Ponga las manos en la cadera y empuje hacia dentro.

Lift your arms above your head like this. / Levante los brazos arriba de la cabeza así.

Now lie down. / Ahora acuéstese.

Face up. / Boca arriba.

I'm going to examine your abdomen. / Le voy a examinar el abdomen (la barriga).

Arrange yourself straight on the table. / Acomódese recto en la mesa.

Relax your muscles. / Relaje los músculos.

Let your head rest. Don't try to lift it. / Descanse la cabeza. No trate de levantarla.

Tell me if it hurts. / Dígame si le duele.

I have to do a rectal examination. / Necesito hacerle un tacto rectal.

Do you know what a rectal exam is? / ¿Sabe Ud. que es un tacto rectal?

I need to examine your rectum with my finger, using a glove. / Necesito examinar su recto con mi dedo, usando un guante.

Roll over onto your left side. / Voltéese a su lado izquierdo.

Bend your knees toward your chest. / Doble las rodillas hacia el pecho.

Bear down as if you were having a bowel movement. / Puje como si estuviera defecando.

Squeeze my finger. / Apriete mi dedo.

I need to examine you for a hernia. / Necesito examinarle para ver si tiene una hernia.

Cough please. / Tosa por favor.

Pelvic Examination / Examen Pélvico

I need to do a pelvic examination. / Necesito hacerle un examen pélvico.

Put your feet in the stirrups. / Coloque los pies en los estribos.

Move forward. / Muévase hacia adelante.

Separate your legs. / Separe las piernas.

I'm going to insert the speculum. / Voy a introducirle el espéculo.

I'm going to do a Pap test. / Voy a hacerle una citología (prueba de Papanicolaou).

The exam is almost over. / Falta poco para terminar el examen.

I need to examine you with my fingers, using a glove. / Necesito examinarla con mis dedos, usando un guante.

Now I am going to examine your vagina and rectum and the tissue in between. / Ahora le voy a examinar la vagina, el recto, y el tejido entre ellos.

Neurological Examination / Examen Neurológico

Close your eyes. / Cierre los ojos.

Do you smell anything? / ¿Huele algo?

What does it smell like? / ¿A qué huele?

I am going to examine your peripheral vision. / Voy a examinarle la visión periférica.

Cover your left eye and with your right eye look in my eye. / Tápese el ojo izquierdo y con el derecho mire mi ojo.

Now tell me "Yes" the moment you see my finger wiggling. / Ahora diga "Sí" al momento que vea mover mi dedo.

Don't look at my finger. / No mire mi dedo.

Keep looking at my eye. / Siga mirando mi ojo.

Close your eyes and don't let me open them. / Cierre los ojos y no permita que se los abra.

Can you hear the sound of my fingers rubbing? / ¿Puede escuchar el sonido de mis dedos frotando?

Close your eyes and tell me the moment you hear my fingers rubbing. / Cierre los ojos y dígame al momento que escuche mis dedos frotando.

On which side does the tuning fork sound louder? / ¿En cuál lado suena más fuerte el diapasón?

Or does it sound the same on both sides? / ¿O suena igual en los dos lados?

Which sound seems louder. This? / ¿Cuál sonido le parece más fuerte? ¿Este?

Or this? / ¿O éste?

(*For additional dialogue concerning the cranial nerves see GENERAL EXAMINATION above.*) / (*Para diálogos adicionales sobre los pares craneales, vea el EXAMEN GENERAL arriba.*)

Stand please. / Levántese por favor.

Walk toward the door. / Camine hacia la puerta.

Now walk to me. / Ahora camine hacia mí.

Walk on your toes. / Camine de puntillas.

Walk on your heels. / Camine con los talones.

Walk in a straight line, putting one foot directly in front of the other, like this. / Camine en una línea recta, poniendo un pie directamente enfrente del otro, así.

Hop on one foot. / Salte en un pie.

Now on the other one. / Ahora en el otro.

Squat down. / Póngase en cuclillas.

Now get up without using your arms. / Ahora levántese sin usar los brazos.

Stand with your feet together and your arms extended in front of you, palms up, like this. / Párese con los pies juntos y los brazos extendidos enfrente, las palmas hacia arriba, así.

Keep your arms extended. / Mantenga los brazos extendidos.

Close your eyes. / Cierre los ojos.

I won't let you fall. / No lo voy a dejar caer.

Sit here please. / Siéntese aquí por favor.

Squeeze my fingers as hard as you can. / Apriete mis dedos lo más fuerte que pueda.

Separate your fingers like this and don't let me close them. / Separe los dedos así y no permita que se los cierre.

Make a circle like this and don't let me break it. / Haga un círculo así y no permita que se lo rompa.

Pull against my hand. / Jale contra mi mano.

Push against my hand. / Empuje contra mi mano.

Harder. / Más fuerte.

Make a fist. / Haga un puño.

Flex your wrist against my hand. / Flexione (Doble) la muñeca contra mi mano.

Raise your arms against my hands. / Levante los brazos contra mis manos.

Extend your leg against my hand. / Extienda la pierna contra mi mano.

Pull it back. / Jálela hacia atrás.

Push your foot against my hand. / Empuje el pie contra mi mano.

Bend your foot upward. / Doble el pie hacia arriba.

Raise your leg against my hand. / Levante la pierna contra mi mano.

Touch your nose with your finger. / Tóquese la nariz con el dedo.

Now touch my finger. / Ahora toque mi dedo.

Keep on touching your nose and my finger, back and forth, as rapidly as you can. / Siga tocando su nariz y mi dedo repetidamente lo más rápido que pueda.

Touch your knee with the heel of your other leg. / Tóquese la rodilla con el talón de la otra pierna.

Now slide your heel down your shin to your foot. / Ahora con el talón recorra la espinilla hasta el pie.

Can you feel the tuning fork vibrating? / ¿Siente vibrar el diapasón?

Now it isn't vibrating. / Ahora no está vibrando.

Can you tell the difference? / ¿Siente la diferencia?

Close your eyes. / Cierre los ojos.

Is it vibrating or not? / ¿Está vibrando o no?

Now? / ¿Ahora?

Can you feel when I touch you with this piece of cotton? / ¿Puede sentir cuando le toco con este algodón?

Close your eyes and tell me "Yes" each time you feel the cotton. / Cierre los ojos y diga "Sí" cada vez que sienta el algodón.

The moment you feel it, tell me. / Al momento que lo sienta, me dice.

I'm going to use this pin to test your sensations. / Voy a usar este alfiler para examinar sus sensaciones.

This is sharp. / Esto es puntiagudo.

This is dull. / Esto es romo.

Can you feel the difference? / ¿Siente la diferencia?

Close your eyes and tell me "Sharp" or "Dull" each time I touch you. / Cierre los ojos y dígame "Puntiagudo" o "Romo" cada vez que lo toque.

Did you feel anything? / ¿Sintió algo?

Do you feel this point? / ¿Siente esta punta?

Do you feel these two separate points? / ¿Siente estas dos puntas separadas?

Close your eyes and tell me "One" or "Two" according to how many points you feel. / Cierre los ojos y dígame "Una" o "Dos" según cuantas puntas sienta.

I am going to check your reflexes. / Voy a examinarle los reflejos.

Relax. / Relájese.

Relax your leg. / Relaje la pierna.

NURSING / ENFERMERÍA

Orientation / Orientación:

Hello. I'm Lee. I'll be your nurse today. / Hola. Me llamo Lee. Voy a ser su enfermera (enfermero) hoy.

Let me show you how your bed works. / Permítame mostrarle como funciona su cama.

This button here raises your head and this other one raises your legs. / Este botón aquí eleva su cabeza y este otro eleva sus piernas.

This works the T.V. / Esto hace funcionar la televisión.

If you need me, press this button here. / Si me necesita, oprima este botón aquí.

If you want to make a call, dial nine first. / Si quiere hacer una llamada, marque el nueve primero.

You need to put on this gown. / Tiene que ponerse esta bata.

You can put your clothes in this drawer. / Puede poner su ropa en este cajón.

Do you have any valuables with you? / ¿Lleva algo de valor consigo?

Do you want us to lock it up? / ¿Quiere que se lo guardemos bajo llave?

I need to take your vital signs. / Necesito tomarle sus signos vitales.

Relax your arm. / Relaje su brazo.

Hold this thermometer under your tongue. / Mantenga este termómetro bajo su lengua.

Please step over to this scale; I need to weigh you. / Por favor, párese sobre esta balanza; necesito pesarlo.

I need to start an IV on you. / Necesito ponerle suero.

Make a fist. / Cierre el puño.

You're going to feel a stick. / Va a sentir un pinchazo (piquete).

Don't forget you're attached to this IV now. / No olvide que ahora está conectado a este suero.

Visiting hours are from nine in the morning to eight in the evening. / Las horas de visita son de las nueve de la mañana a las ocho de la noche.

Comfort / Comodidad:

Are you cold? / ¿Tiene Ud. frío?

Would you like an extra blanket? / ¿Quisiera otra cobija más?

An extra pillow? / ¿Otra almohada más?

Are you too warm? / ¿Tiene demasiado calor?

Are you comfortable? / ¿Está cómodo?

Are you having pain? / ¿Tiene dolor?

How bad is your pain on a scale from 1 to 10? / ¿Qué tan intenso es su dolor en una escala de 1 a 10?

Where is the pain? / ¿Dónde siente el dolor?

What do you usually take for the pain? / ¿Qué es lo que acostumbra tomar para el dolor?

I'll call your doctor and see if he can prescribe something for the pain. / Voy a llamar a su médico para ver si le puede recetar algo para el dolor.

Nourishment / Alimentación:

Here's a menu showing your choices for dinner. / Aquí tiene un menú de lo que puede escoger para cenar.

You can order something from the cafeteria if you like. / Puede pedir algo de la cafetería si gusta.

Are you on any kind of special diet? / ¿Está Ud. en alguna dieta especial?

Are you diabetic? / ¿Es diabético?

Do you have high blood pressure? / ¿Tiene presión alta?

Do you need help eating? / ¿Necesita ayuda para comer?

After midnight you won't be able to eat or drink anything because of the study you are having in the morning. / Después de la medianoche no va a poder comer ni tomar nada debido al estudio que le van a realizar en la mañana.

Try to drink more fluids. / Trate de tomar mas líquidos.

Your doctor doesn't want you to eat in case you need surgery. / Su médico no quiere que coma en caso de que necesite cirugía.

Would you like ice chips? / ¿Quisiera pedacitos de hielo?

You're getting plenty of fluids through your IV. / Está recibiendo suficientes líquidos a través del suero.

Here's a basin in case you need to throw up. / Aquí tiene una riñonera (un recipiente) en caso de que necesite vomitar.

I need to pass a tube through your nose down into your stomach. / Necesito pasarle un tubo por la nariz hasta el estómago.

It will be a little uncomfortable but it shouldn't be painful. / Le será un poco incómodo, pero no debería ser doloroso.

When I tell you, I'm going to want you to swallow. / Cuando yo le avise, voy a querer que trague.

Swallow. / Trague.

Good. / Bien.

Elimination / Eliminación:

Do you have diarrhea? / ¿Tiene Ud. diarrea?

Do you want something for constipation? / ¿Quiere Ud. algo para el estreñimiento?

I need to give you an enema. / Necesito ponerle un enema (una lavativa).

Are you going to be able to walk to the bathroom? / ¿Va a poder caminar al baño?

Do you want me to bring you a bedpan? / ¿Quiere que le traiga una bacinilla (un pato, un cómodo, una chata)?

I can bring you a urinal. / Puedo traerle un orinal (pato).

You need to urinate in this container. / Necesita orinar en este recipiente.

I'm going to need a sample of your stool. / Necesitaré una muestra de sus heces fecales (su popó, su caca).

Let me close the curtain. / Permítame cerrar la cortina.

Your doctor has ordered a catheter. / Su médico le ha indicado (ordenado) un catéter.

I'm going to pass this tube through your urethra, that is, through the opening just above your vagina. / Le voy a pasar esta manguerita por su uretra, o sea, por la abertura justo arriba de su vagina.

I'm going to pass this tube through your penis into your bladder. / Le voy a pasar esta manguerita por su pene hasta la vejiga.

It's not as bad as it sounds. / No es tan malo como suena.

Just relax. / Simplemente relájese.

Be sure not to pull this out. / Asegúrese de no sacarse esto.

Medication / Medicamentos:

What medications do you take at home? / ¿Qué medicamentos toma Ud. en casa?

Are you allergic to any medicines? / ¿Es alérgico a alguna medicina?

Here are your medicines. / Aquí tiene sus medicinas.

Drink this liquid please. / Tome este líquido por favor.

Would you like a pill to help you sleep? / ¿Quisiera una pastilla que le ayude a dormir?

Would you like another injection for the pain? / ¿Quisiera otra inyección para el dolor?

I need to give you a suppository. / Necesito darle un supositorio.

It's a medicine that is placed in your rectum. / Es un medicamento que se coloca en el recto.

Activity / Actividad:

You need to walk around in order to regain your strength. / Necesita caminar para recuperar las fuerzas.

I'll help you. / Yo le ayudaré.

Your doctor wants you to sit up in a chair for a while. / Su médico quiere que se siente en una silla por un rato.

Ask for help before getting out of bed. / Pida ayuda antes de levantarse de la cama.

Do you feel dizzy when you stand up? / ¿Se siente mareado cuando se levanta?

Your doctor doesn't want you to get out of bed. / Su médico no quiere que Ud. se levante de la cama.

You need to rest. / Necesita descansar.

I will be coming in every couple hours to turn you. / Voy a regresar cada dos horas para cambiarlo de posición (voltearlo).

Hygiene / Higiene:

Would you like to take a shower? / ¿Quisiera ducharse (tomar un baño de regadera)?

I'm going to give you a sponge bath. / Voy a darle un baño de esponja.
Here's a toothbrush and toothpaste. / Aquí tiene un cepillo de dientes y pasta dental.
Here's a washcloth and towel. / Aquí tiene una toallita para lavarse y una toalla.
Here is a container for your dentures. / Aquí tiene un recipiente para su dentadura.

Respiratory / Respiratorio:

Are you short of breath? / ¿Le falta el aire?
You need to keep your oxygen mask on. / Necesita mantener puesta su máscarilla de oxígeno.
Take a deep breath. / Haga una respiración profunda.
You're due for another breathing treatment. / Es hora para otra nebulización.
Put this mouthpiece in your mouth and suck in air. / Colóquese esta boquilla en la boca y chupe aire.
Make the ball go as high as you can. / Haga que la bolita suba lo más alto que pueda.
You need to do this every hour or so. / Tiene que hacer esto cada hora más o menos.
I need you to spit into this container. / Necesito que escupa en este recipiente.
There's no smoking in the hospital. / Está prohibido fumar en el hospital.
If you need to smoke, you can use the patio on the second floor. / Si tiene que fumar, puede usar el patio en el segundo piso.

Discharge Planning / Planes para dar de alta:

Who do you live with? / ¿Con quién vive Ud.?
Is there someone who can help you? / ¿Hay alguien que pueda ayudarle?
Do you have a wheelchair at home? / ¿Tiene una silla de ruedas en su casa?
A hospital bed? / ¿Una cama de hospital?
Who prepares your meals? / ¿Quién le prepara la comida?
Your doctor says you can go home now. / Su doctor dice que ya puede regresar a su casa.
You can call your family and tell them to come pick you up. / Puede llamar a su familia y pedirles que vengan a recogerlo.

Miscellaneous / Miscelánea:

You better ask your doctor the next time you see her. / Es mejor que le pregunte a su médico la próxima vez que la vea.
Mr. Gomez, can you hear me? / Sr. Gomez, ¿puede oírme?
Open your eyes. / Abra sus ojos.
Squeeze my hand. / Apriete mi mano.
I'm sorry to wake you up, but I need to take your blood pressure and temperature. / Disculpe que lo despierte, pero necesito tomarle la presión (de la sangre) y la temperatura.
I need to prick your finger to measure your sugar. / Necesito pincharle (picarle) el dedo para medirle el azúcar.
Would you like the hospital chaplain to visit you? / ¿Quisiera que el capellán (sacerdote) del hospital lo visite?

PEDIATRICS / PEDIATRÍA

Your baby is fine. / Su bebé está bien.
He's a little jaundiced, but we can fix that with light treatments. / Se ve un poco amarillo, pero podemos arreglar eso con tratamiento de luz.
Are you going to breast-feed or use a bottle? / ¿Va a darle el pecho o le va a dar biberón (mamadera, pacha)?
You need to burp him after each feeding. / Necesita hacerlo eructar después de cada comida.
Don't dilute the formula. / No diluya la fórmula.
It's not good to put your baby to bed with a bottle of milk. / No es bueno acostar a su bebé con un biberón de leche.
Have you weaned her yet? / ¿Ya la ha destetado?
She is ready to eat solids. / Ya puede comer alimentos sólidos.
Don't give her food that could make her choke, like beans or peanuts. / No le dé comida con la que se pueda atorar, como frijoles o maníes (cacahuates).
Make sure your children aren't eating chips of paint off the walls. / Asegúrese de que sus hijos no estén comiendo pedacitos de pintura de las paredes.
Who cares for your baby when you are at work? / ¿Quién cuida a su bebé cuando Ud. está en el trabajo?
Does your son coo? Squeal? Laugh? Babble? Say any words? Talk? / ¿Hace su hijo sonidos como una paloma? ¿chilla? ¿ríe? ¿balbucea? ¿dice algunas palabras? ¿habla?

Can he lift his head up? Sit up? Crawl? Walk? / ¿Puede levantar la cabeza? sentarse? ¿gatear? ¿caminar?

Don't worry, he's developing fine. / No se preocupe, se está desarrollando bien.

Many children his age can't talk yet. / Muchos niños a su edad todavía no pueden hablar.

Tantrums are normal at this age. / Los berrinches son normales a esta edad.

There's nothing wrong; she's just teething. / No hay ningún problema; solamente que le están saliendo los dientes.

Has she been pulling on her ear lately? / ¿Ha estado jalándose la oreja últimamente?

Ear infections are common among children her age. / Las infecciones del oído son comunes en niños de su edad.

Does she have asthma? Allergies? A heart murmur? / ¿Tiene ella asma? ¿alergias? ¿un soplo cardíaco?

Has he ever had seizures? Eye problems? Pneumonia? / ¿Ha tenido alguna vez convulsiones? ¿problemas de los ojos? ¿neumonía?

Do you have a record of your child's immunizations? / ¿Tiene una tarjeta de vacunas de su niño?

You need to lower the temperature of the water coming out of your faucets. / Necesita bajar la temperatura del agua que sale del grifo (de la llave).

You need to put all poisons out of reach of your children. / Necesita poner todas las sustancias tóxicas fuera del alcance de sus niños.

Do you have a car seat for your child? / ¿Tiene un asiento de seguridad en el carro para su niño?

Is there a working smoke alarm on each floor of your house? / ¿Hay un detector de humo que funcione en cada piso de su casa?

Would you like to attend a class on parenting? A class on cardio-pulmonary resuscitation (CPR)? / ¿Quisiera asistir a una clase para padres? ¿una clase de reanimación cardiopulmonar (RCP)?

Does your daughter know her street address? / ¿Sabe su hija la dirección de su casa?

Can she brush her own teeth? Dress herself? Comb her hair? / ¿Puede cepillarse los dientes ella misma? ¿vestirse? ¿peinarse?

She will probably quit sucking her thumb on her own eventually. / Con el tiempo, es probable que deje de chuparse el dedo.

I wouldn't worry about it. / No me preocuparía por eso.

How long has she been acting listless? / ¿Hace cuánto que ha estado decaída?

Do you think she has been molested? / ¿Cree que ha sido abusada?

How often does your son wet the bed at night? / ¿Con qué frecuencia moja la cama su hijo?

It's normal for him to feel jealous of his younger brother. / Es normal que su hijo tenga celos de su hermano menor.

Have you had trouble disciplining him? / ¿Ha tenido problemas disciplinándolo?

How do you punish him? / ¿Cómo lo castiga?

Has he been missing school a lot? / ¿Ha faltado mucho a la escuela?

To the patient: / Al paciente:

How are you doing in school? / ¿Cómo te va en la escuela?

Do you have trouble paying attention? / ¿Se te hace difícil prestar atención?

What grade are you in? / ¿En qué grado estás?

Do you smoke cigarettes? / ¿Fumas cigarrillos?

Have you tried any drugs? / ¿Has probado alguna droga?

Are you sexually active? / ¿Es Ud. sexualmente activo?..¿Ha tenido relaciones sexuales recientemente?

Do you use birth control? / ¿Usas algún método anticonceptivo?

Do you have any questions regarding sexual matters? / ¿Tienes algunas preguntas sobre asuntos sexuales?

Are you unhappy about your appearance in any way? / ¿Por algún motivo te sientes descontento con tu apariencia?

Do you get along with your parents? / ¿Te llevas bien con tus padres?

Do you feel you can talk to them about personal things? / ¿Sientes que puedes hablar con ellos acerca de cosas personales?

What do they do that bothers you? / ¿Qué hacen que te molesta?

What do you do that makes them angry? / ¿Que haces que los hace enojar?

What do you do during your free time? / ¿Qué haces en tu tiempo libre?

Do you spend a lot of time alone? / ¿Pasas mucho tiempo solo?

Are you involved in sports? / ¿Participas en deportes?

Do you belong to a gang? / ¿Eres miembro de una pandilla?

Have you had any trouble with the law? / ¿Has tenido problemas con la ley?

What do you plan to do after high school? / ¿Qué piensas hacer después de terminar la preparatoria?

DENTISTRY / ODONTOLOGÍA

When was the last time you saw a dentist? / ¿Cuándo fue la última vez que vio a un dentista?

Do you brush your teeth after each meal? / ¿Se cepilla los dientes después de cada comida?

Do you floss regularly? / ¿Usa hilo dental regularmente?

You need to brush more along the gum line. / Necesita cepillarse más en la linea de la encía.

Open really wide now. / Ahora abra bien la boca.

Open part way. / Ábrala un poco.

Bite down. / Muerda.

Close your mouth around this as though it were a straw. / Cierre la boca alrededor de esto como si fuera un popote (una bombilla, un pitillo).

Rinse your mouth and spit. / Enjuáguese la boca y escupa.

Turn your head toward me. / Voltée la cabeza hacia mí.

Are you feeling any pain? / ¿Está sintiendo algún dolor?

You have a loose filling. / Ud. tiene un empaste suelto.

I'm going to replace it with an acrylic filling. / Se lo voy a reemplazar con un empaste acrílico.

You need a root canal. / Necesita una endodoncia (un tratamiento de conducto).

I need to remove one of your teeth and put in a bridge. / Necesito sacarle uno de los dientes y colocarle un puente.

Is there someone who can drive you home afterward? / ¿Hay alguien que lo pueda llevar a su casa después?

Have you ever had to take antibiotics before a dental procedure? / ¿Alguna vez ha tenido que tomar antibióticos antes de un procedimiento dental?

The only part that hurts is when I give you the numbing medication. / Solo le va a doler cuando le ponga el anestésico.

It will only hurt for a minute or so. / Solo le va a doler por un minuto más o menos.

You're going to feel a little stick. / Va a sentir un pequeño pinchazo (piquete).

You may feel a little burning. / Puede sentir un poco de ardor.

Bite down hard. / Muerda fuerte.

When you bite does it feel as though your tooth is too high? / Al morder, ¿siente que su diente está demasiado alto?

You have some staining on your front teeth. / Tiene un poco manchados los incisivos.

Would you be interested in a treatment which would make your teeth whiter? / ¿Le interesaría un tratamiento que le hiciera más blancos los dientes?

Swish this around for a minute and then spit it out. / Enjuáguese la boca con esto por un minuto y luego escúpalo.

You shouldn't eat, drink or rinse your mouth for half an hour. / No debe comer, beber, ni enjuagarse la boca por media hora.

RADIOLOGY / RADIOLOGÍA

Could you be pregnant? / ¿Podría Ud. estar embarazada?

How do you know? / ¿Cómo lo sabe?

When did you last eat? / ¿Cuándo fue la última vez que comió algo?

Are you able to sit up (stand, walk)? / ¿Es capaz de sentarse (levantarse, caminar)?

Stand here. / Párese aquí.

Put your hands on your head. / Ponga sus manos en la cabeza.

Put your chin here. / Ponga su mentón (barbilla) aquí.

Take a deep breath and hold it. / Respire profundo y no suelte el aire.

Don't move. / No se mueva.

Relax. / Relájese.

Go ahead and breathe. / Ya puede respirar.

Get on the table, please. / Súbase en la mesa por favor.

You can get dressed now. / Ahora puede vestirse.

Come this way please. / Venga por acá por favor.

Are you allergic to seafood? / ¿Es Ud. alérgico a los mariscos?

I'm going to inject the contrast now. / Le voy a inyectar el medio de contraste ahora.

You may feel a little warmth. / Puede que sienta un poco de calor.

You may get a metallic taste in your mouth. / Puede que sienta un sabor metálico en la boca.

That is normal. / Eso es normal.

Do you have any metal in you? / ¿Tiene Ud. algo de metal en su cuerpo?

No pacemaker? Hip replacement? Rods or pins? / ¿Nada de marcapasos? ¿prótesis de cadera? ¿grapas? ¿barras o clavos?

Have you ever had brain surgery? Inner ear surgery? / ¿Alguna vez ha sido operado del cerebro? ¿O del oído interno?

Have you ever worked in welding or grinding? / ¿Alguna vez ha trabajado en soldadura o amoladura?

Do you ever get claustrophobic? / ¿Padece a veces la claustrofobia?

Does it bother you to be in a small, cramped place? / ¿Le molesta estar en un lugar pequeño y apiñado?

You're going to hear a lot of noise. / Va a escuchar mucho ruido.

Remove everything metallic from your clothes and your body. / Quite toda cosa metálica de su ropa y su cuerpo.

Like earrings, bracelets, and watches. / Como aretes, brazaletes, y relojes de pulsera.

CODE STATUS DISCUSSION /
HABLANDO DE REANIMACIÓN

Lastly, there is a question I ask of all my patients. / Por último, hay una pregunta que le hago a todos mis pacientes.

What would you like us–the medical team–to do in the very unlikely event that your heart should stop or you should stop breathing? / ¿Qué querría que hiciéramos nosotros–el equipo médico–en el caso muy improbable en que se le pare el corazón o que Ud. deje de respirar?

Would you like us to do everything reasonable to try to resuscitate you? / ¿Querría que hiciéramos todo lo razonable para reanimarlo?

Would you like us to let you go in peace? / ¿Querría que lo dejáramos morir en paz?

If we thought you had suffered brain damage, would you like us to continue resuscitation efforts anyway? / ¿Si creemos que ha padecido daño cerebral, querría que continuáramos con la reanimación?

Would you like us to continue resuscitation efforts as long as we thought there was a reasonable likelihood that you could get back to how you are now? / ¿Querría que continuáramos con la reanimación mientras creámos que hay una posibilidad razonable de que Ud. pudiera recuperarse, como está ahora

Would you like to name a family member or close friend who could advise us regarding your care in case you become unable to communicate? / ¿Quisiera designar a un familiar o a un amigo cercano quien pudiera avisarnos acerca su cuidado en caso de que Ud. se vuelva incapaz de comunicarse?